Culture
and
Childrearing

Culture and Childrearing

ANN L. CLARK, R.N., M.A./EDITOR
Director of Nursing Education
Hawaii Nurses Association
Honolulu, Hawaii

F.A. DAVIS COMPANY • *Philadelphia*

Library of Congress Cataloging in Publication Data
Main entry under title:

Culture and childrearing.

  Includes bibliographies and index.
  1. Children—Management—Addresses, essays, lectures.
2. Family—United States—Addresses, essays, lectures.
3. Pluralism (Social sciences)—Addresses, essays, lectures.
4. Children of minorities—United States. I. Clark, Ann L.
[DNLM: 1. Ethnic groups—United States.   2. Childrearing.
WS105.5.C3 C592]   HQ769.C957 1980   649'.1   80-19481
ISBN 0-8036-1836-0

Preface

The various cultures that immigrate to America bring with them their unique values and their traditional practices and beliefs. Most often, they bring a dream that life will be "better" for themselves and for their children. At the same time, the America they find is an America undergoing great changes through technological progress. These changes impact on the family, and thus dynamic changes are occurring within the family. The American family, once responsible for all aspects of childrearing, now finds that only procreation and early orientation of children remain their exclusive functions.

Health professionals working with children and with childrearing families need to appreciate two things:

First, that the members of the contemporary American family, because of accelerated social changes, are culturally almost on their own as they struggle to find the solution to a number of childrearing issues. This has occurred because of the great distances between their home and the home of their parents; perhaps more importantly because the answers of the *last* generation simply do not fit with the problems of *today. Second,* health professionals need to appreciate that because of social changes family members now look to agencies and individuals outside of the family to assist them in their roles. Institutions such as child care centers, schools, and the church have taken on functions of socializing, teaching, and counseling once filled by parents. Psychologists, speech pathologists, pediatricians, pediatric nurse practitioners, and others are being relied on more and more by childrearing families.

Health professionals need, then, to blend these appreciations with knowledge of the values and practices that families of other cultural groups that immigrate to America hold and to plan their intervention utilizing these wider perimeters. Only then will health care be sensitive, meaningful, and effective.

This book has been written to assist health professionals to bridge the gap between what *they* have come to value (by virtue of their own cultural orientation, their professional preparation, and work experience) and the "real world" of their client/patients, who come to them from a multitude of different cultural orientations.

The following chapters, which explore the childrearing values, beliefs, and practices of the major cultures to be found in America today, have been written almost exclusively by professional nurses who proudly claim the culture as their own. It is anticipated that a study of their chapters will assist health professionals to bring greater sensitivity to their practice and impact on the health-illness experiences of their clients in a positive manner.

Ann L. Clark

Acknowledgments

Very few, if any, published works would ever reach potential readers if it were not for the support services one enjoys. Just "unearthing" the contributing authors of this book took the talents of a number of my friends and colleagues. I am grateful to them for their assistance.

To the contributing authors go my very special thanks. I only knew four of them personally when I began this book, and I still have not met the majority of them. However, during the ensuing months we have exchanged many ideas and solved many problems by telephone and by mail, and we have shared a number of personal experiences as well. In this short period of time, there has been a marriage, several changes in professional position, and a baby has been conceived and born. This all seems appropriate enough, for the book is about families — their joys, their problems, and concerns, their values, beliefs, and practices.

Interest and assistance, often well beyond what one could expect, have been offered by the staffs of Hawaii Medical Library and Hamilton Library at the University of Hawaii. Particularly I wish to single out Ginny Tangi at H.M.L. for her interest and enthusiasm as the book has progressed, and all the staff at H.M.L. for their patient listening to my excitement as well as my despair.

To my friends who helped me to find appropriate illustrations for the text, even taking some of the pictures themselves, I saw mahalo. Their names can be found under their materials. To all the children and their families who permitted us to take their pictures, I hope you enjoy finding your image between the pages of this book. I want to add special thanks to Brad Powell, whose photographs add interest to the cover and to several chapters.

To my husband, who keeps me organized and sometimes protected from the pressures of the outside world and from my own driving, ambitious self, mahalo nui loa.

This, my fourth book with the same publisher, F.A. Davis Company, silently speaks of the concern and assistance nurse authors find in working with this fine publishing company. Judy Kim, past nursing editor, has not only been a colleague in all these endeavors, but a friend as well. Thanks, also to Bruce MacGregor for his editorial assistance.

Finally, I want to thank Beulah Scholl who carefully typed and proofread many of the pages of this manuscript. Without her I would have been lost.

Ann L. Clark

Contributors

Consuelo J. Aquino, R.N., M.P.H.
Adult Medical Nurse Practitioner
Diabetic Nurse Educator
Kaiser Permanent Medical Care Program
Diabetic Nurse Educator
American Diabetic Association
Honolulu, Hawaii

Marie Scott Brown, R.N., Ph.D.
Professor of Nursing
University of Oregon Health Sciences Center
Portland, Oregon

Evelyn L. Char, R.N., M.S.
Acting Director of Alternatives for Women Program
Diamond Head Community Mental Health Center
Honolulu, Hawaii

Ann L. Clark, R.N., M.A.
Director of Nursing Education
Hawaii Nurses Association
Honolulu, Hawaii

Marta Borbón Ehling, R.N., M.S.
Irvine, California

Charles E. Farris, M.S.W.
Associate Professor of Social Work
Barry College
Miami, Florida

Lorene Sanders Farris, R.N., M.S.
Instructor for American Indian Students
Title 4, Part A
Dade County Schools
Miami, Florida

Betty Greathouse, Ph.D.
Associate Professor
College of Education
Arizona State University
Tempe, Arizona

Gloria I. Lacay, R.N., B.S.N.
Public Health Nurse
Maternity, Infant Care—Family Planning Projects
New York, New York

Linda Diep Liem, R.N., B.S.N., M.P.H.
Public Health Nurse
Head Start Program
Honolulu, Hawaii

Nguyen Dang Liem, Ph.D.
Professor of Southeast Asian Languages and Literature
Department of Indo-Pacific Languages
University of Hawaii
Honolulu, Hawaii

Velvet G. Miller, R.N., B.S.N., M.Ed.
Associate Director, Nursing Division
Scottsdale Memorial Hospital
Scottsdale, Arizona

Aimee Emiko Sodetani-Shibata, R.N., M.N.
Instructor of Nursing
University of Texas
Galveston, Texas

Lorraine Stringfellow, R.N., M.P.H.
Assistant Professor of Maternal and Child Health
Department of Community Health Development
School of Public Health
University of Hawaii
Honolulu, Hawaii

Contents

Culture
and
Childrearing

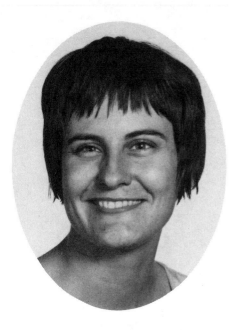

Chapter 1

I was born in Amarillo, Texas, the youngest of three children and grew up primarily in a suburban setting in the Midwest, a typical Nacireman community. My professional education began at Marquette University in Milwaukee, where I received a B.S. in Nursing, and was continued at the University of Colorado, where I received a master's degree in Parent-Child Nursing. At the time of my graduation from that program the first Pediatric Nurse Practitioner Program was beginning. Intrigued by what seemed to me a highly accountable and influential type of nursing, I enrolled immediately. I then practiced as a pediatric nurse practitioner in one of the urban Chicano areas of Denver and became aware of a vast network of alternative health care systems that existed in the heart of the metropolis. Dealing with curanderos and herbal remedies awakened my interests in other ways of providing health care as well as other types of life-styles and belief systems. Soon after that I enrolled in a master's and then a doctoral program in anthropology. I currently hold the latter degree granted from the University of Colorado.

Since that time, I have been involved in clinical practice, teaching, and research relating to primary care of childbearing and childrearing families. I have maintained a particularly strong interest not only in learning about how other people through the ages and in other parts of the world have borne and reared their children, but also in trying to separate out which of our own professional beliefs about childbearing and childrearing are scientifically grounded and which are merely parts of our own professional magical system.

Culture and Childrearing
Marie Scott Brown, R.N., Ph.D.

The concept of holistic medicine has become very popular recently. It includes ideas that are new to many modern-day medical practitioners. They are not, of course, ideas that would be new to the old-time country family doctor. Nor are they ideas that are new to a number of health care professions, particularly to nursing. Although the term "holism" is currently popular, the concept of treating the whole person is a very old one in nursing. The nursing tradition has long prided itself on its eclectic ability to integrate findings from all sciences involved in studying human beings and to apply these findings to improving the health of human beings. The idea of incorporating not only physical sciences but a host of behavioral sciences into the education of nurses is one that has been practiced for many years. Schools of nursing have long taught relatively sophisticated courses in physiology, psychology, and sociology as they apply to human behavior in health and illness.

Recently nursing, joined by other health care professions, has begun to look critically at the information anthropology has to offer it. This book is intended to be a major contribution to that movement, particularly to the subfield of parent-child care. Just what does anthropology have to offer to parent-child care? There are certainly a number of answers to that question. The most apparent and probably the best appreciated answer is that it can help health care professionals clinically when they deal with clients of cultures other than their own. It can help them understand some of the cultural differences that exist; it can help them assess which of these differences are really helpful, harmful, or indifferent in terms of the health of their clients; and, where the differences indicate potential problems, it can help them devise strategies of changing clients' behavior in a manner that is least destructive of their life-style and is most likely to be accepted and followed. The following chapters will look in depth at nine cultures; they will help the reader understand these cultures and the ways that individuals in these cultures rear their children; they will also help the reader devise successful ways of giving care to these families.

Anthropology, however, has other contributions to make, and it is these other contributions that will be discussed in this chapter. Anthropology is "the study of man," that is, it is an attempt to find out what the essential nature of man is. In order to do this, it studies human beings in every possible situation in which they can be studied—in every geographical location in which they can be found and in every possible historical and prehistorical situation about which information can be uncovered. It even studies the behavior of other closely related species (a field more properly called ethology, but one in which many anthropologists are involved). Anthropology attempts to learn what makes human beings human—is it their language? their use of tools? their social behavior? What characteristics of human beings are always present wherever and whenever human societies have existed? Are these characteristics part of what accounts for the essence of humanness? These are some (certainly not all) of the questions with which anthropology concerns itself. It is clear that a real understanding of the essential nature of human beings is also important to a nursing profession that is trying to determine and promote conditions that will result in a healthy existence for such beings.

Health care professionals, particularly in the United States, have been hindered greatly in the study of human behavior in health and illness by being exposed to only a very small sample of human nature. We have said that women should deliver their babies while lying on their back because we have never seen any other ways of delivering babies. We have said that people require a certain amount of protein every day because we never realized that people in many parts of the world survive with a yearly intake of protein roughly equivalent to what we think is essential as a daily intake—and they do so in apparently good health. To those of us used to thinking that crawling is a necessary and important part of child development, it may come as a surprise to realize that in the Balinese culture, children never crawl. There are many things we have assumed are "givens" in family life and child-rearing that are not at all universal in the experience of our species, many of which, in fact, are quite unusual and specific only to our own culture. It might help us, for instance, in dealing with the woman who does not want to wean her child until 2 or 3 years of age if we realized that from the point of view of mankind as a whole her idea is quite common; in fact it is our idea of weaning during the first year that is quite rare and unusual from a broader historical and geographic perspective. This chapter, then, will be an attempt to take a broader look at human behavior in bearing and rearing children. It will look at this behavior as it has occurred and still occurs throughout the entire world and throughout the history and prehistory of our own species, and, occasionally, it will compare this with what is known about other species as well. The benefits to be gained from this kind of comparative study are many. Specifically, the following advantages can be gained in this way:

1. *It should help us free ourselves from some of our ethnocentrism.* Essentially, ethnocentrism is the idea that the way we ourselves live and the way we do things is, of necessity, the best way, simply because it is our way. In fact, there may be many things that we do that really are the best way, but this is not so simply because we do them, and until we are able to give up this notion, there will be no way for us to objectively evaluate which of our own ways are better, which are simply more familiar, and which, perhaps, are worse.

2. *It should help us gain a more accurate perspective of how our practices compare with those of the rest of our species.* Interestingly enough, we will discover that the way we bear and rear our children is, in many respects, quite atypical of how most human beings have done so. That it is unusual does not mean that it is necessarily worse—or better—than other ways, but it does mean that it is probably worth looking at more closely. It may be better because for some reason it is more congruent with the rest of our culture (which, in itself is quite atypical of most of humanity), or it may be better because we have been able to capitalize on the experience of the rest of mankind and make an improvement. On the other hand, it may be that the reason almost no other cultures have ever adopted our way is because their ways are better. Or, finally, it may be that our way is neither better nor worse, but simply different. Whatever the case may be, the perspective obtained should be helpful in giving us some objectivity when evaluating our own childbearing and rearing methods.

3. *By first discovering phenomena in other cultures, it may help us discover the same phenomena in our own culture, which have never been realized before because they had been so much a part of our way of thinking.* This is the case, for instance, with the couvade, a custom in which the man takes on some of the pregnancy, labor, and delivery behavior of his wife. This is a phenomenon first reported from other more "exotic" cultures. These reports stimulated researchers to look for this same phenomenon in our own culture. The discovery that it does indeed exist in our culture has allowed us new and valuable insights into fatherhood during the prenatal period as it is experienced by our own clients.

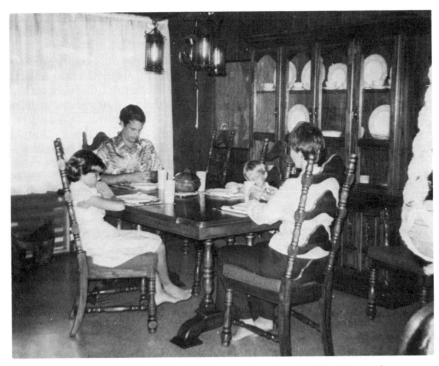

Figure 1. The nuclear family in America saying grace before the meal.

4. *It may provide us with new solutions to universal problems that are better than those we currently employ.* When studying the many positions that women the world over use to deliver their babies, for instance, it is apparent that delivering a baby while the mother lies on her back is a very atypical method. A little thought reveals that it is obviously quite unanatomical for the woman, however convenient it may be for the obstetrician. Similarly, to deliver a baby in a strange situation with no known significant others is quite aberrant in terms of how most cultures handle this situation. This is an example of how the study of other cultures may suggest better ways of doing things than we currently employ.

These, then, are some of the advantages that it is reasonable to expect when looking at childbearing and childrearing from a cross-cultural and even a cross-species perspective. With these objectives in mind, this chapter will review some of the available anthropological material that is related to a number of topics important to parent-child care. These will include:

1. Marriage and the family
2. The role of woman, particularly in regard to the family

3. Preparing for the child and the actual coming of the child
4. Infancy and toddlerhood
5. The middle childhood years
6. Adolescence

MARRIAGE AND THE FAMILY

A cross-cultural view of the family quickly makes apparent the fact that our own cultural ideas of marriage and family are quite unusual. Western society, for the most part, idealizes monogamy and the nuclear family: one father, one mother, and children (Fig. 1). These nuclear families may have attachments to other families (grandparents or great-grandparents on both sides), but they are usually relatively independent in terms of fulfilling subsistence needs and affectional needs. This relative isolation of such a small number of people into one residence is quite unusual from a cross-cultural perspective.

An anthropologist looking cross-culturally at the institution of the family will ask several questions: Is the family universal? Are there different forms of family life? If so, are certain forms more suited to certain types of cultures? Are there inherent strengths and weaknesses to each form of family life? What accounts for some of the very

5

unusual forms of family life? These are questions that should be highly relevant to nursing as well, particularly in an age when family life is changing rapidly, traditional family values are being questioned, and new family life-styles are emerging, both as planned and unplanned alternatives to the traditional American family. Let us look at each of these questions.

Are marriage and the family universal? The answer to this question depends on how the term family is defined. Broadly defined, the answer is yes, although there are cultures in which this institution looks very unusual to the Western observer. The Tibetan family with two or three husbands and one wife, the African family with two or three wives and one husband, and the Kaingang family with several husbands and several wives are all examples of families that might appear very peculiar to the Western observer, yet are actually more typical of the way human beings usually marry and form families than is our own practice of monogamy. Nonetheless, all these groups have a unit that does fulfill the basic definition of a family: "a social arrangement based on marriage and the marriage contract, including recognition of the rights and duties of parenthood, common residence for husband, wife, and children, and reciprocal economic obligations between husband and wife."[1] There are a few situations in which some anthropologists believe the family does not exist, but these are quite rare.

There are basically three types of marriage and three forms of family structure. Marriage between one man and one woman as we have in our own culture is typical of only 20 percent of the recorded cultures of the world.

The vast majority of cultures in the world prefer (even though economic restrictions often prevent many individuals in the culture from participating in) polygamous marriages. Polygamous marriages are of two types: polygynous (i.e., one husband with many wives) or polyandrous (one wife with several husbands). The second type is quite rare and often associated with an even more rare type of marriage, group or plural marriage with many husbands and many wives all cohabiting together. In all these situations, there is one clearly important difference from the nuclear family—in each there is a relatively large ratio of adults to children residing in close proximity. Almost nowhere else in the world is a single adult confined to continuous and almost exclusive interaction with small children

in the way many American housewives are. In many situations, particularly those of polygynous societies in which the women reside in the same household, the childrearing duties are shared among all the wives; in these situations, the child is freed from the unmitigated input of a single adult and the adult's social interaction is alleviated with adult company as well as the company of children. Because there are greater numbers of children (since there are more childbearing women), there also appears to be a greater potential for peer socialization, and many of these cultures employ the older children (sometimes only 4 or 5 years old) as caretakers for the infants and toddlers, relieving the women for much of the agricultural work that must be done. This family structure has obvious advantages for rearing children: there is more help for the mother, there is more peer support for the mother, and there is more peer interaction for the children.

It also has some disadvantages. Reports of strains between the co-wives are numerous. Although there are many ethnographic case studies indicating that the co-wives do indeed frequently form a coalition against a dominant husband, there are also innumerable reports of very intense jealousies. One interesting study[2] discovered that the closer the co-wives lived, the greater the strain of hostility. Andreski in 1970 collected 26 autobiographies of women living in polygynous households. With the exception of head-wives, there is nothing but complaints about the system. Interestingly enough this strain of jealousy appears to be less marked where sororal polygyny is practiced (i.e., where a man marries several sisters); the common interpretation of this finding is that sisters have, early in life, arrived at mechanisms for handling jealousy and, for this reason, are better able to do so in marriage. There are other disadvantages as well. The fathering in this situation is typically very limited, since one father often relates to 15 or 20 children and seldom lives with any of them consistently. This has very clear repercussions, at least for the boys who, upon reaching adulthood, often have difficulty achieving a clear male identity. This is a topic that will be further explored under the section on adolescence. Another disadvantage is that of the young caretakers. Although there are obvious advantages to peer socialization, to entrust a large majority of the daily care of a baby or toddler to a preschool-aged child certainly would appear to be less advantageous than the caretaking of a mature adult with a special investment and interest in the child (e.g., the parent).

Polyandrous and group marriages both are very rare and often exist in the same societies. The Tibetans, the Marquesans, the Toda, and the Kaingang are practically the only groups ever reported to have practiced these forms of marriage. Because the ethnographic reports are somewhat limited, it is difficult to assess the influence of such marriages on the childrearing practices. They would appear to have some of the same advantages as the polygynous systems since many adults would be in the same household; in addition, one would expect fewer children since there is only one childbearing woman in the home, in most cases. It would seem that this could considerably dilute the strain of being the only adult responsible for the childrearing chores and responsibilities. On the other hand, it is quite unclear how much of the childrearing the fathers participate in. The strains of jealousy between husbands seem probable, but the ethnographic accounts are quite variable regarding this.

There are basically three distinct forms of families, each with many variations. The nuclear family is the form most familiar to our own culture. It is typically composed of a married man and woman with their children. The second family form is the extended family, again a form relatively familiar to most health professionals. Although it is not predominant in our major culture, a number of ethnic groups within this culture practice some form of extended family (e.g., many recent immigrants from Mexico and Puerto Rico do so). The extended family is composed of several nuclear families and formed by joining the nuclear family of an individual married couple to that of the parents of either the husband or wife. Finally, the polygamous family is a series of nuclear families that are extended not through the generations as is an extended family (i.e., mother's mother or father's father), but through the husband-wife axis (i.e., either polygyny, polyandry, or plural or group marriage).

The extended family has many of the same influences on childrearing as does the polygamous family, for example, the workload and responsibility of childrearing is never solely the responsibility of one adult. In addition to this, there is always an available older woman who is experienced in rearing children and often responsible for the important decision-making related to childrearing. The advantage to this is obvious. The disadvantage is, of course, the same one experienced by many young families in our own culture when mother-in-law comes to visit—having someone else tell you how to raise your children can and often does cause considerable interpersonal friction.

It is clear then, in surveying the way the majority of cultures throughout time and space have organized their marriages and family life, that our own system is quite unusual. It is probably neither better nor worse, but it is important to realize that it has both advantages and disadvantages to more typical human ways of handling the situation. It would seem that one lesson that this kind of cross-cultural comparison could teach us is that it is very unusual to expect a single or even two adults to take full responsibility for their children (Fig. 2). There is a growing awareness in the women's movement and the studies of homemakers that this situation does, in fact, subject many women to an inordinate amount of stress. To be relatively isolated from adult company, to be constantly interacting with and responsible for (in a way no other culture imagines) every aspect of a child's development, and to be largely cut off from the mainstream of this culture's reward system may be a very unhealthy situation for both the mothers and children in this culture. At least this hypothesis bears close scrutiny.

WOMAN'S ROLE

Throughout all known cultures, the person in closest, most continuous contact, and for that reason probably the most influential person in the life of a young child, is a woman, most often the mother (Fig. 3). Because of her central position in the childrearing process, it is important to look closely at the woman's role and status. Surely the cultural significance and self-esteem of such a person will influence how effectively she is able to provide a healthy environment for the development of her children. What other stresses her culture and environment impose on her will affect the time and energy that remain for her childrearing role. The respect that is given to her motherhood role is likely to influence how much she invests in this role and how much consequent role satisfaction she derives from it.

This section will look cross-culturally at two aspects of women's lives that are likely to affect the way they relate to and influence their chil-

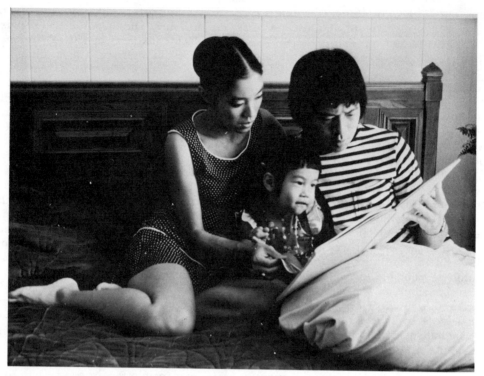

Figure 2. Throughout the world, two adults taking full responsibility for their children is an unusual pattern. (Photograph by Brad Powell)

dren: cultural status and self-esteem.

From a cross-cultural perspective, it is clear that the female role has certain common aspects in all cultures. The current women's movement has brought to our attention the "second class citizen" status of women in our own culture. Interestingly enough, this status is quite universal and even more accentuated in nonWestern cultures. The myth of an evolutionary stage of matriarchy when women were supremely powerful and the myth of the Amazonian women are just that—myths. There is absolutely no anthropological evidence to suggest that either of these two cultural phenomena ever occurred. Although cultures are organized around different kinship and locality patterns, in none of these patterns could women as a group be considered to have equal status with men.

In a matrilineal society (i.e., one in which the kin group traces its family tree through the woman rather than the man) one might anticipate that women would enjoy a higher status than men. This is not so. Even though the lineage may be traced through the woman, it is still the man who wields the power, in this case the

mother's brother. In regard to raising children, the avunculate is a frequent cultural pattern (i.e., the system in which the mother's brother rather than the biological father is the male who relates most closely with the child—legally, affectionally, socially, and often financially). Matrilineality is a rather unusual organizational pattern for a culture—in Murdock's World Ethnographic Sample only 84 out of the 565 reported cultures practice matrilineality.

A system even more unusual, but more advantageous to the woman's status is matrilocality, a system in which a newly married couple resides with the wife's relatives rather than the husband's clan. In this situation, the woman retains the strong clan support and familiarity of her childhood; it is the man who must adjust to being the "newcomer." This is certainly the situation in which the woman is most likely to enjoy a relatively high social status. This is quite a rare situation, however, and exists in less than half of the matrilineal societies and in very few patrilineal societies.

The term matrifocal family refers to one in which the woman does indeed enjoy a higher

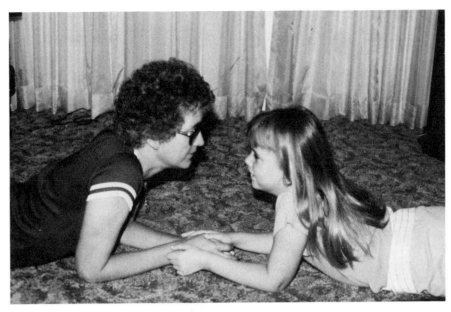
Figure 3. Probably the most influential person in the life of a young child is a woman, most often a mother.

cultural status than the man. It does not exist as a major family form in any society, but does tend to occur in the lower socioeconomic groups of large complex societies such as our own. It is usually an outgrowth of a situation in which men of lower socioeconomic status are less able to get a job than women in the similar social class. This results in considerable status for the woman within the given family, but it still occurs in a larger society in which men enjoy the higher social status. In addition to this, it is a situation that is often transient. When the family income level rises, it is likely that a more culturally typical marriage will ensue and the more usual patrifocal family will emerge. Even when the woman is in this relatively powerful situation, it is always accompanied by considerable economic stress, since she is both the caretaker and the provider (a situation of many of our own lower income families as well as most middle-class single parent families in our culture). It would seem that this additional stress to the woman would be likely to negate any positive affects from the increased social status.

Most societies in the world have been both patrilineal and patrilocal. In this situation, women are at a severe disadvantage in terms of cultural prestige. They typically leave the social group of their childhood at marriage to become the "mistrusted stranger" in a rival clan. The men in this clan have grown up together and have learned to achieve male solidarity. It is often difficult for the women to achieve a similar solidarity since they come from a variety of backgrounds, and, although there do occur strong female groups, they are seldom culturally prestigious or powerful.

Cultural prestige as discussed above derives primarily from nonfamilial power. The other aspects of women's cultural roles that should be looked at are their work roles (which may or may not be in a familial context) and their role in the family. Almost all cultures have a clear dichotomy between the work roles of men and women. Precisely what one group does and does not do, however, seems to vary rather widely, and, in many situations seems quite arbitrary. Mead, for instance, reported that the Arapesh women carried heavy loads on their heads, but men never did so, the cultural belief being that women's heads were stronger than men's.[3] The Kota group from India also believed that women have stronger heads than men, but that men have stronger arms than women. For this reason, women carried heavy loads on their heads while men carried similar loads in their arms. There are, however, some almost universal divisions of labor. Hunting and warfare, for instance, are almost always men's work. The explanation that these require greater strength does not seem ten-

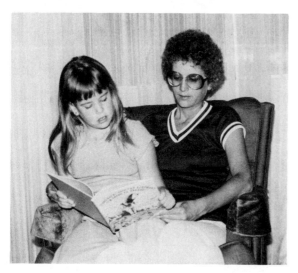

Figure 4. American mothers have complete responsibility for their children.

able in light of modern understanding of the physical differences between men and women. The more probable explanation is that women's most important job is considered to be childrearing, and since this requires relative stability in terms of mobility and a type of work that is interruptible, hunting and warfare are seldom possible. Women do perform some hunting tasks, usually those that can be done closer to home, and a considerable amount of cultivation, as well as crafts and marketing. It seems clear, however, that the most culturally valued role for women everywhere is motherhood. It is the only available role to the vast majority of women during most of our history and prehistory and even in most contemporary cultures. Few cultures have any role available for the unmarried woman, and situations in which the woman is barren in a marriage are almost always grounds for divorce as well as an extreme cultural disappointment.

Little is known about the use of contraception from a cross-cultural viewpoint, largely because the majority of the ethnographies have been done by men who used very few female informants. Some groups, like the Marquesans, in which the women had only the greatest disdain for the role of motherhood, developed very effective contraceptives, in this case resulting in high rates of infertility from repeated nonsterile abortions. In most situations, however, the most effective contraception was probably the many sexual taboos. Long (several years) postpartum taboos

were present against sexual intercourse throughout most of the tropics. This seems to be associated with low protein environments in which an infant who is weaned before the second year in order to accommodate a sibling is likely to suffer or die from protein malnutrition. Taboos on sexual intercourse are also associated with a wide variety of other activities; many cultures forbid the man from having intercourse for several weeks to several months before many "manly" activities, such as war and hunting. In addition to this, the high infant mortality resulted in surprisingly small numbers of children per woman in most cultures.

Regardless of how much the role of mother is culturally valued, however, where women share an important part of the responsibility for subsistence (which is often the case), the children come second to this activity. DuBois'[4] account of the Alorese points out the extreme drain the woman's economic responsibilities put on her motherhood. In most cases, the majority of childcare was left to very young girls (4 or 5 years old), with the mother supplying primarily the breastmilk, but little of the affection. This kind of economic strain on women has very clear implications in all the ethnographic literature on the culture's childrearing practices, and it is one often seen in our own society in situations in which women are not only the chief childrearers, but also the primary providers for a family.

In addition to the drain of economic pursuits, the motherhood expectations of most societies are quite different from those of our own. Nowhere else in the world is the woman expected to be so solely and completely responsible for every aspect of her child's development (Fig. 4). This is partially because in other cultures many adults are involved in the child's care and partially because other cultures do not have the strong cultural dictum that stresses the importance of the adults' interaction with children. As Murphy and Murphy state in their ethnography of the Mundurucu:

> The reasons for this have less to do with devotion than with the circumstances of life. Mundurucu mothers do not have to prepare their children for school and supervise their studies because there are no schools. Mothers do not watch their children cross streets or caution them against traffic because there are neither streets or cars. Women do not warn the young about "strange men" because there are no strangers. They are not obsessed by the life chances of their children because the course of life is pre-

determined. Piano lessons, orthodonture, Little League, and all the other means by which the modern mother bedevils both herself and her children are absent. By the time the child is six or so, the burden of its protection and socialization shifts to the household, the peer group, and to the community-at-large. Mundurucu women are not "eaten up" by their young, as are American women, and child rearing is less work.[5]

Certainly the self-concept of women is derived largely from the value the culture places on them. As we have seen, they are most often valued as "second best," and the culture tells them this in many ways. Cultures in which female infanticide is practiced (there is no known record of male infanticide) must surely convey to their female members that they are second-class citizens. Cultures in which the bride price acts as a purchase for a woman much as a purchase for cattle certainly impart the same message. The Eskimo culture in which the men lend their wives to other men as a personal favor is in a similar position. Freuchen describes the situation like this: "It should be clearly understood that . . . it is strictly an arrangement made between the men. The wives have little to say in the matter."[6] Similarly, the levirate, or custom in which a widow is automatically inherited as a wife to the deceased man's brother is, again, a testimonial to the fact that the women are, at least in many respects, property of the men. Roden quotes the following Egyptian lullabies as an overt description of the relative value of men and women:

Lullaby for a Son
After the heat and after the bitterness, and after the sixth of the month,
After our enemies had rejoiced at her pain and said, "There is a stone in her belly!"
The stone is in their heads! And this overwhelms them.
Go! O bearer of the news! Kiss them and tell them, "She has borne a son!"

Lullaby for a Newborn Girl
When they said, "It's a girl!"—that was a horrible moment.
The honey pudding turned to ashes and the dates became scorpions.
When they said, "It's a girl!" the cornerstone of the house crumbled.
And they brought me eggs in their shells and instead of butter, water.
The midwife who receives a son deserves a gold coin to make earrings.

The midwife who receives a son deserves a gold coin to make a ring for her nose.
But you! O midwife! Deserve thirty strokes of the stick!
Oh! You who announce a little girl when the censorious are here![7]

When studying societies such as these, however, it may mistakenly be assumed that the women completely believe in the cultural norm of their relative worthlessness. There is considerable evidence, however, that this is not true. They are not completely subdued, and even in cultures that severely repress women, it is interesting to note the variety of ways in which women do force the culture to allow them some means of self-expression. In fact, it is quite common in these cultures to have a rather overt expression of sexual antagonisms, the so-called "sex-war." For the women's part, this appears to stem from resentment at their role; for the men, it appears to stem from the ever-present fear that this resentment will erupt to do them damage. It is very common for the men to be quite careful not to "contaminate" themselves with female substances. Women are frequently feared to be witches and their bodily fluids (particularly those associated with "womanly" functions such as menstruation, postpartum lochia, and vaginal fluids) are thought to be the means of transmitting spells. Menstrual huts in which women must seclude themselves during menstruation are often constructed some distance from the village; special birthing places are similarly segregated to avoid contamination of the men. The taboos on sexual intercourse with a woman before war or hunting usually exist for the express purpose of preventing the man from becoming "weakened" by the female influence. Men's societies to which women are not admitted often center around a Men's House with secret men's symbols. Such men's cults are commonplace in societies with high levels of sexual antagonism and low social status of women. Long and very secret initiation rites for men often occur in these same societies. Interestingly enough, strong as such cultural pressure must be, the women do not entirely accept the idealized male superiority. As Murphy and Murphy describe it:

Male cults symbolizing sex antagonism are widespread. They are expressive of male superordination: only adult men have direct access to supernatural power; only they may own, handle, or even see the sacred objects; only they may perform the sacred rituals. The women's primary function is negative: they are to keep their distance, to be awed and frightened by the mysterious rites. In general, they are supposed to be thoroughly intimidated by the apotheosis of male power. This is how the men see it, but there is some doubt as to the women's attitudes. It is very clear that at least Mundurucu women know all about the cult and its practices from which they are so excluded, yet . . . they were neither mystified nor cowed. It is as if they had investigated the secret sources of men's power—and had found absolutely nothing.[8]

and later:

If the men's house symbolism has any function at all in Mundurucu society, it is to conceal from the men the fragility of their own superiority; it perpetuates an illusion. Their position is a vulnerable one. . . . Perhaps Margaret Mead summed it up best when she said, in a passing remark: "If the men really were all that powerful, they wouldn't need such rigmarole."[9]

For the woman's part, her resentment is often very open, and many cultures in which women occupy particularly low status appear to structure certain "venting systems" for the women. These serve as culturally approved methods of expressing these sexual antagonisms. In certain African societies, for instance, on specific days it is expected that the women may scream obscene insults and even hurl physical objects at any man in sight with total impunity. Another example of institutionalized catharsis is the Zar Cult of Ethiopia. Ethiopia is one of those African countries in which women occupy an extremely low status. Women, predictably, are the most frequent victims of mental illness, usually hysteria, often precipitated by an incident of neglect by their husbands. When a woman is stricken with the illness of the Zar, she is immediately enrolled in the Zar Cult, a group of women formerly victims of the disease. A long and elaborate ceremony is performed with this woman as the center of much attention. At some point she is possessed by the spirit of the Zar who speaks through her, demanding various luxuries from her husband. It is unthinkable that the husband should refuse the spirit of Zar, and thus he produces the demanded luxuries, which then become the property of his wife. With the group support, the ritualistic catharsis, and the remunerative gifts, the woman soon recovers. Similar cults are described in a variety of Brazilian cultures. It is interesting to note that as women become less of

an oppressed group, more lower class and/or deviant men begin to become part of these cults, adding to the evidence that they are indeed a means of expressing discontent with social position.

Another very important cultural asset that exists at least in most matrilocal groups is a strong female support group. Because most women in these societies depend on each other for help in childrearing, in their economic activities, and for adult-to-adult socialization, they often form very effective support groups, which help considerably to enhance their self-esteem as well. This is, unfortunately, an asset that has never been available to the American woman. Not only does she miss the advantages from close association with other women in terms of direct help with childrearing, but she also misses the less tangible, but perhaps more important help that comes from a very close interdependent peer group in terms of emotional support. The resulting isolation of the American woman stranded in a nuclear family is described by Murphy and Murphy in this way:

The American woman, on the other hand, suffers acutely from sheer loneliness and boredom. This was brought home to us vividly one day when a woman asked Yolanda (the American ethnographer) where she went to draw water in her village in America. Yolanda explained that we do not go to a stream, but bring water through a hollow tube, like a long piece of bamboo, right into our houses. The women were not impressed, only dismayed. "But if you don't go with the other women to get water and to bathe, aren't you lonely?" Yolanda thought about it a moment and answered, "Yes, we are."

The modern American woman often confesses to a feeling of entrapment and anomie. She is not only cut off from realizing some of the central values of the culture, such as they are, but she is also cut off from the association of others. Caught in a nuclear family household and in the constant company of small and demanding children, by the time the growth of the young gives her free time, her abilities are irrelevant to the changing world. And she finds not freedom but abandonment in the departure of the children. . . . The culmination of the long and, for the woman, isolating childrearing process is that the couple discovers suddenly that they have each other, and only each other, on their hands. This is one reason why so many American marriages break up after twenty or twenty-five years. The American family is self-destructing; it preserves little continuity and it has few extensions.

Unlike the Mundurucu woman, her American counterpart has few bases for structuring relations with other women. The middle-class woman may join clubs or become active in one or another form of community service, but these are of a wholly voluntary nature. She may find pleasant company and quite useful work, but it has none of the strong and compelling economic qualities of Mundurucu female cooperation. . . . And in her interaction with the husband, she has little support from others. Her family of origin is scattered and preoccupied with its own concerns; besides, it shares the American view that such problems are best left to the principals. As for other women, she may find a bit of sympathy or counsel, but little in the way of active and practical help. They, too, are locked into their own little worlds of house, husband, and children.

Certainly, nothing even remotely comparable to the unity of Mundurucu women exists to sustain the American woman. For all the low official status of the Mundurucu woman, there is far less wife beating among them than in the average American suburb, and, indeed, there is far less direct domination and coercion of wives by husbands. The Mundurucu females are protected by their unity, while ours are, at best, separate or, at worst, pitted against one another.[10]

Many other instances of the resentment of women at their low status are evident in the ethnographic literature. The resultant sexual antagonism has clear implications for childrearing, because it undermines the partnership of the mother and father in the childrearing process, and because it poses particular problems for the little girl in achieving a positive self-image and for the mother-son relationship, which creates a particular kind of problem that will be discussed further under adolescence.

In a day in which we are trying to restructure woman's role in our society, it would seem wise, then, to take several lessons from this kind of cross-cultural survey:

1. Women under severe stress from heavy economic as well as domestic responsibilities have difficulty finding the time or emotional or physical energy for optimal childrearing.
2. Most other cultures provide childrearers with some relief from the constancy of childrearing by having other adults who both share the responsibilities and provide an opportunity for adult socializing.
3. Societies that program a lower status for women and an antagonism between the sexes are likely to engender a number of childrearing problems: the father's role is more likely to be distant and undermined by the mother, little girls will have more difficulty achieving a positive self-concept, and the mother-son relationship will be fraught with particular kinds of problems.

PREGNANCY*

All reported cultures show some kind of recognition of the state of pregnancy. Almost always, recognition is most obvious in the magical belief system surrounding this condition. Malinowski, an early anthropologist, observed that magical practices tend to be most prominent in situations associated with uncertainty.[11] This appears to be true with regard to pregnancy. Groups everwhere seem to feel a certain lack of control regarding the outcome for both mother and baby and apparently try to increase their control by prescribing specific tangible things they can do to increase their chances of success. In relation to pregnancy, these magical beliefs are both positive and negative: certain positive actions or rituals are prescribed to insure a successful outcome. Certain negative sanctions are also involved. These sanctions are usually present in the form of taboos.

Positive actions that the mother or others can take to increase the chances of a happy outcome for herself and her baby are quite varied. Often specific items of clothing are worn, such as the muneco worn by the Spanish-speaking people of the Southwest. This is a cord worn beneath the breasts and knotted directly over the umbilicus. It is thought to insure a safe delivery and prevent morning sickness. Medications are also often thought to be beneficial to the pregnant woman and her unborn child. These may be for the immediate easing of symptoms, such as the spearmint or sassafras teas used by Mexican women to ease their morning sickness or the Benedictine used in our own culture. They may, on the other hand, be taken as an insurance for a good delivery and healthy baby, as are the iron pills in our own culture or the various cathartics used during the last month or two prior to delivery by many expectant Spanish-American women in the Southwest.

Much more common are the negative sanctions or taboos. Stephens classifies these taboos into three categories: food taboos, activity taboos,

---

*The ideas presented in this section were originally written for the article, A cross-cultural look at pregnancy, labor and delivery. J. Obstet. Gynecol. Nurs. Sept./Oct., 1976. Reprinted here with permission.

and sex taboos.[12] Food taboos are the most nearly universal and in one study[13] they were found to exist in 33 of the 35 cultures observed. These taboos often consist of prohibiting foods whose physical characteristics resemble certain possible characteristics of the child. In Polynesia, for instance, women never eat double fruit or eggs with double yolks for fear of a twin pregnancy. In our own culture the eating of strawberries is associated by some people with the so-called "strawberry" birthmark. Even in our medical culture the long-used prohibition of salt is beginning to look like it should be classified as an unscientific food taboo. The same is true of the general restriction of food so common 8 or 10 years ago when one main goal of obstetrics was to reduce the mother's weight gain to a bare minimum.

Activity taboos are somewhat less common, but do exist in many cultures, including our own. Particularly common seems to be the idea that a pregnant woman should not look at certain things, such as snakes, other particular animals, or the full moon. In the Southwest, Spanish-speaking women have traditionally feared the moon, whose rays may deform or cripple the unborn child. In many cultures the unborn child is expected to take on certain characteristics of animals seen by the mother—the swiftness of the antelope or the ferocity of the bear, for instance. In some cultures, the mother is prohibited from killing snakes or preparing certain foods. In our own culture many women refrain from various types of physical activities; some of these prohibitions seem sensible, some seem superstitious.

Most of these taboos stem from the fear of injuring the unborn child, but many emanate from the fear that a pregnant woman has supernatural, most often evil powers, and these may harm others, particularly men. For instance, if a man eats food prepared by the hands of a pregnant woman, he may become ill. In cultures in which this belief is held, there almost always exist a similar belief concerning menstruating women. Women are sometimes simply prohibited from doing certain activities that might injure men. As mentioned before, in some situations they are actually physically isolated from men in a special menstrual or pregnancy hut. Seldom does this go on for the entire pregnancy, but it often holds true for the menstruation period, the actual birth, and as long as 2½ years of the postpartum period. In our own culture, the common exclusion of the husband from the delivery room is reminiscent of the menstrual hut. Perhaps the idea in this country that a woman should not be President for fear she might wage war during her menses may also have overtones of the evil power associated with womanly functions.

Sexual taboos are also quite common, probably more so than activity taboos. Not surprisingly, they are usually associated with polygamy, the situation in which the husband has access to other women. These taboos may start as early as the second month and last as long as 2 years postpartum. Again our own medical culture shares, as you know, in many of these taboos. Obstetricians in this country frequently suggest limited sexual activity for extended periods of time toward the end of pregnancy, even though there is very little scientific basis for this.

These taboos are most often incumbent on the woman, but may also restrict others in the culture, particularly the husband. In a group called the Lepcha, for instance, the father-to-be must be exceedingly cautious during his wife's pregnancy.[14] He may not build a fence or the delivery will not be safe. He may not remove a fish from the rivertraps or the child will be born with his nose stopped up. He may not put anything into a box or the child will not be delivered until the box is opened. He must not touch a horse's bridle or both the mother and the child will die. He must not look at a solar eclipse or the child will be stillborn. He must not watch the birth of puppies or his child will be born with one eye smaller than the other. The custom of having the father observe certain precautions during the pregnancy is a very widespread one and often continues during the labor, delivery, and postpartum period. It is a practice that has many implications for health care and will be discussed further in the following section.

Labor and Delivery

Although the biological process of labor and delivery is basically the same for all cultures, it is handled differently and surrounded by different attitudes in different cultures. Many other cultures have quite sophisticated systems of childbirth, including oxytocics,[15] Caesarean sections,[16] and various kinds of herbal medicines.[17-19]

Most non-Western labor positions are upright. Out of 76 cultures studied by Naroll and associates,[20] 62 used kneeling, sitting, or squatting positions. Even our own culture has adopted the supine position only recently. In the early 1900s the lateral Simms position was more common, as it is today in Britain. Research on this subject has suggested that the supine position we use may indeed be disadvantageous to spontaneous delivery.[21,22] Perhaps this is one of the areas in which we could learn from other cultures.

Not only do the physical approaches to labor and delivery differ between cultures, but the psychological attitudes toward it differ as well. Newton and Newton suggest several dimensions in which such attitudes may be compared.[23] Included in these are the attitudes toward the privacy of the delivery and the attitude of what they call "achievement vs. atonement."

The value of privacy in relation to labor and delivery varies from the situation of the Talamancan tribe in South America, where the woman delivers completely alone even if there are complications, to the seclusion of the woman from the men of the tribe as practiced in many of the Oceania tribes, to the very open and frank occurrence of birth as seen in the Navajo tribe, where all who pass by the hogan are expected to come in and offer encouragement and moral support. In the Pukapuka culture, in fact, birth is such an open topic that one of the favorite games of the young children is playing at having babies. First the boy and girl pretend to have intercourse, then the little girl puts a coconut in her dress and imitates the labor behavior she has seen so many times in the older women, and finally she simulates the birth by producing the coconut from under her dress.

Newton's and Newton's concept of "achievement vs. atonement" refers to a culture's attitude toward whether the birth process is defiling or praiseworthy. It also includes the question of whose achievement a birth is, and who is the beneficiary of this achievement. In some groups the father is considered to be the beneficiary of the woman's trouble, and he must "pay" his wife's family for this service. In other groups the child is considered the beneficiary and must always be grateful to his mother for having given him birth. In still other groups it is the society that must be grateful, as in the case of the Ila of Rhodesia, in which all the community shout thanks to the new mother.

The opposite attitude (i.e., that it is the mother who is the beneficiary) is also present in some cultures. In many of these, the woman is considered "unclean" and must atone for this uncleanliness through various rituals. The Laotians, for instance, have the mother go through such a rit-

ual named "You Kam," translated to me as "to submit to penitence." Atlee feels that our culture is one in which the woman must atone for the birth rather than consider it an achievement.[24] The obstetrician is more likely to be seen as deserving of thanks than the mother. Gifts are seldom given to the mother as is the case in many cultures. They are almost always directed toward the infant.

One of the most fascinating features of a cross-cultural study of pregnancy and childbirth is the custom of the couvade. This refers to the practice in which the child's father shows symptoms resembling those of pregnancy and sometimes of delivery. Trethowan has made a useful distinction between the couvade syndrome and the couvade ritual.[25] The ritual is a very common one practiced by many groups around the world. In it the child's father goes through a ritual in which he pretends to be delivering a baby at about the time his wife is due to actually deliver. The syndrome is different from the ritual in that there is no pretense involved. The man actually suffers from real physiological or at least psychological phenomena that resemble pregnancy and childbirth. The couvade syndrome is less extensively found than the couvade ritual, but is not uncommon, particularly in South America. It has been reported from all parts of the world, however, and has received some study in our own culture.

Mention was first made of this for our own culture in 1955 by Curtis, who studied 55 expectant fathers in the armed services.[26] Twenty-two of these developed symptoms such as constipation, morning sickness, changes of appetite, and heartburn, which Curtis associated with their wives' pregnancies. Unfortunately, he did not study a control group, so his results were difficult to evaluate. A later study by Bardhan in 1964 gave similar results, but again was uncontrolled.[27] These studies provided the impetus for a larger and more scientifically conducted study by Trethowan and Conlon in 1965.[28] The investigators studied 327 expectant fathers as well as a similar number of married men, matched for various sociological variables, whose wives were not pregnant. The results were not only statistically significant, but rather striking. Of all the symptoms studied, those that were statistically more frequent in the husbands of pregnant women were nausea, vomiting, loss of appetite, and toothache. The first three of course are common symptoms of pregnancy. The origin of toothache remains obscure, but it is a very common couvade symptom in all cultures. In certain groups in Chili, for instance, a woman's pregnancy is usually first suspected and sometimes diagnosed by the fact that her husband has a toothache. In old England, this was also a common belief, and even the playwrights of the time often made reference to such things as "breeding a child in the teeth." Perhaps this belief is connected in some way to the old idea that a woman loses a tooth for every pregnancy, but this is unclear.

The frequency of these symptoms in expectant fathers in our own culture is usually surprising even to maternity nurses. In the studies cited, one in five expectant fathers have some kind of morning sickness. This is about twice as often as it occurred in the control group. Interestingly enough, it was not always associated with the woman's morning sickness; in many cases, the woman herself had no symptoms while her husband did. Appetite changes were also common. Usually this consisted of a loss of appetite, sometimes an increase in appetite, and in a few cases cravings for unusual foods. Toothache affected 25 percent of the expectant fathers, but only about 10 percent of the nonexpectant husbands. About 25 percent of the husbands experienced some type of digestive problems, most often heartburn. Actual abdominal swelling in the husband, as well as perineal soreness after a wife's episiotomy, has been reported, although these are rare. Also in the literature are situations in which the man complains of abdominal cramping simulating labor pains at the time of his wife's confinement. Most often these symptoms (except nausea and vomiting) occur during the latter part of pregnancy and labor and delivery. They are more likely to occur during first pregnancies and occur most often in couples experiencing considerable anxiety over the anticipation of a child.

Various explanations have been proffered for this phenomenon: (1) some feel that it indicates a reaction-formation in a man whose feelings toward his wife and unborn child are quite ambivalent; (2) others feel it indicates an envy of the female ability to bear a child (i.e., the so-called "parturition envy"); (3) still others feel it is an externalized attempt to establish paternity.

This seems a very clear case of how a close look at cross-cultural practices can help us better understand certain behaviors in the childrearing practices of our own culture. This phenomenon would probably never have been suspected in this country if reports from more exotic groups had not prompted the inquiry. The findings that couvade is not uncommon here should, I think, make us as health professionals more cognizant of the fact that expectant fathers may be in need of as much care as mothers. Hopefully, the current trend toward including the father in the delivery room and other parts of the birth process is an indication that we are moving in this direction. Attempts to include him in prenatal care and education as well as postpartum follow-through are also important.

There are some important lessons to be learned by looking at other cultures and how they react to and approach the management of pregnancy, labor, and delivery. In certain cases, we may find that other methods seem more sensible than our own (the position for delivery, for instance). In other situations, such as the couvade, we may find that things first apparent to us when looking at another culture are also present in our own. And in all cases, the knowledge of how people with differing backgrounds and experience approach this part of the life cycle helps us to expand our knowledge and understanding of pregnant couples.

EARLY CHILDHOOD

Because cultures tend to preserve their value systems at all costs, and because these value systems are most successfully preserved through childrearing practices, most individuals in a culture come to accept the way they raise their children as the only way, or at least as the very best way (Fig. 5). This is no less true in our own culture. Even though we are a diverse culture with seemingly many different variations of lifestyles and childrearing practices, and even though our culture seems to be changing rapidly and appears to be open to all forms of new and different ideas, this appearance may be a delusion. In fact when we look at childrearing from a cross-cultural perspective, we find that our culture is quite deviant from the world-wide norms of early childrearing and we are really quite narrow in the spectrum of diversity we accept. As people interested in these phenomena, we should attempt to get a broader perspective encompassing as wide a spectrum of time and place as possible. In addition to such a cross-cultural perspective, the period of early childhood is one in which even a cross-species investigation proves helpful in broadening our understanding of this

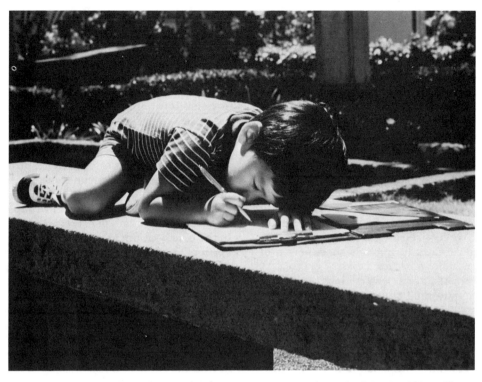

Figure 5. Culture patterning is obvious at an early age. (Photograph by Brad Powell)

stage of the life-cycle. Not only can we learn from how other people in other times and places have raised their children, but the ethologists are currently making available a great deal of information concerning how other closely related and not-so-closely related animals rear their young. Investigation of this kind of information should always be preceded by a caution: many species evolve behaviors that seem more similar to our own than they really are. To jump to conclusions from animal data about human behaviors and conditions that may or may not be conducive to the healthy childrearing of humans is erroneous. These data can, however, be useful in terms of providing hypotheses. It is important to remember, though, that these are just hypotheses—they need to be studied specifically in regard to human beings, who differ in many important respects from other animals.

The purpose of this section, then, is to look at what information is available about the early childrearing practices and experiences of other species as well as other cultures.

One example of an ethological application that can be useful in understanding human child-

rearing experiences has been made popular by the work of Kennell and Klaus.[30] They cite many of the ethological studies that served as an impetus for their own research on early human maternal-child interaction patterns. Critical to an understanding of their work is an understanding of the ethological term "critical period." This term, used in the strictly ethological sense, means a period during which a certain set of circumstances must occur for the young animals to respond in a certain way. For animals this period is often quite short—a few minutes or days. It is important to note here that there is really no known critical period of such short duration in human beings. One of the distinguishing marks of our species is its extreme maleability—it is doubtful that we will ever find a critical period in humans in the same sense that it appears in lower animals; human beings appear to be much more plastic and adaptable than that. It is likely, however, that humans have many "sensitive periods," that is, periods in which it is easier to elicit certain responses than at other times during the life span. It is a common observation, for instance, that many things are learned more easily during childhood than during adulthood (e.g., a second language, and probably certain fine and gross motor skills); these things are not impossible to learn later, they are just more difficult. This is an important distinction, for failure to appreciate it has resulted in some serious misinterpretations of the work of Klaus and Kennell. Klaus and Kennell were specifically interested in a very short period of early childhood—the time immediately after delivery of the new infant. In studying this period in other animals, they found many accounts of a critical period occurring at that time. This critical period referred to a very short period of time during which the mother animal would "bond" or "attach" to her infant. In order to do this, it was necessary for her to see her infant during this short period of time.

In goats, for instance, this critical period appears to occur immediately after delivery and lasts for about 5 minutes. During this time if the mother is unable to see and interact with her kid, she will, if united with him later, show aberrant patterns of mothering. She will butt him away and fail to nurse him in the usual manner. Similar behavior occurs in rats and cattle with such early separation. The exact timing of this critical period differs from species to species but appears to occur in some variation for all species studied and reported.

Another area that intrigued Kennell and Klaus was the studies showing specific maternal behavior patterns that began immediately after delivery. One fascinating study was that done by Birch on the perinatal behavior patterns of rats.[31] During pregnancy, the mother frequently licks herself, particularly in the anogenital region. When the baby rats are born this licking behavior is extended to them. Birch constructed special collars for the necks of the mother rats to prevent them from licking themselves during pregnancy and their offspring after delivery. Distorted, bizarre mothering patterns occurred in these rats. Once the collars were removed, they actually ate many of their own litter and refused to nurse the remaining young. It would seem then, that at least in many species there appears to be a specific critical period following shortly after delivery in which it is essential that maternal-infant interaction take place. Interruption of this normal process leads to aberrant maternal behavior with subsequent failure of normal growth and development of the infant.

Still another area of ethological research on maternal behavior that generated hypotheses for research with humans is the rat research done by Rosenblatt and Siegel.[32] They attempted to discover whether immediate postpartal maternal behavior was the result of "innate releasing mechanisms" within the newborn (i.e., physical or behavioral characteristics of the infant that "release" nurturing behavior in the mother) or of hormonal changes within the mother. A lengthy series of experiments involving the attempt to get virgin mice or males to "attach" to newborns and the injection of virgin rats with the plasma of near-delivery pregnant rats resulted in the conclusion that, at least in rats, there appears to be a release near delivery of estradiol, which remains in the blood stream after delivery and which may "prime" a mother to attach to her infant. This substance and its subsequent disappearance may account for the sensitive period during which attachment seems much more likely and easily accomplished. It does not seem to be completely determining, however, since virgin rats and male rats could also be coaxed (although not as easily as a newly delivered mother) to attach to newborns.

All of these studies further prompted Kennell and Klaus and their group at Case Western Reserve to further investigate the importance of early human mother-child interaction. They began by studying the development of interactional patterns between mothers and premature babies. They noted that these mothers followed the same predictable sequence of interaction as had been shown earlier to exist with mothers of full-term infants, but they did so at a slower rate. That is, they began by touching the infants' extremities with their fingertips, gradually proceeding to touch more of the infant's body, first with their whole fingers and later their palms, so that by 8 minutes of age, mothers of full-term infants were caressing their babies' entire bodies with the palms and fingers of their hands. This sequence also occurred in mothers of premature infants, but would often not be complete until 3 to 5 days of age. In studying this difference they decided to test the hypothesis that it was not only the fact that the prematurity itself was worrisome and disruptive to the parents, but that it might well be the many medical and hospital barriers we erect to the normal early mother-infant interaction that was causing a faulty initial attachment process, and that this poor attachment resulted later in an increased incidence of mother-child behavioral problems.

To test this hypothesis, the group at Case Western Reserve began a study involving 28 women having their first babies. These women were divided into two groups. The first 14 mothers constituted the control group, which received the usual hospital care during their delivery and postpartum days. In this hospital, as in most, that meant that they saw their child very briefly after delivery, once again at 6 to 12 hours, and then every 4 hours for about 20 minutes until discharge. In addition to the usual time with their infant, the experimental group was given 1 hour's contact during the first postpartum hours and then an extra 5 hours each afternoon for the 3-day hospital stay. These mothers and infants have now been followed for 2 years, and startling differences between the groups have appeared. Mothers who had increased early interaction with their infants were significantly more soothing to their babies according to several measures: they tended to pick them up more often when they cried, they stood closer to them when they were examined by the physician, they spent more time cuddling their infants, they more often used an "en face" eye contact (that is, their eyes were on the same axis as the baby's eyes), and they reported missing or thinking about their babies more often when away from them. These measures all occurred within the first year. A 2-year follow-up study looked specifically at speech patterns of mothers addressing their children.[33] Again, significant differences appeared. Those mothers who had early and increased interaction time with their infants showed, 2 years later, very different ways of talking to their children. They used significantly more adjectives, questions, and total number of words than did the mothers with the traditional amount of early contact. They also issued fewer commands than did the other group. The fact that an additional 16 hours of mother-infant contact in the early postpartum period could result in significant changes on such a wide variety of measures and lasting over a period of 2 years is rather startling.

It is important to reiterate at this point that extreme caution must be used in interpreting these results. The studies on animals were carefully controlled and used large samples. Studies on human beings cannot be that carefully controlled nor were large samples used. This must be remembered when making clinical applications. Although it is more than reasonable to change delivery room procedures in such a way as to make early bonding of mother (and father) with the baby easier, it is important to remember that bonding can occur at other times. Because this research has been highly publicized in the lay press, it is not surprising that many mothers who for some reason were unable to interact with their baby immediately after delivery are voicing guilt feelings and fears of having ruined their relationships with their children permanently. This is a good example of how animal data, combined with very small human studies, can be used indiscriminately to do considerable damage. It is quite clear, as stated before, that for human beings there are no short critical periods, and it is unreasonable to assume that parents' cannot bond or attach to their child at a later time even if the immediate postdelivery time is not available to them.

Other types of animal studies are also interesting in terms of possible similarities to human behavior. Lorenz's early work on the gray-necked goose is, of course, well known for revealing that some early interaction is necessary for the gosling of this species to develop normal behavior patterns.[34] It is during this time that the gosling "imprints" the form of his mother in his mind and will follow only that imprint. In normal situations this means he is then able to follow only his mother. In Lorenz's studies, when he separated the mother-infant pair and the goslings saw him instead of their mother, they imprinted to his form and would follow only him. In fact, when it was a box they first saw, they would follow only the box. Another interesting aspect of this imprinting phenomenon in geese is that in the adulthood of these geese, they mated with a form similar to that which they had followed during infancy. For some of these geese, it meant they were only able to exhibit mating behavior toward Lorenz or toward a box. Observations on the similarity of this phenomenon to the human phenomenon of wanting to marry "a gal just like the gal that married dear old dad" are frequently made.

Harlow's studies of chimpanzees are also interesting in this respect.[35] These well-known studies indicate that early mother-infant interaction is necessary for later acquisition of normal chimpanzee behavior. Being deprived of such early interaction results in later difficulty in relating to other chimpanzees, particularly to mates of the opposite sex. Adult females who did not receive the normal early mothering were later unable to copulate in the normal chimpan-

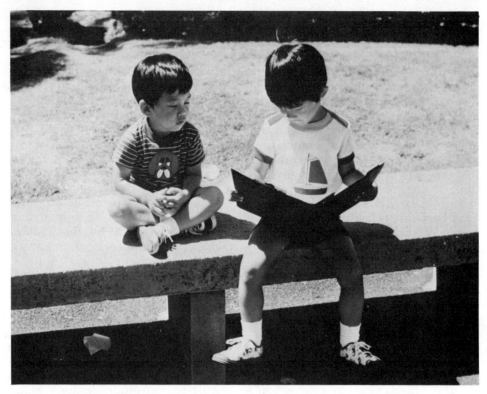

Figure 6. All children throughout the world do not have similar childhood experiences that assist them in learning about their world. (Photograph by Brad Powell)

zee manner, and even more interestingly, if they were impregnated, they were unable to perform normal chimpanzee mothering behavior themselves. Equally interesting, however, was the fact that although they did not perform these normal mothering behaviors with their first offspring, they were able to learn these mothering skills and performed quite adequately with their second offspring—again evidence of the fact that species higher in the evolutionary tree tend to exhibit sensitive rather than critical periods. This kind of primate study has been useful not because it can be applied directly to human beings, but because it helps to suggest hypotheses that are currently being studied in relation to human parenting behavior, particularly of parents who were battered as children. It is well known that such individuals frequently batter their own children, but the idea that this behavior is not totally determined at childhood, but can be changed during adulthood, is a very useful one clinically. Another interesting finding of Harlow's studies is that peer interaction for the mon-

keys who were deprived of normal mothering helped to overcome some of the more aberrant behaviors exhibited by motherless and peerless monkeys (e.g., head-banging and extreme aggression).

It is clear, then, that looking at early childhood experiences from a cross-species point of view can widen our horizons to possible explanations for our own behavior, and, if this information is used with due caution, it can serve as the grounds for very fruitful hypotheses concerning the best environmental conditions for our own young.

In addition to looking at early childhood experiences from a cross-species vantage point, cross-cultural comparisons can also be useful (Fig. 6). Until recently the only tool available to anthropologists who do cross-culture comparisons was a file called the Human Relations Area File; this file consists of information on all the cultures of the world that have been reported. One difficulty with this source is the fact that although many primitive groups and a fair number of civilized groups are represented, there

20

are very few peasant or kingdom groups. This may bias the sample in such a way that we are really comparing our childrearing methods not to the rest of the world but primarily to the tribal groups. Such comparisons, however, are useful in that they help give us an idea of how other people have handled some of the universal problems of childrearing. Currently, more appropriate data banks are being made available. They represent 136 cultural areas; each of these areas is represented by a culture judged to be "typical" of that culture area. They include primitive, peasant, and kingdom groups as well as more modern groups. These should make more accurate research possible in the near future. Even the comparisons we have currently available (i.e., those based on the older Human Relations Area Files), which compared our culture as it was 20 years ago with other groups of people living at that time or before, show us interesting things and help us put some practices of early childrearing in perspective. One of the more surprising findings from such a comparison is that, as a group, we are much less warm with our infants than are most people. Whiting and Childe, who did such a comparison, found that 75 percent of the cultures in their sample showed more nurturance and warmth to their infants than we did.[36] Indicators used for this were nursing, body contact, and general attention. In the length of time we nurse our children, we are quite deviant. In 1953, when the study was done, they found that the average length of time spent by American mothers nursing their infants was 6 months. The average world-wide time was 2½ years; often children in other cultures will be nursed until their teen-age years if no new sibling is born.

Body contact in our culture is also unusually limited. Much more common is the situation in which the child sleeps with his mother for all his infancy and is almost constantly carried by his mother or siblings during the day. A typical example is the Ifaluk:

> . . . the infant is exposed to the faces and arms of many people. For the westerner, the amount of handling the infant receives is almost fantastic. The infant, particularly after it can crawl, is never allowed to remain in the arms of one person. In the course of a half hour conversation, the baby might change hands ten times, being passed from one person to another. This transference of the infant is not due to the fatigue of the person who is holding it at the time, but is done at the request of the others. The

adults, as well as the older children, love to fondle the babies and to play with them, with the result that the infant does not stay with one person very long. . . .

> Infants are not only greatly desired, as we have already seen, but they are given the greatest care and indulgence possible. The infant is idealized to the point that its over-indulgence and pampering become phantasies from the standpoint of Western standards. We have seen that no infant is ever left alone, day or night, asleep or awake, until it can walk. To isolate a baby would be to commit a major atrocity, for if a baby is left alone, "by and by dies, no more people."

> Should an infant cry, it is immediately picked up in an adult's arms, cuddled, consoled or fed. Thus the baby is in a state of almost complete dependence on the adults about it. This oversolicitude extends to the two- and three-year-olds as well, assuming that another baby has not entered the household. Should the baby fall, and begin to cry, he is immediately picked up. . . .

> To claim that the infant is king in Ifaluk is not to exaggerate the situation at all. The infant is in control of a social situation and easily dominates the adults, bending them to his will.[37]

In most non-Western groups, however, the weaning time is markedly less warm. It is usually abrupt and traumatic; it most often occurs at the birth of a new sibling. The older child goes rapidly from a role in which all his needs were met immediately and completely into a role in which he fends pretty much for himself. Whiting describes a typical weaning process in Kwoma:

> When a child is weaned he may no longer sit in his mother's lap by day nor lie by her side at night. This is apparently felt as the most severe frustration experienced at this period of life. No longer is it possible to attain the vantage point from which all drives have hitherto been satisfied. . . .

> With weaning, then, many of the demands which the Kwoma child has learned to make during infancy become no longer successful. His mother no longer responds in the same helpful way to many of his requests. His demands to be taken into her lap, scratched, patted, or warmed, are now ignored. When she no longer heeds his demands, he becomes more vociferous. Unless he is in serious danger, she still does not cater to him. . . .

> If a child is too vociferous and persistent in his demands, he is actually punished. . . .

> Weaning greatly increases a child's experience of anxiety. His desire to sit in his mother's lap and his fear of being pushed away and scolded for it, the desire to suckle and the belief that there is a marsalai [monster] in his mother's breast, the wish for

his demands to be heeded and the punishments he receives for crying, all are anxiety-producing sources of conflict. . . .

In the realm of prestige, the Kwoma child during the period of weaning plunges from the top to the very bottom of the social hierarchy.[38]

Whiting and Childe did one of the more complete comparisons of cultures in terms of their severity in childrearing practices.[39] On the two types of socialization that they compared during the early childrearing years, our culture came out as relatively severe. They compared oral socialization, including both early nursing and weaning, and found that American socialization was somewhat more severe than that in the average society. Interestingly enough, they also found that in societies in which early oral socialization was severe, adults tended to seek oral remedies for their ills. Certainly this appears to be true for our pill-swallowing society. It is almost as if because we were unable to get our fill of oral satisfaction as children, we have been left with the illusion that if we only had enough oral satisfaction as adults, all our ills, physical and psychological, would be cured.

In the other type of early socialization studied by Whiting and Childe, that of toilet training, our culture was found to begin socialization earliest and to be the second most severe of all those societies reported.[40]

In summary, it is interesting to note that a culture that is so impressed with the lifelong effects of early childrearing experiences on the adult personality is, in the perspective of a cross-cultural panorama, quite nonnurturant and severe in the socialization practices it employs during early childhood. It may be that some of these practices are not as "natural" or healthy as we have believed, and careful consideration of some hypotheses derived both from cross-cultural and cross-species behavior may result in ways in which we could considerably improve this phase of the life-cycle in our culture.

MIDDLE CHILDHOOD

Like the studies in our own culture, the cross-cultural studies of middle childhood are much fewer than those of other stages of childhood. They have tended, for the most part, to relate either to how a culture socializes children during the middle childhood years to handle aggression and sexuality or to how cultures inculcate children of this age with various values; the most studied values are competitiveness, achievement, and self. This section will briefly review some of the cross-cultural work available on each of these topics.

Socialization of aggression in our society starts earlier and is done in a more severe manner than is true for most societies. This is probably related to the fact that more organized, interdependent, and densely populated groups can tolerate less expression of aggression than can smaller groups, particularly those for whom the economy is based on individually completed tasks such as hunting and gathering rather than complicated tasks necessitating complicated kinds of cooperation. A health professional dealing with the mental health problems of our adults and the currently felt need for "assertiveness training" cannot help but wonder, however, what toll this takes from the individual. How can we as a society foster enough freedom for the individual's mental health but enough cooperation for the good of the group?

Our sex training appears to be rather severe as well. We rated more severe in socialization of sexuality than three fourths of the Whiting and Child sample taken in 1953. An example of one of the less severe groups is the Kaingang of Brazil. Here is the ethnographer's report of their practices of childhood sexuality:

The sexuality of little boys is stimulated by their mothers by manipulation of the genitals before they can walk. . . . Yet with all this I never saw or heard of intercourse among children. . . . The children receive so much satisfaction from adults it is hard to see why they should bother with one another. They are at the beck and call of anyone who wants a warm little body to caress. As Monya, age two, wobbles by on fat uncertain legs Kanyahe calls to him. He slowly overcomes the momentum of his walk, turns about, smiles and wobbles obediently over to Kanyahe. Children lie like cats absorbing the delicious stroking of adults. The little children receive an enormous amount of adult attention and one never sees them caress one another or lie down together. It is impossible to keep track of children around the campfire. By choice and from necessity they literally sleep all over the place. They like to cuddle next to an uncle, aunt, or step-mother. In the winter when there may be only one blanket to shelter a family, the little ones are driven to crawling under the cover of someone else who welcomes the additional warmth of the little bundle. This wandering around often culminates in the sexual experience to which the grown-ups are eager to introduce the child, and he is generally enjoyed first by a person much older than he. Some married men have nicknames that bear a humorous reference to their experience in trying to deflower young girls. Hakwa was called, "You pierced your mother" because he had deflowered a young girl who had the same name as his mother. Kovi received a nickname because his first cousin clawed his penis when he tried to deflower her. The growing child's sexual experience is primarily humorous, often illicit, administered by adults, and apt to be violent in the case of girls.[41]

A comparison of this description with our own method of socializing children about how to handle their sexuality cannot help but impress us with the extreme difference. Perhaps this was due, in the past, to the fact that our children would have to go through a long period of sexual abstinence during a very prolonged adolescence if the society was to assure its ideal two-parent family to new babies. Although our period of adolescence continues to be extremely prolonged compared with other societies, the advent of very effective contraceptives may be changing this societal situation. It appears that this availability is changing adolescent and young adult patterns of sexuality considerably; it will be interesting to see if these changes are reflected in our sexuality teaching during middle childhood as well.

The values that different societies inculcate in their children during the middle childhood years is another area that has received some cross-cultural investigation. Probably one of the better studied of these values is competitiveness versus cooperation. Our society is so ingrained with the value of competition that it is sometimes difficult for us to realize that this value is extremely unusual from a cross-cultural perspective. It may come as a shock to many Western readers that there are many cultures, such as those in the Philippines, in which the traditional childhood games are games in which there are no winners or losers—imagine playing a game purely for the enjoyment of the game alone! Equally surprising to Western schoolteachers who entered the Philippines to teach in the school system was that the traditional methods of encouraging competition among the students in order to elicit the best performance of each was totally ineffective with Filipino children. To be singled out by the teacher as the best reader or speller was, to the Filipino child brought up in an atmosphere of cooperation, an extreme embarrassment. The cultural norm forbids flaunting your achievements or good fortune in any way. Some cross-cultural ex-

periments have been devised to investigate this phenomenon. Madsen designed a marble-pull game in which two children were positioned at opposite sides of the table.[42] The objective was for them to pull on a string that was attached to a marble-containing cup. Since both children's strings were attached to the cup by magnets, if they both pulled at once, the cup would fall and neither child would get the marble. If they were able to take turns, each child would obtain the marble when it was his or her turn. Interestingly enough, even when given explicit instructions on how to obtain the marble, American children were seldom able to cooperate, while Mexican children did so almost 100 percent of the time. Further investigations on other cultures tried this experiment with Mexican, Israeli, and Canadian rural and urban children. The conclusion was that children from any culture's urban area were significantly less able to cooperate than were those from the rural area. Societies with highly urban populations were much less able to cooperate than those with largely rural populations. Exactly what implications these findings have for structuring a mentally healthy environment for our largely urban society is not totally clear, but with the type of emphasis our culture puts on winning, we should look carefully at the effects on the losers—who by definition will almost always be in the majority. What about all our school children who are not the best artists or basketball players or scholars? What implications does this cultural value have for them during their middle childhood years—and later?

Another value that has been studied rather extensively is achievement (Fig. 7). Starting with the many studies of McClelland and associates in the early 1960s,[43] this area of study has emerged as one of the more thoroughly investigated. Studies began to investigate "achievement-oriented" individuals (as manifested primarily by their TAT stories). Correlations between this characteristic and a variety of other factors (e.g., high social mobility and successful economic endeavors) were found. Later, entire cultures were investigated in regard to how much they valued this achievement-orientation. Folktales, children's stories, and even poetry designs were analyzed in much the same way the TAT scores had been. Not surprisingly, the best cultural correlation was between a culture that placed a high value on achievement and that achieved a high degree of capitalism. Perhaps more relevant to health professionals

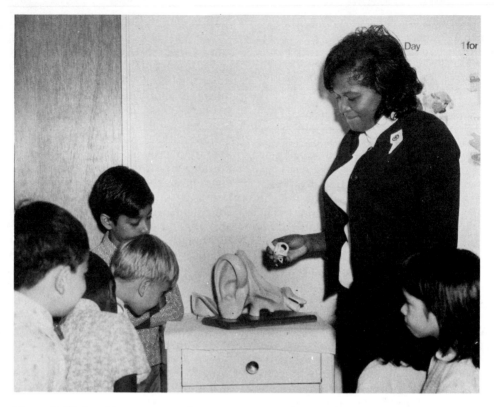

Figure 7. High achievement is valued in America. (Photograph courtesy of Houston Independent School District, George E. Watters, photographers)

working with children, however, was the high correlation between such cultures and a particular type of family structure and childrearing practice—clearly, the cultures that had highly patriarchal lineage systems with strongly authoritarian male-dominated family life were associated both with very rigid methods of childrearing during the middle childhood years and with low achievement scores. Children in these cultures were taught first and foremost to learn and honor the traditional ways of their forefathers. Innovative thinking was actively discouraged and achievement was never seen as something the individual could accomplish by himself. In more egalitarian family structures, childrearing during middle childhood seems to be more flexible and encourages the development of the individual achievement motivation. Not surprisingly, many of these societies are the same ones that value competitiveness, often at the expense of cooperation. Again the implications for the mental health of our own culture and our

children are not clear-cut, but they certainly seem to merit investigation.

The final value that has had a reasonable amount of investigation from a cross-cultural perspective is self-orientation. As Munroe and Munroe point out, the idea of the importance of "self" is a new one even in Western culture.[44] They note that self-prefixes (e.g., self-esteem and self-concept) did not even exist in our language until the seventeenth century. The growth of individualism and the idea of the importance of the self has increased dramatically since that time. A variety of studies have looked at this phenomenon cross-culturally, and in all cases, Western culture has been found to be extraordinarily deviant in this regard. The value studies of Kluckhohn and Strodtbeck found Western cultures significantly higher in orientation to self, while several American Indian groups were far more group-oriented.[45] The Six Cultures Study by Whiting and Whiting rated the behavior of 3- to 11-year-old children from six cultures on what

24

they called "egoistic" behaviors.[46] There was a significant spread among the six cultures on this variable, but most striking was the fact that American children were a full 40 percent higher than the second highest ranking children on indices of self-orientation. An even more interesting finding to emerge from this study was the fact that the major variable that appeared to correlate highly with self-orientation was the complexity of the society and the resultant small work load for the mother. Apparently, in situations in which the mother's workload does not tax her extensively, she either has more time to foster a sense of self in her children or she relies on them less for help with her own workload, in this way freeing them to develop their own sense of self.

This self-orientation has both positive and negative aspects to it. One disadvantageous phenomenon that seems to be associated with it is high rates of depression.[47] Apparently one needs to have a relatively strong sense of self in order to experience oneself in any tragic sense. There are also some aspects of personality correlated with this sense of self that seem, at least in many cultures, to be advantages. One of these is the ability to accept responsibility for one's own behavior and to regulate it accordingly. The ability to delay gratification, for instance, seems to be more highly developed in the person with a strong sense of self. This ability is obviously at the heart of capitalistic societies. Certain cognitive abilities to differentiate ideas from one another, the so-called "context-free" thought, are also abilities apparently dependent on a strong differentiation of self from the social context. These are abilities that the Western cultures clearly go to great lengths to develop in their children during the middle childhood years. Finally, the idea of empathy seems to be related to the idea of self. If one cannot experience one's self, it is difficult to imagine how another being feels. Empathy can, of course, be both positive and negative. If a person can imagine how another person with whom he has a positive relation feels, he may be able to facilitate his friend's ability to feel better. If, on the other hand, a person can vividly imagine what enemies may feel under certain conditions, torture, atrocities, and sadism also become possibilities.

It is clear, then, that Western culture is quite deviant in certain respects regarding how child-rearing occurs during the middle childhood years. We have traditionally socialized aggression and sexuality quite severely, although it

would appear that we are changing in this regard. On the other hand, we stress achievement, competition, and sense of self far more than most cultures. Exactly what implications these peculiarities of Western culture have for the mental health of our children and our adults bears close scrutiny.

ADOLESCENCE

In all cultures throughout the world and throughout time, there is some stage in the life-cycle in which the child becomes an adult. In any given culture, that means that the individual must relinquish whatever benefits and disadvantages that culture deems belong to childhood and assume those that the culture establishes as belonging to the stage of adulthood. But exactly what this transition entails differs greatly between cultures. Although the rare ethnography, such as Margaret Mead's description of Samoa,[48] states that this transition occurs very smoothly with no turmoil, the vast majority of cultural reports discuss a variety of difficulties encountered during this period. Probably the best-studied aspect of this period is how the adolescent achieves whatever the culture defines as the appropriate sex role identity. These studies may be able to give us some useful insight into this developmental task—one that is changing very rapidly in our own culture.

The anthropological interest in this period of the life-cycle was probably started by the frequent and startling accounts of very severe male initiation rites in Africa and New Guinea. A typically striking example of one of these early accounts of a male initiation rite, for instance, comes from Junod's description of the Thonga:

> When a boy reaches the age of 10 to 16 years he is sent to the circumcision school which is held every four to five years. They are marched to the "yard of mysteries" en masse, and when they arrive, eight at a time are chosen and sent forward to begin the rites by running through the gauntlet, after which they are seized by four men and stripped of their clothing. Their hair is then cut and they are seated on eight stones facing three fierce looking men covered with lion manes. At this point they are struck from behind, and when they turn to look, the "lion-men" seize their penis, and perform both a circumcision and a very painful subincision. The initiate is now secluded for three months during which time more trials are undergone. The first of these is the numerous beatings. There is a daily ritual in which the boys are severely kicked and beaten on the shoulders. At other times during the day, they are beaten on the

slightest pretext, particularly if they do not eat quickly enough. At night they are said to suffer tremendously from the cold since the ceremony is held during the coldest three months of the year, and no covers are allowed at night when the initiates must lie flat on their backs on the ground. An added difficulty at night is the white worms which swarm over the ground and continually bite the boys. Another severe trial for the boys is thirst. For the entire three months, the initiates are not allowed any water whatsoever. The final trial is that of the nauseating meals. Unsavory porridge is served over which the men frequently pour the half digested grass found in the bowels of antelope. The boys are then required to eat as rapidly as possible and are beaten if they are too slow. Junod says it is not infrequent for the boys to vomit on the porridge, but it must be finished just the same. Punishments for infractions of the initiation rules are also severe. For a serious offense: "The boy must present his hands, put them against each other and separate the fingers. Sticks are introduced between the fingers and a strong man, taking both ends of the sticks in his hands, presses them together and lifts the poor boy, squeezing and half crushing his fingers." Death also is not infrequently caused by failure of the boy's wounds to heal properly.[49]

Many similarly striking accounts followed and questions began to be raised about what cultural phenomenon could possibly account for such an apparently inhumane custom. One thing was quite clearly expressed in the male initiation of all cultures, that is, the purpose of the initiation was to rid the boy of "womanliness," so that he could become a man and perform the culturally appropriate "manly" functions in that society. Why should some cultures apparently need to go to such drastic measures to ensure that their boys become men while other cultures seem to simply expect that such maturation would occur? Why were the vast majority of such initiation rites reported for only boys? Why did it seem so essential to rid the boys of their womanliness? These were some of the questions that led to one of the most interesting of the cross-cultural theories related to human maturation.

Whiting and Childs began to correlate a number of cross-cultural variables with severe initiation rites, and from the information derived from these correlations, they began to construct a theory to explain these correlations.[50] The theory that resulted is one that should probably be looked at closely by health professionals in our own culture who must deal with a number of sexual identity questions. In the study a number of interesting variables were found to be associated with severe male initiation rites: tropical environments, polygyny, prolonged mother-infant sleeping arrangements, and long postpartum taboos on sexual intercourse. The explanation proposed for this by Whiting was that in tropical environments, the resources for supplying the protein for a young growing brain are quite small. There are seldom large game available. For this reason, prolonged availability of mother's milk may be essential to the survival of the infant. In cases such as this, a prolonged taboo on postpartum intercourse would be useful since this will prevent a second birth from occurring too quickly and making the milk unavailable to the first child. Polygyny is a logical family type in this situation since a man who must refrain from intercourse with his wife for several years is likely to desire other sexual outlets. In a polygynous situation, particularly with a nursing infant or toddler, it is commonly most efficient to have each woman in her own home with her own children while the husband circulates and spends each night at a different house (but none at the house where a wife is nursing and the postpartum taboo is in effect). In most such situations the nursing child continues to sleep with his mother. Even after nursing is finished, the mother continues to be the most important adult in the child's life. Other adults may also be important, but they are almost always other women. Male role models are relatively inaccessible, so that as the little boy matures and begins copying the behavior of the adults he emulates, these adults are most likely to be women. Perhaps equally important, the women whom he copies are also likely to be in the type of culture described previously as being characterized by extreme antagonisms between the sexes. If the adults who teach the growing boy most of his behavior and attitudes are also women who resent men, it is likely that they will also teach him some of their disdain for men. In Whiting's hypothesis, it is not surprising, then, that as the young boy becomes an adolescent, he has very little incentive to become a culturally appropriate man. In cultures such as the traditional African ones, this could be a very costly problem, since many of these cultures depend for their very survival on some of the most culturally "male" activities, particularly warfare. The culture, then, must institute a device that will motivate these recalcitrant young boys into becoming men. This device is the male initiation.

Furthermore, the hypothesis continues, the more recalcitrant the initiate, the more severe the initiation. This contention seems to be borne out repeatedly by the ethnographic description of these rites.

The next question to arise was why these severe male initiation rites were restricted to New Guinea and the African cultures. What about the South American cultures that were equally tropical, polygynous, had prolonged nursing and long postpartum sexual taboos, and extended mother-infant sleeping arrangements? These cultures had no reported rites of male initiation. Whiting's answer to this question was that these are cultures in which a strong male identity is not culturally crucial—they were not cultures that depended heavily on protecting themselves by warfare. They could afford to allow their men to maintain some ambiguity in their adult sexual identity. They backed up this argument with another interesting statistical correlation—that between the couvade and a tropical culture that did have prolonged nursing, mother-son sleeping arrangements, and postpartum taboos on sexual intercourse but that *did not* depend on warfare skills. The explanation was that men in such a culture did not need strong male identities. Indeed, the culture could afford to allow them such an ambiguous sexual identity that they could even attempt to participate in the most female of all behaviors—parturition. All these statistical correlations discovered in the Whiting/Child hypothesis have been shown to be accurate. The explanation of how these are correlated is only a theory, but a very plausible one. The application to our own culture is certainly not direct, but it does give us some interesting data to consider, particularly in the light of the increasingly common single parent family (a good number of which are mother-son families). How do the boys in such situations achieve an appropriately male identity when they reach adolescence? Or, in a society such as our own where sex roles are becoming less sexually stereotyped, do we need to have boys achieve any particularly "manly" attributes as they achieve adult status?

The opposite question is equally interesting, although the cross-cultural data are less illuminating in regard to it: What happens to the little girl who grows up with minimal adult male involvement? Miller once theorized that in the traditional Black family of the 1940s, the system was the matrifocal one described earlier.[51] Miller felt that because there was no strong male with whom to identify, the boy had a very difficult time achieving an adult male identity. Two cultural options were open to alleviate this situation. One was the army, which Miller felt served as a Western male initiation rite. The other was the gang, another class-specific male initiation rite. Interestingly, corroborative evidence is presented by Rohrer's work, which seems to indicate, as do many other studies, that a great deal of ambivalence and cross-sex identification persisted into the adult life of the urban Negro male in the 1940s.[52] In a study of the gang itself, the same conclusion is evident. As Rohrer says, "The feelings of inadequacy of the gang members are specifically related to sexual confusion. Extensive homosexuality is institutionally part of gang life, and the subsequent insistent masculinity protests too much to be anything other than a necessary reassurance against self doubts. Such feelings date from a childhood in which being a male in a matriarchal home is equated with being unworthy." Whether this particular application to a subculture within our own culture is appropriate or not, the larger issue of looking carefully at what adult sexual identities are important for a culture to maintain, and what potential obstacles to that development are programmed into the childbearing patterns, remains an important issue for health professionals in our own culture to study.

Other important adolescent tasks seem less crucial in other cultures than our own. The assumption of the adult work-role is, in our highly complex society, becoming a very important difficulty for adolescence. Which of the million available potential occupations a particular adolescent will find satisfying to him, how to learn about its existence, how to become prepared to do it, how to be sure it will remain a viable job after he learns it, and how to gain employment in it—all these are problems specific to our culture. As discussed under the section "Middle Childhood," almost no other culture allows an individual to reach adolescence without a very thorough exposure to the training he will need for his lifelong vocation. Nor is there the fear that the job market will change during an individual's life-span. Few adolescent groups in other cultures must deal with these particular problems.

The question of legitimate outlets for the emerging physical drives of sexual maturation is also one in which our culture is markedly deviant. In few other cultures is there such a long lag between physical maturation and the availability of culturally approved means of expressing sexuality. Often, these means are early marriages, sometimes contracted during infancy, but almost always contracted and begun before the end of adolescence. In cases in which a marriage is not arranged at this time, there is almost always another culturally approved method of expressing sexuality. In many African cultures, for instance, a cultural practice of "taking by stealth" consists of a practice in which the adolescent boys sneak into the adolescent girls' communal sleeping quarters and have intercourse (usually without penetration—the so-called interfemoral intercourse) while the girls pretend to remain asleep. The obvious recognition of a culturally approved outlet for adolescent sexuality soon after it becomes manifest is one that our culture, at least until recently, has been unusual in ignoring. Psychiatric case studies are replete with evidence that this restriction, enforced by culturally induced guilt feelings, has been the cause of considerable mental health problems in our own culture. Perhaps realization of how unusual we are in this respect as well as an opportunity to study what other cultures do about this potential problem may be instructive.

SUMMARY

We have looked, then, from a cross-cultural and occasionally a cross-species perspective at six aspects of the life-cycle: marriage and the family, the role of women and mothers, childbearing, early childhood, middle childhood, and adolescence. Throughout each of these discussions we have concentrated on allowing ourselves to achieve a broader and more freeing perspective, so that we will be able to look more objectively at our own culture. In light of this objective, this chapter will conclude with one final piece of ethnographic description, this time of a cultural group first studied by Ralph Linton—the Nacirema. Although Linton describes some of the general practices of this group, he did not investigate their childbearing and rearing practices to any great extent. The following is my own ethnographic description of these people, one that has been made from my revisit to the group in the late 1970s. Perhaps a look at some of the magic and customs of these people can give us a better perspective on just what extremes human beings are capable of when they bear and rear their children.

AN ETHNOGRAPHY OF THE NACIREMAN PEOPLE

Upon discovering she is pregnant, the Nacireman woman immediately visits the medicine man or occasionally a specialized practitioner, the vestal virgin, bringing with her a sample of her first morning excrement. The practitioner then ritually mixes this urine with a secret magic potion, swirling the mixture around on a magical cardboard in a series of highly stylized gestures. At the appropriate time, the vestal virgin performs her magical divination, pronouncing whether the woman is indeed pregnant or not. If she is pregnant, she is then instructed in a highly complex series of protective magic steps, which she is to begin immediately. The negative taboos will be discussed later; here it is important to make mention of the large number of positive magical interventions advised to insure a safe delivery for mother and child. First and foremost is a series of frequent visits to the medicine man or vestal virgin, which become more and more frequent toward the time of delivery. Each visit is accompanied by a vast array of ritual. First, a special rubberized tubing is wrapped snugly around the woman's arm and the pressure increased to a point of bare tolerance. A magical divination rod is then inserted into the woman's first morning urine, which she faithfully brings with her at each visit. She is then laid down on the ritual table where the medicine man or vestal virgin begins a series of magical manipulations, massaging gently the ankles and wrists to ascertain any hidden poisonous fluid that may have been secretly injected into the woman's body by an unknown enemy—probably by having her unknowingly ingest a malignant substance known as salt with her food. The unborn child is similarly massaged and divination is made regarding its position and whether this position is propitious for a safe delivery; the child is then ritually assessed by a magical measuring device and pronounced to be growing well or not well. Finally, a piece of odd-looking regalia specific to the trade of the medicine man or vestal virgin is placed on the practitioner's head. The practitioner inserts one end of the device in his or her ears and the other on the mother's abdomen. After a short period of concentration, the practitioner announces that he or she has indeed communicated with the unborn child who is doing well at this time, but demands that the mother follow carefully all the practitioner's suggestions to insure continued good health. Among these suggested practices is the daily ingestion of a vast array of specific types of food. The practitioner, however, being often of the paranoid personality type, does not always trust that his client will follow his directives and for this reason further prescribes a daily ingestion of a magic substance concocted by the large Medical Concoction Companies of the culture and purchased at great expense. This particular concoction is ferrous gluconate or another similar substance that the particular practitioner prefers. For women divined to be particularly weakened and vulnerable to malevolent forces, an additional substance known as folic acid is prescribed.

The mother is then instructed to attend a specialized session taught by the vestal virgins in which the secrets of the childbirth rites are revealed to her. Occasionally her husband is also allowed to attend these secret sessions. She is further instructed in another series of protective magical manipulations directed primarily at her bodily properties and their preparedness for the delivery. A very complex and ritualized set of movements and gestures are taught—some of the more common ones being known as the "squatting position," the "leg raising exercises," and the "Kegal maneuver." Special breathing magic to ward off the Evil Spirits of Delivery are also taught. Special manipulative procedures related to the woman's nipples are also said, if practiced faithfully, to ward off future trouble with nursing.

These rituals and instructions are highly prized by the woman who promised to pay a great price at the end of her delivery. She seldom refuses or even considers refusing this price, although it is not infrequent at the end of the delivery for her to have difficulty paying the amount agreed upon.

Delivery

The woman is carefully instructed by the vestal virgins as to the most propitious moment to come to the birthing hut—a special room carefully secluded from the rest of the culture in a large and fearsome building called the latipsoh and feared by all the inhabitants of the culture as the Place of Death. She is instructed to come alone, or occasionally with her husband. When she does so, careful interrogation reveals whether she did indeed wait until the most propitious moment to arrive—if not she is sent home again. But if the time is right, the medicine men and vestal virgins

then begin a long, complicated, and, to the uninitiated eye, quite barbaric set of magical procedures meant to ward off the Evil Spirit of Delivery. First, the woman's pubic hair is scraped off her skin with a blunt instrument to insure that no evil spirits are hidden there waiting to attack the newborn infant. Also in an attempt to forestall any intrusion by evil spirits, a long tube-like apparatus is inserted into the woman's anus; magic fluids are then introduced into her body, resulting in a massive bowel movement that takes with it, the medicine men proclaims, all the evil forces that reside in the gastrointestinal tract. To further protect the newborn (whom the culture views as extremely vulnerable to evil forces), a vast array of magical cleansing procedures are performed over the woman's vaginal area.

A number of other magical measures are employed. A sharp, thin, hollow metal tube is inserted into the woman's arm, through which is introduced whatever portion the medicine man deems appropriate for protection during delivery. During labor, the vestal virgins assume their positions around the woman, leading her in a variety of magical incantations with rhythmic breathing to blow off the magic spirits of pain. Finally, when the time of delivery is near, the vestal virgins position the woman in one of the most torturous of the culture's institutions, a special apparatus used only at the time of birth. In it the woman is made to lie flat on her back with her legs and feet raised at a 90-degree angle and bent at the knee. It is thought that if a woman is able to deliver her baby in this almost impossible position, she will have passed the first initiation rites of motherhood.

Immediately prior to the delivery, the most barbaric (to the uninitiated observer) of the demon-ridding procedures is performed. The medicine man produces two pronged, razor-sharp instruments and proceeds to cut into the woman's perineum. The rationale for this procedure is the assurance of an opening wide enough for any baby's head. When the baby is delivered, he or she is taken quickly away so as not to be contaminated by the parents, who are uninformed as to the appropriate magical interventions that are needed to assure continued good health of the baby. The medicine man attends to repairing the woman's perineum in much the same way as the seamstresses of the culture repair ripped garments. The vestal virgins immediately begin a series of rituals directed toward the baby—he is placed in a magical transparent box where it is felt that the evil spirits of Cold are not allowed access. A variety of bundling and washing maneuvers are performed. He is not allowed to be fed, even if the mother's breasts are leaking, since early introduction of food is thought to make him vulnerable to a series of malevolent forces. The baby is completely covered less the parents see too much of him and contaminate him by their powerful glance, but they are allowed a quick look at the eyes and head. He is then returned to the more competent care of the vestal virgins, who continue to do the majority of care until the woman is pronounced to be safe enough to return to the society. The mother is then sent home with the child, whom she has frequently seen only 2 or 3 hours a day since birth. She is given a series of long and detailed instructions about the appropriate rituals to be followed to ward off the Evil Spirits of the Cord and other malevolent forces. She is instructed as to proper feeding, bathing, and other techniques, but she is seldom able to comprehend the complexity of these rituals since she is not initiated into them until immediately before she returns home, a time at which she is usually quite anxious.

Early Childhood

Upon returning home, the woman and her husband are left quite alone by the society. Although there are a variety of visitors who come to pay their respects and bring offerings to the newborn, only the luckiest of the Naciremans receive any substantial help. They live in a neolocal society where the small nuclear family seldom has close ties with either the matrilineal or patrilineal kin. Since the families tend to be small, in most cases the parents have never had any experience with childrearing, even during their own childhood. The early childhood years are thought to be trials by which the parents may prove themselves. The cultural ideal is that the parents will completely mold the infant to become a laudable member of the Nacireman society; if any flaws appear in the child now or throughout his entire life, the culture makes it quite clear that it was the ineptitude of the parents during the early childhood years that caused the problem. Most Nacireman parents say that it is the first 2 weeks that are the most trying. They are unaccustomed to the baby's crying and constantly in fear that they have done something wrong to allow the evil spirits to enter his body, but are in great fear of

calling the Medicine Man, knowing that he will then realize that they are indeed inadequate parents. The culture does provide some literature meant to help the parents in an anonymous manner so that their inadequacies are not exposed to the rest of the culture. These books tell the parents how to feed, burp, clothe, and bathe their baby, and how to tell when evil spirits are gaining control and they must call in a Medicine Man.

In general the culture could be characterized as quite cold with their infants. They cuddle them occasionally, but seldom carry them about. In fact, an observer has the impression that they hardly love their children at all, their cultural customs are so peculiar. The child is frequently allowed to "cry it out" at night so that he will quickly learn that no help is coming and that he must learn to be independent at nighttime. This is apparently to preserve the strength of his parents, who must invest their energies in pursuits other than the care of the baby. The culture has devised an amazingly vast array of artifacts, apparently constructed with the express purpose of freeing the parents from carrying the child. Infant-sized seats that swing, jump, roll, or just remain still are available in every conceivable style. Large netted or barred boxes are available in which the baby can be safely stored while the parents are free to work. The culture has also produced some highly peculiar customs in relation to feeding. Some mothers nurse, but the majority of them nurse, not according to when the baby is hungry, but according to the dictums of a Clock God, who allows the child to be fed only at preordained times. In fact, many women even choose not to nurse their infants, apparently in an attempt to teach them early the culture's value of independence. These infants are provided with special containers, the tops of which are rubberized and shaped to resemble a woman's breasts. Although the parents hold the infant while feeding them in the early months, it is hoped that this container will encourage the infant to become able, at an early age, to feed himself. It is a most unusual sight for the anthropologist to witness very tiny infants quite independently holding these containers themselves and drinking at will. Weaning in this culture is done at an extraordinarily early age, sometimes as early as 6 months! A variety of containers meant to encourage this early independence training are available.

The sleeping customs for infants of the culture are also quite unusual. They are almost never allowed to come into the parents' bed. In fact, some parents do take the young infants into their bed or at least near their bed during the early weeks when the child is still waking during the night, but they almost never reveal this secret to the Medicine Man or vestal virgins for fear of severe reprisal. The cultural disapproval of this practice apparently relates to an almost paranoid fear of early incest. Sleep patterns are also unusual. As mentioned before, children are strongly encouraged, in many cases almost forced, to sleep through the night whether they are hungry or not. The common practice in other cultures of simply feeding the child whenever he is hungry during both day and night is almost unheard of in the Nacireman culture.

Bowel control in this culture is taught relatively early and quite severely. Indeed, it appears to be a focus of central interest to the culture. Much casual conversation relates to how early various children gain such control. Censure for children slow to gain such control can be severe. The amount of time and energy that is put into this training by the parents is impressive to the observer. To an outsider it would appear that almost the entire day's conversation in a family of this age child relates to how many times, when, how, and where the child has evacuated. Even specially constructed receptacles are made in child-sizes for this life-stage, the thought again being that early encouragement of this procedure will make the child more independent, as well as result in less work for the parents.

The very rich habitat and high economy of this culture results in a most unusual system of childrearing. Because it is seldom necessary for the mother to participate in a substantial way in the economy, her primary job is to insure that the child matures properly. To this end she puts all her energies. Since she has had very little experience in childrearing herself, and since she seldom has access to an older, more experienced woman, she begins by reading the available literature and discussing issues with other women in similar situations. The vast amoung of time, energy, and motivation invested in this job are made evident by the incredible array of rituals she devises for insuring that her child matures into a Nacirema High Chief. She reads voluminous literature about how to stimulate each of his senses appropriately, exactly how and when and what to feed him, what exercise is appropriate for babies, toddlers, and older children, exactly what social attitudes they should display, what mate-rials are needed to develop proper fine and gross motor skills, and what social experiences should be engineered by the mother. Indeed, the woman's entire life appears to be totally consumed with designing the child's physical, psychological, and social world. This behavior is considered most laudable for the mother, although occasional informants have suggested that this intense investment of the mother in the child has certain cultural disadvantages for the mother herself, and epidemiological evidence does suggest a certain amount of poor mental health manifested by these women later in life and symptomatized in excessive alcohol consumption and relatively high suicide rates.

Middle Childhood

Because the early formation of the child's personality and intellect are considered so important, the culture has devised certain interesting institutions to insure that children are subjected to interaction with the Wisest Sages of the culture, who are located in institutions called the Loohcs. These loohcs are usually housed in a large structure, one of the more ornate in the culture, and each child is expected to spend the majority of his waking hours in the Loohcs interacting with the Wise Ones and with a variety of cultural artifacts. It is hoped that both his cognitive and affective developments will be positively influenced in this way.

Each child in the Loohcs is expected to master an almost impossible array of magical and ritual information related to all aspects of Naceriman life. Vast amounts of time and energy are devoted to mastering their language—both spoken and written. This is not an easy task since the language is one of the less coherent ever to be developed by a human group. In addition to this, considerable energies are devoted to inculcating the Naceriman value system into each child. The value system is in itself quite unusual, and the observer cannot help but wonder how this culture has managed to survive with some of the extraordinarily antisocial values it teaches its children. Although the loohcs maintain that they expose the children to the many ritual learnings so that each child will have an optimum chance for enjoying life in this culture, it is quite clear to even a casual onlooker that the mechanisms for inculcating these learnings are anything but social. In spite of the obvious riches of the culture, the Wise Ones repeatedly emphasize, both overtly and covertly, that there are a limited amount of benefits available in the society and that these will be given to only a select number of the children. This is thought to motivate the children to learn the Sacred Mysteries. It apparently does so, but it also appears to teach them an intense rivalry unheard of in any other culture in history. The Naciremans appear to believe that it is impossible for any individual to enjoy life unless he has the most and the best of every conceivable natural and cultural resource that exists. It is truly amazing that a culture that has inculcated its children to such heights of competition is even able to maintain a coherent social whole.

The extent to which the Wise Ones go to stimulate this intense competition is amazing. Even the loohcs compete with each other, organizing groups of children to devote great amounts of time and energy to learning a wide variety of totally nonsensical games and then to play against each other. The winners are greatly lauded, and the motivation to achieve in these behaviors, which appear to the outsider as totally senseless, is remarkable. Needless to say, the result is children who are highly competitive and self-centered, but also very productive. The most successful of these children are sent to the Highest Loohcs of the land, where the Wisest of the Sages are housed and the Most Sacred and Secret Mysteries are taught.

Extreme disappointment ensues if an individual child is judged not capable of attending such a Loohcs. Great shame is brought to himself and his parents (particularly his mother), who are made to feel extremely guilty since it is assumed that the child's inability to learn all these rituals is the result of a lack of culturally approved stimulation during the early years.

Adolescence

The adolescence of the Naciremans is also most unusual. Rather than the typical year or two, it is prolonged to an almost unheard of 9 to 10 years. The culture's insistence that the full granting of adult social status be prolonged this much past physical maturation appears to create a number of problems for it. Puberty is recognized, but little attention is paid to it since true adult status is yet many years away. Culturally approved sexual outlets for the emerging pubertal child are simply not available. The result is that the majority of children do engage in some form of sexual experience, either heterosexual, homosexual, or masturbatory, but they seldom admit to it, and

the culturally induced guilt seems to lead to a variety of mental health problems during adolescence and often persisting throughout the individual's life. Equally unusual is the lack of assignment of a useful work role for the adolescent. Because of the complexity of the society, the means of production are highly specialized and it is felt that much experience in the Loohcs is necessary before an individual can contribute meaningfully to the society's economy. This puts the adolescent in a particularly dependent position, even though the society constantly stresses the value of independence. As a result, a considerable degree of anxiety and resentment seems to develop in adolescents—so much so, in fact, that they frequently form subgroups that totally reject the major values of the culture. Although these subgroups generally subside when the culture finally admits the individual to full participation in adult status, it is still striking that they persist with the strength that they appear to have. Most older Naciremans, in fact, frequently state that this is the most difficult and trying stage of the life-cycle in Nacirema—both for the individual and for those around him or her.

An Overview

Although it is a cursory overview of the Nacireman culture's childbearing and childrearing practices, this description at least provides us with some interesting insights into the extreme plasticity of human nature. For a cultural group to be able to bear and rear their children in such a totally deviant manner from the rest of mankind and yet to maintain for hundreds of years a viable culture does indeed attest to the strength of the species. It will be interesting for future anthropologists to follow the course of this unusual group. One cannot but wonder what the long-term effect of these unusual approaches to childbearing and rearing will be.

REFERENCES

1. Stephens, W.N.: *The Family in Cross-Cultural Perspective.* Holt, Rhinehart, & Winston, New York, 1963, p.8.
2. LeVine, R.A.: *Witchcraft and co-wife proximity in southwestern Kenya.* Ethnology 1 (1): 39-45, 1962.
3. Mead, M.: *From the South Seas: Studies of Adolescence and Sex in Primitive Societies.* William Morrow, New York, 1939.
4. Du Bois, C.: *The People of Alor: A Social-Psychological Study of an East Indian Is-*

land. The University of Minnesota Press, Minneapolis, 1944.

5. Murphy, Y., and Murphy, R.F.: *Women of the Forest*. Columbia University Press, New York, 1974, p.224.

6. Freuchen, P.: *Book of the Eskimos*. World Publishing Co., New York, 1961, p.67.

7. Roden, C.: *A Book of Middle Eastern Food*. Alfred A. Knopf, New York, 1972, pp.387-388.

8. Murphy and Murphy, p.141.

9. Ibid., pp.219-250.

10. Ibid., p.226.

11. Malinowski, B.: *Magic, Science and Religion*. Beacon Press, Boston, 1948.

12. Stephens, p.9.

13. Ayres, B.C.: *A Cross-Cultural Study of Factors Relating to Pregnancy Taboos*. Doctoral thesis, Radcliffe College, Boston, 1954.

14. Gorer, G.: *Himalayan Village*. Michael Joseph, London, 1938.

15. Beals, R.L.C.: *A Sierra Tarascan Village*. Publication No. 2, Smithsonian Institute of Social Anthropology, Washington, D.C., 1946.

16. Wright, J.: *Collective review—the view of primitive peoples concerning the process of labor*. Am. J. Obstet. Gynecol. 2:206, 1921.

17. van der Eerden, M.L.: *Maternity Care in a Spanish American Community of New Mexico*. Catholic University of America Press, Washington, D.C., 1948.

18. Koenig, S.: *Beliefs and practices relating to birth and childhood among the Galician Ukranians*. Folklore 50:272, 1939.

19. Lowie, R.H.: *The Cros Indians*. Farrar and Rinehart, New York, 1935.

20. Naroll, F., Naroll, R., and Howard, F.H.: *Position of women in childbirth*. Am. J. Obstet. Gynecol. 82:943, 1961.

21. Mangert, W.F., and Murphy, D.P.: *Intraabdominal pressures created by voluntary muscular effort*. Surg. Gynecol. Obstet. 57:745, 1933.

22. Vaughn, K.O.: *Safe Childbirth: The Three Essentials*. Bailliere, Tindall, and Cassell, London, 1937.

23. Newton, N., and Newton, M.: "Childbirth in cross-cultural perspective." In Howells, J.G. (ed.): *Modern Perspective in Psycho-Obstetrics*. Brunner-Mazel, New York, 1972.

24. Atlee, H.B.: *Fall of the Queen of Heaven*. Obstet. Gynecol. 21:514, 1963.

25. Trethowan, W.H., and Conlon, M.F.: *The couvade syndrome*. Br. J. Psychiatry 111:57, 1965.

26. Curtis, J.L.: *A psychiatric study of 55 expectant fathers*. U.S. Armed Forces Med. J. 6:937, 1955.

27. Bardhan, P.N.: *The fathering syndrome*. U.S. Armed Forces Med. J. 20:200, 1964.

28. Trethowan and Conlon, p. 57.

29. Brown, M.S.: *A cross-cultural look at pregnancy, labor, and delivery*. J. Obstet. Gynecol. Nurs. Sept.-Oct. 1976, pp. 35-38.

30. Klaus, M., and Kennell, J.: *Maternal-Infant Bonding*. C.V. Mosby Co., St. Louis, 1976.

31. Birch, H.: *Sources of order in the maternal behavior of animals*. Am. J. Orthopsychiatry 26:279, 1956.

32. Rosenblatt, J.S., and Siegel, H.I.: *Hysterectomy-induced maternal behavior during pregnancy in the rat*. J. Comp. Physiol. Psychol. 89:685-700, 1975.

33. Ringler, N.M., Kennell, J.H., Jarvella, R., et al.: *Mother to child speech at 2 years—effects of early post-natal contact*. J. Pediatr. 86:141–144, 1975.

34. Lorenz, K.Z.: *King Solomon's Ring*. Time Incorporated, New York, 1962.

35. Harlow, H.F., Harlow, M.K., and Hansen, E.W.: In Rheingold, H.R. (ed.): *Maternal Behavior in Mammals*. John Wiley and Sons, New York, 1963.

36. Whiting, J.W.M., and Childe, I.L.: *Child Training and Personality*. Yale University Press, New Haven, 1953.

37. Spiro, M.E.: "Ifaluk ghosts: an anthropological inquiry into learning and perception." In Hunt, R. (ed.): *Personality and Cultures*. Natural History Press, New York, 1949, pp. 89-94.

38. Whiting, J.W.M.: *Becoming a Kwoma*. Yale University Press, New Haven, 1941, pp. 33-36.

39. Whiting and Childe, p. 202.

40. Ibid.

41. Henry, W.E.: *The thematic and apperception technique in the study of culture-personality relations*. Genet. Psychol. Monogr. 35:3-135, 1947.

42. Madsen, M.C.: *Developmental and cross-cultural differences in the cooperative and competitive behavior of young children*. J. Cross-Cultural Psychology 2:365-371, 1971.

43. McClelland, D.C., and Winter, D.G.: *Motivating Economic Achievement*. Free Press, New York, 1969.

44. Munroe, R.L., and Munroe, R.H.: *Cross Cultural Human Development*. Brooks/Cole Publishing Co., Monterey, 1975.
45. Kluckhohn, F.R., and Stordtbeck, F.L.: *Variations in Value Orientations*. Row, Peterson, Evanston, Illinois, 1961.
46. Whiting, B.B., and Whiting, J.W.M., in collaboration with Longabaugh, R.: *Children of Six Cultures: A Psycho-Cultural Analysis*. Harvard University Press, Cambridge, 1975.
47. Wittkower, E.D. *Perspective in Transcultural Psychiatry*. Int. Psychiatry 8:811-824, 1969.
48. Mead, M.: *Coming of Age in Samoa*. William Morrow, New York, 1928.
49. Junod, H.A.: *The Life of a South African Tribe*. MacMillan Co., London, 1913, p.84.
50. Whiting and Childe, p.205.
51. Miller, N., and Dollard, J.: *Social Learning and Imitation*. Yale University Press, New Haven, 1941.
52. Rohrer, J.H., and Edmonson, M.S.: *The Eighth Generation*. Harper & Row, New York, 1960.

BIBLIOGRAPHY

Atlee, H.B.: *Fall of the Queen of Heaven*. Obstet. Gynecol. 21:514, 1963.

Ayres, B.C.: *A Cross-Cultural Study of Factors Relating to Pregnancy Taboos*. Doctoral thesis, Radcliffe College, Boston, 1954.

Bardhan, P.N.: *The fathering syndrome*. U.S. Armed Forces Med. J. 20:200, 1964.

Beals, R.L.C.: *A Sierra Tarascan Village*. Publication No. 2, Smithsonian Institute of Social Anthropology, Washington, D.C., 1946.

Birch, H.: *Sources of order in the maternal behavior of animals*. Am. J. Orthopsychiatry 26:279, 1956.

Brown, M.S.: *Anthropology, nursing and mental health*. J. Psychiatr. Nurs. 12 (1):7-11, Jan.-Feb. 1974.

Brown, M.S.: *Mother-child relationship has lasting effects*. Can. J. Psychiatr. Nurs. XVI (5):10-12, Sept.-Oct. 1975.

Brown, M.S.: *A cross-cultural look at pregnancy, labor, and delivery*. J. Obstet. Gynecol. Nurs. 35-38, Sept.-Oct. 1976.

Brown, M.S.: *Child rearing in crosscultural perspective*. Health Values 1 (2):77-81, March-April 1977.

Curtis, J.L.: *A psychiatric study of 55 expectant fathers*. U.S. Armed Forces Med. J. 6:937, 1955.

Du Bois, C.: *The People of Alor: A Social-Psychological Study of an East Indian Island*. The University of Minnesota Press, Minneapolis, 1944.

Freuchen, P.: *Book of the Eskimos*. World Publishing Co., New York, 1961.

Gorer, G.: *Himalayan Village*. Michael Joseph, London, 1938.

Hammond, D., and Jablow, A.: *Women in Cultures of the World*. Cummings Publishing Co., Menlo Park, California, 1976.

Harlow, H.F., Harlow, M.K., and Hansen, E.W.: In Rheingold, H.R. (ed.): *Maternal Behavior in Mammals*. John Wiley and Sons, Inc., New York, 1963.

Henry, W.E.: *The thematic and apperception technique in the study of culture-personality relations*. Genet. Psychol. Monogr. 35:3-135, 1947.

Junod, H.A.: *The Life of a South African Tribe*. Macmillan Co., London, 1913.

Klaus, M., and Kennell, J.: *Maternal-Infant Bonding*. C.V. Mosby Co., St. Louis, 1976.

Kluckhohn, F.R., and Stordtbeck, F.L.: *Variations in Value Orientations*. Row, Peterson, Evanston, Illinois, 1961.

Koenig, S.: *Beliefs and practices relating to birth and childhood among the Galician Ukranians*. Folklore 50:272, 1939.

LeVine, R.A.: *Witchcraft and co-wife proximity in southwestern Kenya*. Ethnology 1 (1):39-45, 1962.

Lorenz, K.Z.: *King Solomon's Ring*. Time Incorporated, New York, 1962.

Lowie, R.H.: *The Cros Indians*. Farrar and Rinehart, New York, 1935.

Madsen, M.C.: *Developmental and cross-cultural differences in the cooperative and competitive behavior of young children*. J. Cross-Cultural Psychology 2:365-371, 1971.

Malinowski, B.: *Magic, Science and Religion*. Beacon Press, Boston, 1948.

Mangert, W.F., and Murphy, D.P.: *Intra-abdominal pressures created by voluntary muscular effort*. Surg. Gynecol. Obstet. 57:745, 1933.

McClelland, D.C.: *The Achieving Society*. Van Nostrand, Princeton, 1961.

McClelland, D.C.: *Achievement and entrepreneurship: a longitudinal study*. J. Pers. Soc. Psychol. 1:389-392, 1965.

McClelland, D.C.: *Motivational Trends in Society*. General Learning, New York, 1971.

McClelland, D.C., Atkinson, J.W., Clark, R.A., et

al.: *The Achievement Motive.* Appleton-Century-Crofts, New York, 1953.

McClelland, D.C., Sturr, J.F., Knapp, R.H., et al.: *Obligations to self and society in the United States and Germany.* J. Abnorm. Soc. Psychol. 56:245-255, 1958.

McClelland, D.C., and Winter, D.G.: *Motivating Economic Achievement.* Free Press, New York, 1969.

Mead, M.: *Coming of Age in Samoa.* William Morrow, New York, 1928.

Mead, M.: *From the South Seas: Studies of Adolescence and Sex in Primitive Societies.* William Morrow, New York, 1939.

Miller, N., and Dollard, J.: *Social Learning and Imitation.* Yale University Press, New Haven, 1941.

Munroe, R.L., and Munroe, R.H.: *Cross Cultural Human Development.* Brooks/Cole Publishing Co., Monterey, California, 1975.

Murphy, Y., and Murphy, R.F.: *Women of the Forest.* Columbia University Press, New York, 1974.

Naroll, F., Narrol., R., and Howard, F.H.: *Position of women in childbirth.* Am. J. Obstet. Gynecol. 82:943, 1961.

Newton, N., and Newton, M.: "Childbirth in cross-cultural perspective." In Howells, J.G. (ed.): *Modern Perspective in Psycho-Obstetrics.* Brunner-Mazel Publishers, New York, 1972.

Roden, C.: *A Book of Middle Eastern Food.* Alfred H. Knopf, New York, 1972.

Rohrer, J.H., and Edmonson, M.S.: *The Eighth Generation.* Harper & Row, New York, 1960.

Rosenblatt, J.S., and Siegel, H.I.: *Hysterectomy-induced maternal behavior during pregnancy in the rat.* J. Comp. Physiol. Psychol. 89:685-700, 1975.

Spiro, M.E.: "Ifaluk ghosts: an anthropological inquiry into learning and perception." In Hunt, R. (ed.): *Personality and Cultures.* Natural History Press, New York, 1949, pp.89-94.

Stephens, W.N.: *The Family in Cross-Cultural Perspective.* Holt, Rhinehart, and Winston, New York, 1963.

Trethowan, W.H.: "The couvade syndrome." In Howells, J.G. (ed.): *Modern Perspectives in Psycho-Obstetrics.* Brunner-Mazel Publishers, New York, 1972.

Trethowan, W.H., and Conlon, M.F.: *The couvade syndrome.* Br. J. Psychiatry 111:57, 1965.

van der Eerden, M.L.: *Maternity Care in a Spanish American Community of New Mexico.* Catholic University of America Press, Washington, D.C., 1948.

Vaughn, K.O.: *Safe Childbirth: The Three Essentials.* Bailliere, Tindall, and Cassell, London, 1937.

Whiting, J.W.M.: *Becoming a Kwoma.* Yale University Press, New Haven, 1941, pp.33-36.

Whiting, J.W.M., and Childe, I.L.: *Child Training and Personality.* Yale University Press, New Haven, 1953.

Whiting, J.: "The function of male initiation ceremonies at puberty." In Maccoby, E.E., et al. (eds.): *Readings in Social Psychology.* Holt, Rinehart, and Co., New York, 1965.

Whiting, B.B., and Whiting, J.W.M., in collaboration with Longabaugh, R.: *Children of Six Cultures: A Psycho-Cultural Analysis.* Harvard University Press, Cambridge, 1975.

Wittkower, E.D.: Perspectives in transcultural psychiatry. Int. J. Psychiatry 8:811-824, 1969.

Wright, J.: Collective review—the view of primitive peoples concerning the process of labor. Am. J. Obstet. Gynecol. 2:206, 1921.

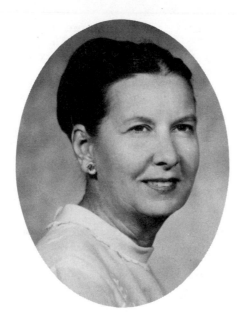

Chapter 2

I was born in Maryland of "old American stock." My family is of English Quaker descent, having already been in America for nine generations when I arrived on this earth. Thus, like most Americans my family were immigrants from the Old World. They arrived in Pennsylvania with the William Penn expedition in 1682, having left England to escape religious persecution. Here they sought a new land with new opportunities to worship God in their own way and in peace.

I am the oldest of two children and experienced loss early in life (at age four) when our mother died after a protracted illness known as "consumption" in those days. Our father remarried before I became 6 and we were raised by a warm and loving step-mother, so that we had five living grandparents and three very large extended families.

No question about it, ours was a patriarchal family. Father made all of the major decisions and most of the family purchases, as well as meting out the necessary rewards and punishments to his children. We learned early to answer "yes sir" or "no sir." "Because I said so" was all the reason my father felt was necessary for him to give. I'm sure my parents never heard of Watson's theories of childrearing, for which I am thankful, and they were, I suspect, never at a loss as to what was the appropriate child-

rearing technique for them to use. Father was both kind and strict. We were clear on the rules and also on the penalties for transgressions. He wanted us to have an education, which had been denied him. We were also expected to help ourselves—there would be no "bailing us out." Poor grades in school were not tolerated. "Saving for a rainy day," "waste not, want not," "cleanliness is next to Godliness," and "a good reputation is more to be valued than gold" are values that were an early part of my training.

We enjoyed a number of traditional celebrations as children that involved our very large extended family. Christmas dinners at grandmother's, Thanksgiving at our home, and summer crabbing parties at the shore are some examples. It was, however, always apparent to me that my father, who was the oldest in his family, was given a somewhat "senior-looked-up-to" status in the family, and somehow this role status reached his children. We children also understood, subconsciously, that we were to be competitive and "do better." Moreover, the pride of our parents was evident when we did experience success.

We were free to make major decisions about our lives. That I chose another religion before I became a teen-ager was acceptable to my parents. Decisions on vocation were discussed within the family, too, and although they would

36

Childrearing in Matrix America

Ann L. Clark, R.N., M.A.

have preferred that I become a teacher, they whole-heartedly supported my decision to go into nursing.

I entered nursing in a diploma program, took a baccalaureate degree at Seton Hall University and a master's degree from New York University. I have followed a profession that has spanned more than 4 decades and focused entirely on maternal and child health. Early in my career I was in nursing service and nursing administration. The latter half of my career has been in nursing education. I have held professorial appointments at Rutgers University, University of Hawaii, and Arizona State University. I am presently in a half-time position as Director of Nursing Education at Hawaii Nurses Association, developing and teaching continuing education programs throughout our island state. This half-time position gives me some free time to pursue writing, research, and some speaking engagements.

I reside with my husband, Marshall, in Honolulu.

This chapter will focus on the manner in which the dominant American culture has been and is going about rearing its young. In the process of doing so, it will explore family life and roles within the family and the changes American families have experienced and are experiencing today. To do this, one must also examine the influence that childrearing experts have and still are having on parents, as the parents search for answers to the baffling tasks they find themselves facing. The chapter will conclude with a look at childrearing in the seventies and eighties.

Matrix America

It seems appropriate that a book on culture and childrearing in America would, out of necessity, attempt to obtain some perspective on how matrix America rears its children, even though the author is aware of the pitfalls of attempting to do so. However, it is in this matrix culture that other cultures that immigrate to America continue the rearing of their children. All the cultures impact with each other and slowly there are changes in each. The immigrating cultures cling to certain values (termed *cultural persistence*), but it is the immigrating culture that makes the greater accommodation when entering the American way of life. Cultural differences become more diffuse with each succeeding generation,[1] but there is a powerful mainstream tradition. The minority groups have themselves acknowledged as much by gradually approximating the cultural norms with the passage of each succeeding generation. Thus, according to Demos, "a scholar may still claim to speak of the American family in general as if such a thing actually existed!"[2]

Ideas for this chapter come, for the most part, from a search of the literature. They are not derived from a clinical study, as are some of the chapters to follow. Because the literature and the clinical research on which much of this literature is based focus on the middle class, this chapter will, for the most part, reflect the manner in which middle-class Caucasian parents, whose roots go back to the Old World, raise their children. This chapter sets the stage for the following chapters, which explore other cultures' child-rearing practices.

As we study the composition of the culture that is labeled "American," we find that Americans of Spanish origin constitute 6 percent of America, Blacks 13.6 percent, American Indians 0.5 percent, and Orientals 0.6 percent.[3] More than 79 percent are Caucasians, who thus make up the majority class. Others coming to this mix in America are accommodated and acculturated to varying degrees into the American way of life. It therefore seems appropriate to assume that the Western culture, certainly with considerable degrees of modification of their ancestors' values, makes up to a large degree the matrix culture of America. The manner in which this culture rears or should rear its children is often the focus of the mass media. Books on childrearing and advice offered by childrearing "experts" are meant, for the most part, for the matrix middle-class American. America has often been called a multicultural melting pot. If that is so, we are still simmering on a back burner of the societal range, as this book will show. Even though we espouse cultural pluralism, it is not yet a reality.[4]

This author assumes that an exploration of the differences between the various groups, without any attempt to evaluate or even to label or pigeonhole, can help health professionals to develop a renewed awareness that can assist them in bringing to their practice a greater depth of understanding and make this intervention appropriate and more meaningful.

The native Americans, with their numerous tribes and various family life-styles, sparsely covered the New World when western Europeans began to arrive in America. The American Indian, however, did not become the matrix society

into which the immigrants acculturated. It is interesting to speculate why this was so. It could have been because of the sheer numbers of the immigrants, or perhaps because the cultures were so very different, but it was more likely because the American Indian wished and still wishes to remain Indian, not to assimilate and not, according to McLain, to "melt in the pot and come out culturally white."[5] So, the pioneers from the Western world, beginning in the seventeenth century, set the matrix culture of America in place. From the nineteenth century, and for years to follow, a vast tide of immigrants from all parts of the Western world flowed into America. They brought with them a wide variation of family life-styles and they differed greatly in their values, beliefs, and practices, in their religions and their cultures. These immigrants and the American Blacks over the last 2 centuries have had the most impact on American life as we know it today. From them have come the basic tenets about family and the functions of the family. These common elements of our culture compose the basis for comparing our culture with any other culture.[6] America *is* the very archetype of diversity.[7]

It is a fact of nature that the child grows to become man (or woman), and according to Mead,[8] Americans go to great extremes to emphasize the contrasts between that child and the adult he or she is to become. For example:

- —Children do *not* make any labor contributions to our industrial society
- —Discipline is exacted "because of love"
- —Respect is culturally prescribed and is a different form of relationship when one becomes an adult
- —Children are seen as sexless (sex information is dangerous and wicked and to be kept from children)
- —Children should be protected from the ugly facts of life
- —Modesty is to be valued
- —Food is to be served regularly three meals a day
- —Children should obey

COMPARATIVE STUDIES

American childrearing has been extensively documented, but most of the studies of childrearing, according to Devereux,[9] provide no comparative framework to give perspective to our own particular styles or deviance. Indeed, the whole history of childhood is plagued by a paucity of documentary sources about actual child-rearing practices in America.[10] Studies of child-rearing literature throw light on explicit and changing ideals of the adult culture, but only to a limited degree on the practices to which children are subjected.[11] There are, however, a number of studies that compare the parenting by Americans with that of other cultures and from these one can obtain, to a degree, the flavor of American child-rearing and the kinds of children these practices produce.

Devereux's study of authority and moral development among German and American children indicates that German children show more conformity to adult values and greater anxiety and guilt for misdeeds than do American children.[12] Wesley studied German and American mothers, comparing opinions and educational attitudes.[13] American mothers, in his study, expect a high degree of self-reliance on the part of the child by the time he reaches 6 years of age. American mothers rank affectionate behavior, responsibility, and curiosity high on a list of desirable traits for their children to attain. These traits are not even mentioned by German mothers. German mothers rank obedience and honesty as desirable traits. On the American mothers' lists, obedience ranks fifth and honesty twenty-first! Traits of helpfulness and politeness, which rank high on the German mothers' lists, do not appear at all on the American mothers' lists.

A comparison of childrearing in England and in America by Devereux shows that there are some similarities, but there are also many significant differences.[14] English children were found to be less sociable, less sensitive, less conscientious, more assertive, and more tense, while American children were found to be characterized by friendliness, affection, enjoyment, and mutual understanding. Peer relationships among the English children contained significantly more dominance and compliance. Devereux explains that the English children's behavior is an outcome of discipline, which "focuses more on the needs and convenience of the adult and his world. The 'good' child is clean, quiet, formally polite, does not interrupt nor intrude in adult centered activities."[15]

A visiting Englishman expounded on his view of American children in the November 14, 1965, issue of the *New York Times* with the following explosion: "American Kids! * % # &." He then documented this view by stating that they are "undisciplined, rude, and do not know their

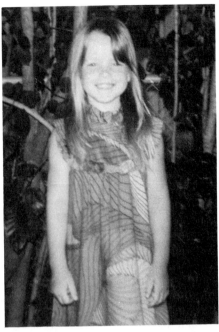

Figure 1. American children are unrepressed and bubble with childish spontaneity.

place." If one expects American children to be silent and respectful, then no doubt he is right (Fig. 1).

Devereux's conclusion was somewhat different:

American children no doubt *are* noisier and perhaps naughtier as well, especially in public places where adults may observe them. But, as American mothers point out, what is taken as bad manners by our foreign visitors may be mostly an expression of unrepressed childish spontaneity and probably represents no ill will or desire to offend. The American child rearing system seems to produce in children a kind of expansive good will toward fellow creatures, including adults. We suspect it may also foster a fairly solid commitment to the fundamental values of moral conduct, once they get them straight.[9]

Pancultural factors of childrearing practices in Sicily and the United States indicate that Sicilian parents are much more strict than are American parents.[16] Detailed comparisons of elemental variables show differential controls to be exercised mainly in regard to sexual and aggressive behavior. American mothers and fathers are much more lenient in tolerating direct aggression toward parents than are Sicilian parents. This holds true for peer-directed aggression as well. American parents define aggression as "standing up for one's rights," a self-defense measure. Thus, according to Peterson, aggression is probably conceived by American adults as part of the training for independence and autonomy of a rugged individualistic kind.[17]

American tolerance for overt sexual behavior seems, on the surface, a bit surprising in view of the common stereotypes regarding Latin sexuality and American prudery, but, no question about it, American children are allowed considerably more sexual freedom than are Sicilian children throughout the major period of sexual socialization. Think about it—the coeducational schools, early dating patterns, and free heterosexual associations for American children *are* different. Sicilian children and adolescents have no such freedom.

> American parents are more strongly inclined . . . to use praise and isolation as disciplinary procedures . . . love oriented approach to child rearing, evidently preferred by American parents, is again consistent with the emphasis on training for autonomy and independence . . . which seems so much a part of the middle class American value system. Parents in the United States disagree more on policies of child rearing . . . possibly because behavorial codes are less well defined in the United States. There is simply more room for disagreement and verbal dispute on all issues.[18]

There are, of course, cultural differences in childrearing even in the early days of life. A study by Rebelsky and Abeles[19] compares the care that infants receive in American homes with that which Dutch babies receive. Dutch babies are kept in cool rooms and dressed with many heavy garments. Further, Dutch mothers spend a limited amount of time with their babies and provide them with a minimum of auditory and visual stimulation. The feeding time is shorter and more rigidly structured and scheduled. In comparison, American mothers dress their babies lightly, keep them in warmer environments, and provide them with considerable visual and auditory stimuli. The feeding schedules are kept flexible for American children. What is the outcome of these different childrearing practices? As early as 3 months, there are marked differences in the infants' responses. Dutch babies do more thumb sucking than do American babies, and American babies make more pleasant vocal sounds than do the Dutch babies.

Studies of differences in childrearing in the United States and in the Union of Soviet Socialist Republics are difficult to find. Bronfenbrenner's study is an exception.[20] He reports that the major difference lies in the contrast between a collective-centered system in Russia and a family-centered system of childrearing in America.

Turning to an Oriental culture, we can find some excellent comparative studies by Caudill and his associates.[21] Normal family life in Japan emphasizes an interdependence and a reliance on other family members. In America emphasis is on independence and self-assertion.[22] These differences in basic philosophy have compelling implications for childrearing and are obvious in infancy with the care the mother gives to her infant and the infant's response to her care. The Japanese baby is a passive child lying quietly except for an occasional unhappy vocalization. His (or her) mother does a lot of lulling, carrying, and rocking of her child. She seems to be mostly trying to soothe and quiet the baby. Her communication with the child is of a kinesthetic nature rather than of an auditory one. In comparison, the American mother does more looking at and more chatting with her baby. She seems to be bent on stimulating the baby to physical activity and to vocal response. As a result, the American baby is more active and happily vocal and is an active explorer of his environment. From the first days of life, here are mothers, by design, fitting their children into the culture to which they belong and in which they must hope to succeed.

There are cultures throughout the world, perhaps most cultures, in which there is constant physical contact between the infant and its mother—basically a kinesthetic contact; this is not true for the American baby. An example of the above can be found in the contact-comfort experienced by the Zambian infant. The baby is carried in a sling on the mother's back, nursed on demand, and sleeps with its mother at night. While the bodily contact is high, the opportunity for face to face contact between the Zambian infant and its mother is minimal. She seems to attach no specific importance to the feeding situation as a social event, according to Goldberg.[23] What is more, vocalization with the infant is kept to a bare minimum. Goldberg believes that the outcome of this low vocalization and mutual gaze, coupled with a constant physical contact between mother and child, results in an infant (the Zambian) taking longer to learn the self-other distinction.[24]

Watching the Zambian infant in his sling, it becomes obvious that he must, almost from the first, make use of a developing muscular control as he "hangs in there" to assume a cooperative relationship with his mother. The Zambian infant also experiences much more intense stimulation in the not-so-gentle way in which he is greeted, handled, and played with. Perched high on his mother's back, the Zambian baby has an early wide and varied contact with the world at large, but his experience with child-centered activities is rare in comparison. This tends to lead to passiveness and unresponsiveness on his part. Goldberg describes Zambian babies as "unbelievably 'good.' Perhaps this general lack of responsiveness and activity . . . indicates some retardation of development as a result of a lack of stimulation. It may also indicate early learning of obediance and conformity in the presence of adults, a highly valued behavior pattern for Zambian children."[25]

Munroe also looks at obedience levels of East African children and compares them with American children.[26] The East African children are also more fully obedient as a group than are the American children. Strong compliance training, to which subSaharan societies subject their children, is seen as a basis for this difference.

These comparative studies and others give us insight into some of the differences as well as some of the similarities of childrearing practices of Americans and representatives of other cultures. They also explain some of the differences in the children that are a result of their culture's childrearing practices.

American parents, however, are in a sense a new breed. Some of the practices in decades past were very like those of other cultures and have been modified as our society has changed. Bronfenbrenner notes that "we in America have moved to greater tolerance of the child's impulses and desires, freer expression of affection, and increased reliance on 'psychological' methods of discipline, such as reasoning and appeal to quiet, rather than physical punishment."[27]

Freed from the traditions of Europe, we in America have certainly been more experimental with childrearing patterns than almost any other culture. This may, in part, explain why America is often viewed as a child-centered society.

Our social and family system also helps to explain the differences. According to Whiting[28] there are two independent cultural features that are predictive of the social behavior of children. They are the complexity of the socioeconomic system and the composition of the household. Children brought up in a nuclear household, which largely is the picture of America today, are more sociable and intimate and less authoritarian and aggressive (Fig. 2). Children brought up in complex cultures, such as America, tend to be more independent and dominant and less responsive to nurture than children brought up in a simpler culture.

It may be worth noting also that, according to Bronfenbrenner,[29] the differences in goals and methods of childrearing appear to be narrowing between the social classes, with lower-class parents beginning to adopt the values of the middle class. Parental socialization procedures in America have become increasingly homogeneous, and there is less parental authority over children in America in all classes. The next section of this chapter will explore how this has come about.

FAMILY LIFE IN AMERICA

Evolution of the Family

First, what are the *functions* of the American family? Here is Duvall's description:

The family is a unity of interacting persons related by ties of marriage, birth, or adoption, whose central purpose is to create and maintain a common culture which promotes the physical, mental, emotional, and social development of each of its members. Modern families fulfill the promise of this definition through at least six emergent, nontraditional functions:

—affection between husband and wife, parents and children, and among the generations;
—personal security and acceptance of each family member for the unique individual he is and for the potential he represents;
—satisfaction and a sense of purpose;
—continuity of companionship and association;
—social placement and socialization;
—controls and a sense of what is right.[30]

The family is subject not only to the changes that the life-cycle imposes, but it is also subjected to the sociological pressure of our society. Particularly, technological pressures are significant to our contemporary families. Indeed, these social pressures have brought about dramatic changes in the family throughout history.

The most evident and perhaps most funda-

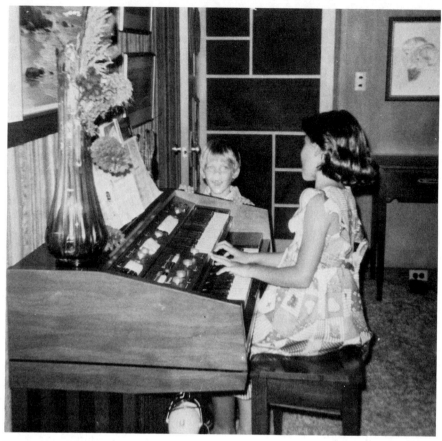

Figure 2. American children are more sociable and intimate and less authoritarian and aggressive.

mental change occurring in the American family was the emergence of the urban family out of the traditional rural family. This section will explore family life and the resulting care of children through colonial America, rural America prior to World War II, and urban America.

The colonial American family was patriarchal. It consisted of a group of people, bound together by blood ties, marriage, and adoption, who lived, worked, and socialized together. The entire family was well organized and existed in semi-isolation, dependent on itself for most of its needs. It had to be resourceful, loyal, and helpful to all its members.[31] By the 1900s, the farm family was still family centered (there were some developing community facilities), but the organization, although still highly interdependent, was becoming less rigid.

Parents were married for life, with separation and divorce rarely known. This, however, did not

assure the children an unbroken parenting experience, for death of young adults did occur with some frequency. When a death did occur, the extended family would then close ranks and fill the void caused by the death, so that children would continue to be cared for.

Members of the farm family all worked hard. The child, as soon as he was able, worked in the fields and the mother, with few or no technological aids, spent a hard life bearing and rearing the children, growing and preparing the food, and caring for the home. The children received a minimum of schooling, since their education was viewed, for the most part, as less necessary than the cultivation of the farm lands. The parents filled the role of teacher to their children, at least to the extent their own limited education would permit.

Families were large in colonial America. The first census (1790) showed that 36 percent of

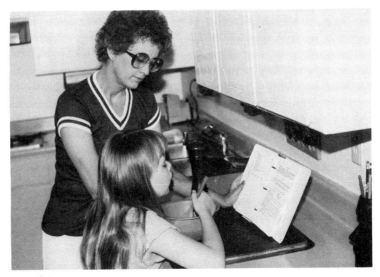

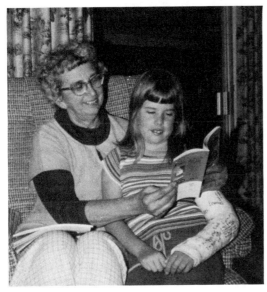

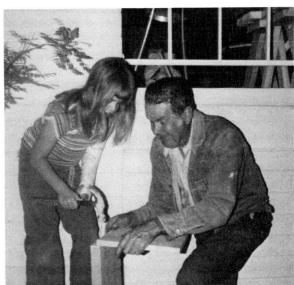

Figure 3. A number of children in America are growing up in single-parent families. Grandparents fill the gap when one parent is missing.

American households consisted of seven or more persons.[32] Prior to the industrial revolution, families could expect to lose more than half of the children born to them owing to infections and other pestilence, for little was known about sanitation and immunizations were yet to be developed.

The greatest changes occurred in the family following the industrial revolution, when families moved to cities. The economic unity of the agricultural prototype disappeared. The family size was reduced and children were reared within families with fewer relatives present. Gradually the nuclear family developed, so that by 1975 only 1 percent of couples lived with relatives.[33] In 1974 the average family consisted of 1.86 children and the big household had virtually vanished.

Family Life Today

There are those who view the family as an "endangered species" and question whether the traditional nuclear family, created by the legal act of marriage, can survive. It certainly has changed and no doubt will continue to change owing to pressures both inside and outside of the family system. Let us look at how these changes are affecting the children.

Children today have access to a large number of people as they mature. They have much less time with father, who now works in a plant or office, often far from the family's residence. The mother, now freed of the household drudgery, has more time to pursue self-actualization, and with the economic crunch of the seventies, more and more women are seeking full-time or part-time employment outside the home. By 1975, among women 20 to 24 years of age who were married and living with their spouse, more than half were members of the labor force. Forty-seven percent of women 25 to 29 years of age were working mothers. In March 1975, more than half of school-age children and nearly 40 percent of mothers with children under the age of 6 were either working or looking for work.[34] It is estimated that at least a million children of working mothers take care of themselves when they are not in school, including some who are under 6 years of age. Many other children of preschool age are being cared for in child-care centers or in other persons' homes while the mother is employed.

Twenty million of our children are living in families disrupted by separation, divorce, or widowhood or in families of unwed mothers (600,000 babies are born to teen-agers). This results in one out of every six children, under the age of 18, living in a single-parent family.[35] However, some of these children find other adults who modify the impact of this experience (Fig. 3).

America is also a mobile nation, where, on an average, family residence is changed every 5 years. Again, the economic and social structure of our society fashions how and where a family will live, for many of these moves are necessitated by the father's employment. This often means that the children are born and reared in places far separated from the extended family and where lack of environmental support increases the stress with which families must cope. It also means that the children are uprooted and must adjust to new peers, new schools, and new customs, not once, but often a number of times during their childhood.

Roles of family members have changed drastically over the last couple of decades, with the bearing of children apparently the one role function that has not changed. Indeed, roles are no

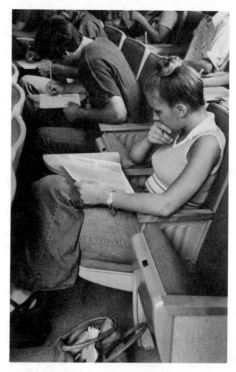

Figure 4. Extended vocational preparation has resulted in a prolonged adolescent period. (Photograph courtesy of Public Affairs Office of The College Board)

longer as clear as they once were. As noted earlier, women assume some major role in the provider aspects of the family. Within the home both parents often assume the blended role of homemaking and of parenting. Finding identity and role function in today's society is complex, which results in more stress and more demands placed on the family unit.[36]

Parents, today, have less and less impact on their children's lives, with specialized institutions such as schools and social agencies filling a role for which the family originally was singularly responsible. In the past, parents were solely responsible for influencing, directing, teaching, and indoctrinating their children, but this is no longer true.

Educational opportunities and society's requirement for extensive educational preparation for a vocation have lead to an extended period of dependency on the part of young people. Adolescence is a relatively new stage of development (Fig. 4). The adolescent of the last century went to work, married, and began to rear a family. Today he most likely remains in the family, but is not subject to the same discipline he experienced as a child. Peer pressure now assumes a larger role in his development. This and the fact that the adolescent has taken on the role of teacher and "trend setter" within the family have led to a severe generation gap, with resulting alienation in many families. In spite of all this, the family remains the most constant element offering security to and influence on the developing child.[37] The value and the quality of life for families and for children in America have undoubtedly improved over the past 200 years, and they continue to improve. Children have a much greater chance to survive to adulthood. The child death rate has been reduced by 50 percent since 1950.

An Historical Look at Childrearing in America

Although childrearing has changed considerably, it may be useful to review the past, for traces of a number of beliefs and practices, not only alien to us but repugnant as well, can still be seen in contemporary childrearing.

In medieval times the child was openly viewed as chattel. Parents had complete control over their children, even to the extent of putting them to death for wrongdoing or even supposed wrongdoing. Children had no rights as we understand them today. Children, as soon as they could assume major care for themselves, were apprenticed out to a master craftsman or worked in the fields with the other laborers.

In colonial America strict discipline of children, from the beginning of life, was the order of the day. Discipline was seen as necessary to save the child from his inherited sin. The Reverend John Robins, a leading preacher of the pilgrims, wrote, "Surely there are in all children . . . a stubborness and state of mind arising from natural pride which must in the first place be broken and beaten down so the foundation of their education being laid in humility and tractableness, other virtues may in time be built thereon."[38]

Children were believed to arrive in the world in sin, inherently corrupted. Parents were urged to "break the will" of the very young. At a very early age there was a vigorous attempt to inculcate religious principles. In Cotton Mather's diary is to be found this scene with a 4-year-old: "I took my little daughter Kathy into my study and then told the child . . . when I am dead to remember everything now said to her. I set before her the sinful condition of her nature and charged her to pray in secret places each day that God for the

sake of Jesus Christ, would give her a new heart."[39]

Laziness, slowness, and lack of attention in school were all viewed as evidence of sin. Religious schools of the day believed that to spare the rod would indeed spoil the child. Physical punishment was liberally used to "beat the devil" out of the child.

Colonial America barely recognized childhood as we view it today. Children were viewed as small adults. It was not until 1800 that children even had clothing that was distinctly their own.

Understanding something of Puritanism, Rationalism, and Romanticism will give us a better understanding of how our childrearing practices have evolved.[40] Many of these philosophical movements relate to our present-day notions about parents and parenting, even though these notions are now more benign and in more variant forms than they were originally intended to be.

PURITANISM

The doctrine that mankind is of evil nature was a fundamental tenet of faith for the Puritan family, and the moral aspect of a child's personality occupied all the parents' attention. Doctrines of evil nature were taught early, along with the ABCs:

> "In Adams fall/we sinned all"
> "The idle fool/is whipt at school"
> "Youth forward slips/death soonest nips"
> "Job fells the rod/yet blesses God"[41]

As seen above, positive judgments were rarely used and control of behavior was maintained by instilling fear. The parent was viewed as an authority figure, not only by the child, but by society as well. There was no parent-child relationship as we know it today. The parent was responsible for controlling the devil in the child and making the child a moral subject for the corporate Puritan community as well.

Today we can still witness parents judging their child as "bad" if his behavior is disturbing, and we can still observe the use of fear to control behavior. Here are some examples with those same Puritan overtones:

> "You are a bad boy"
> "God will get you for that"
> "Wait till your father
>   hears about this"
> "God is watching you"

RATIONALISM

Rationalism can be characterized by the assumption that life and the universe are rational and there is a solution to every problem. Human nature is neither good nor bad. Reason is the significant human characteristic. These beliefs were held by most of our Founding Fathers. The child is viewed as an empty vessel with predetermined traits of human nature. Rationalism is deeply entrenched in our American value system and is said to be the very cornerstone of the ethos of the achievement-oriented, professional, upper middle class;[42] as such it has a powerful influence on parenting today. Listen to some modern-day parents validating this statement:

> "Look it up in the encyclopedia"
> "Give it a try and see"
> "You ought to go to college and
> prepare yourself for life"

ROMANTICISM

Romanticism holds that the child should be allowed to find his own inner voice untrampled by the institutions of society. Romanticism emphasizes *feelings* and recognizes no limit to the child's capacities or to the parents' patience, for that matter. Romanticism says to the parent, in essence, "Let your child find his true soul, his own flash of genious." Feelings are the paramount criterion on which behavior between the parent and child is judged. This philosophy is pervasive in America today, and the mass media's drama tends to propagate its spread. Parents are encouraged to have an attitude of hope and positive feelings while they "attempt to understand," "communicate freely," and "believe and trust" in their children, without any way to evaluate if this trust is warranted.[43]

One of the most striking changes from the nineteenth to the twentieth century in American thinking about children and how they should be reared is the radical alteration in the conception of the child's nature. From the view that a child's nature is one of depravity, which is to be feared, and innate impulses, which are to be curbed at any cost, the child is now believed to have a nature that is not only totally harmless but beneficent as well.[44] Certainly childrearing today can be more casual, more relaxed, and more fun with the disappearance of those evils of nature. But those lingering experiences of upbringing of previous generations will always continue to have their effect on parents.

Childrearing Experts

The history of childhood is plagued by the paucity of documentary sources about actual childrearing practices in America. Perhaps two books, Locke's *Some Thoughts Concerning Education* (seventeenth century) and Spock's *Common Sense Baby and Child Care* (twentieth century), best reflect the middle-class liberal notions of their times.

Parenthood has probably never been left unguided. In past centuries, as today, parents did not rely merely on instinct or on unspoken tradition. Whether the main sources of information and influences were "old wives' tales," proverbial wisdom, or the advice of grandmothers or nurses, the way a child was treated seems to have been more the result of cultural influence than instinctual promptings, according to Stern.[45] The confusing things for parents have been the changing philosophies (sometimes drastic changes) and the conflicting advice they receive. We have only to go back to 1928 and see how our grandparents of today may have been raised. The preponderant theory of the day, à la Watson, went like this:

> There is a sensible way of treating children. Treat them as though they were young adults. Dress them, bathe them with care and circumspection. Let behavior always be objective and kindly firm. Never hug or kiss them, never let them sit in your lap. If you must, kiss them on the forehead when they say good night. Shake hands with them in the morning. . . .
>
> The infant at eight months of age onward, should have a special toilet seat into which he can be safely strapped. The child should be left in the room without toys and with the door closed. When broken (the rule) it leads to dawdling, loud conversation, in general to unsocial and dependent behavior. . . .
>
> Don't believe anyone who tells you that such insistence on routine tends to steam roll the child and to reduce the growth of his own "inward life and powers." "Spontaneity," "inward development" and the like are phrases used by those too lazy or too stupid or too prejudiced to study children in the actual making.[46]

For more than 100 years now, parents have been given specific advice on how to raise their children, first by ministers, physicians, and educators, and more recently by psychiatrists and psychologists, who have added their threats to the dire consequences of not following their favorite brand of advice. And their advice has undergone a 180-degree shift. "Good" advice of some decades ago would now make for unpardonable mistakes.[47] From bad children of the twenties, the experts now seem to be saying that there are no bad children, only bad parents. The trend of advice in a nutshell looks something like this:

Watson
The environment is all-important.

Gesell
Growth comes from within; heredity is important.

Freud (via Spock)
Permissiveness is to be valued.

Piaget
Early learning and a stimulating environment are important.

A toy shop window summarized childrearing advice over 7 decades thusly:

Woe to the parent who turns to the experts.
1910 spank them
1920 deprive them
1930 ignore them
1940 reason with them
1950 love them
1960 spank them lovingly
1970 to hell with them?

Sears' concerns are stated as follows:

The trouble with experts' opinion is that it rests with the private experience of the expert. There is no substantial public evidence to which either a skeptic or a believer can turn to decide whether or not the opinion is correct. One expert is as good as another, and neither of them can prove the validity of what he recommends. . . .

During the past half century we have had many writers giving advice to mothers. Some have been truly expert and have relied heavily on the growing body of child development research. Others have followed fads and prejudices and have probably done more harm than good.[48]

The United States Children's Bureau began publishing a bulletin entitled *Infant Care* in 1914. It is fascinating to follow through the changing advice given to parents over the intervening 66 years. In 1914 parents were instructed to control the child's impulses (thumb sucking and masturbation) promptly and rigorously, and if they failed to do so the impulses would grow

beyond control and permanently damage the child.[49] The child, while in bed, was to be bound down hand and foot, so that he could not suck his thumb, touch his genitals, or rub his thighs together! By 1929 to 1938 autoerotism seemed less dangerous, and by 1942 to 1945 the child was viewed as remarkably harmless, in effect devoid of sexual or dominating impulses. Autoerotism was now seen as an incidental by-product of body exploration. In 1951 there was an attempt to continue this relaxed response, but not without some conflicts. Thumb sucking was viewed as a substitute (albeit not a good one) for being held and talked to. And masturbation was barely mentioned; it was suggested that if it bothered the mother she could give the child a toy to busy his hands.

In the 1973 issue of *Infant Care* masturbation was not mentioned and the advice given for thumb sucking was, "most babies get their thumbs and fingers in their mouths and suck on them. Many seem to find it especially enjoyable and do it often. It causes no harm and can be ignored. Some mothers don't like the looks of thumb and finger sucking and substitute a pacifier. . . ."[50] A suggestion not to substitute a pacifier for needed attention was advised.

Instructions for bowel training have also had an interesting history. According to the 1929 to 1938 issues of *Infant Care,* training is to begin early (by 3 months) and carried out with great determination. This instruction is accompanied by a pervasive emphasis on regularity, doing everything by the clock. This guidance was relaxed over the next 2 decades and in the 1973 issue it was not even mentioned, from which we may assume it is not a topic for discussion during the first year of life.

Weaning, bladder training, and preferred method of neonatal feeding have all gone through a change, either increasing or decreasing in severity. What is interesting to speculate on is a mother's dilemma in raising a number of children over a time span, when such conflicting attitudes are to be found. One might ask, What is she to do with her own attitudes and conflicts?

Quoting Le Masters, "perhaps the low point in American expertise on child rearing came in 1974 when Dr. Benjamin Spock, whose book on infant care went through 58 printings in various editions and sold over 15 million copies, apologized to American parents who had used his book."[51] Spock now feels he helped raise a generation of "brats."[52]

The Contemporary American Parent

The major changes in parental behavior as suggested above and as discerned by analysis of data can be summarized as follows:

1. Greater permissiveness toward the child's spontaneous desires.
2. Freer expression of affection.
3. Increased reliance on indirect "psychological" techniques of discipline (e.g., reasoning or appeals to guilt) as opposed to direct methods (e.g., physical punishment, scolding, or threats).
4. In consequence of the above shifts in the direction of what are predominately middle-class values and techniques, a narrowing of the gap between social classes in their patterns of childrearing.
5. More affection and less authoritarian behavior on the part of fathers and more disciplinary behavior on the part of mothers.

TRADITIONALISTS AND THE NEW BREED

General Mills' consumer center recently commissioned a research study on parenting. The results of 2000 interviews with parents in all parts of the United States is reported in *The American Family Report 1976–1977* and is entitled "Raising Children in a Changing Society."[53] It details how parents are coping with the problems of raising their children in a period of rapid social change. The focus of the study is the family unit:

—The Parents: Fathers and mothers and their views, values, satisfactions, concerns, and outlooks on raising their children.
—Their Children: Boys and girls between the ages of 6 and 12, speaking for all the younger children in the family, on their views and feelings about themselves, their parents, and their own immediate world.

Basically the study examines the changing lifestyles and re-examines many of the traditional values that parents, for many years, have used to guide them in raising their children. It details the development of new sets of values with emphasis on greater sexual freedom, self-fulfillment, the blurring of male/female roles, less conformity, and more openness and frankness.

The study indicates that there is a "New Breed" of parents today (43 percent of the study families) who have rejected many of the traditional values by which they were raised: marriage as an institution, the importance of religion, saving and thrift, patriotism, and hard work

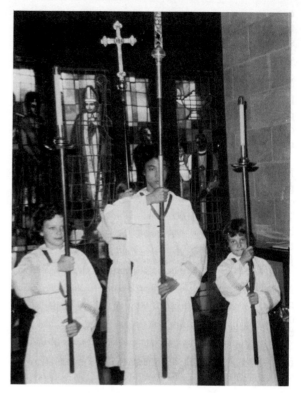

Figure 5. The majority of American parents continue to support some of the basic values by which they were raised.

for its own sake.[54] And they have adopted a new set of attitudes toward being parents and the relationships of parents to children. New Breed parents question the idea of sacrificing in order to give their children the best of everything and are firm believers in the equal rights of children and parents.

Compared to previous generations, the New Breed parents are less child-oriented and more self-oriented. They regard having children not as a social obligation but as one available option, which they have freely chosen. Given the chance to rethink their decision, nine out of ten would still decide to have children.

By contrast, there are the Traditionalists who still represent the majority of all parents (57 percent). Traditionalists continue to support the basic values by which they were raised (Fig. 5), but they, too, have been influenced by the new values and are trying to reconcile these newer concepts with older theories and beliefs. As parents, Traditionalists are stricter disciplinarians and more demanding of their children than New Breed parents. And while Traditionalists have a certain nostalgia for the simplicity of the past, they are not prepared for the same kind of self-sacrificing approach to childraising common in their parents' time.

New Concepts of Parenting

In this new environment, many concepts about parenting have evolved.[55] Some are already accepted by the majority of all parents, others primarily by the New Breed:

Willingness to Sacrifice. Almost half of the New Breed parents (46 percent) feel strongly that parents should not sacrifice in order to give their children the best, while only 16 percent of the Traditionalists share this view. On the other hand, both groups agree by a two-to-one margin that unhappy parents should not stay together just for the sake of their children.

Lives of Their Own. A solid majority of both New Breed (68 percent) and Traditionalists (64 percent) agree that parents have lives of their own even if it means spending less time with their children.[56]

Pleasure Now. Unlike parents of former generations, today's mothers and fathers are strongly "now" oriented. Over half the parents (53 percent) expect to receive their main pleasure from their children now rather than in the future.

You Don't Owe Us Anything. Less sacrificing on the part of the parents means freedom from obligation for the children. Among the New Breed, 73 percent agree that children have no future obligation to parents, regardless of what the parents have done for the children.

Raising Boys and Girls. One of the issues most sharply dividing the New Breed and Traditionalist parents is the difference in their attitudes toward raising sons and daughters. Two out of three of the Traditionalists (68 percent) agree strongly or partially that boys and girls cannot be raised using the same rules, while only 31 percent of the New Breed agrees at all with this concept. The same outlook spills over to other areas. Traditionalists are more likely than the New Breed to believe that it is more important for boys to be good at sports than for girls to be. With their own children, Traditionalists stress the importance of masculinity for boys and femininity for girls, while again, the New Breed advocates more blurring of the sex roles.

Mothers' and Fathers' Roles. Only 32 percent of New Breed parents are willing to accept the role of the man as the main provider, while 48 percent of the Traditionalists support this idea.

Yet in terms of their own lives—and how they handle parental responsibilities—there is less difference in practice than in theory between the two groups of parents. It is still the mothers in both New Breed and Traditionalist homes who have the main responsibilities for cooking, cleaning, shopping, taking children to the doctor, and staying home when children are sick. What may be a change from the past is the fact that the mothers rather than the fathers appear to be the main disciplinarians.

Discipline. The issue of discipline is far from resolved among today's parents. For the most part, mothers and fathers are divided into three groups: the permissive (23 percent), the temperate (51 percent), and the strict (26 percent). A majority of the New Breed parents are members of the permissive group, while the Traditionalists take a temperate or strict view of discipline.

The Laissez Faire Outlook. Involved with self and self-fulfillment, New Breed parents are not only more permissive with their children but many follow a rather laissez faire approach to childraising. There are sizable numbers of parents who believe that children should be allowed to dress as they want, eat whatever is desired (as long as they are healthy), play with the kinds of toys they want, and do pretty much whatever they want to. But in spite of this, New Breed parents are as likely to spank their children when they misbehave as are Traditionalist parents.

Acceptance of Differences in Performance. If a permissive and laissez faire approach to childraising is one characteristic of the New Breed, acceptance of differences among children, including differences in levels of achievement, is another identifying factor. Parents are now split between those who do not push their children, because "it's their lives and let them be" (39 percent), and those who still demand a lot because they feel there is no other way to raise successful adults (56 percent).

The Transmission of Values

Here, then, are two groups of parents with very different sets of basic beliefs, yet curiously they are both trying to pass on to their children the same set of traditional values.

For the Traditionalists, it is an easy decision, for they are carrying on the traditions by which they were raised and the values to which they subscribe.

For the New Breed, the decision is more complex and difficult because it represents a com-

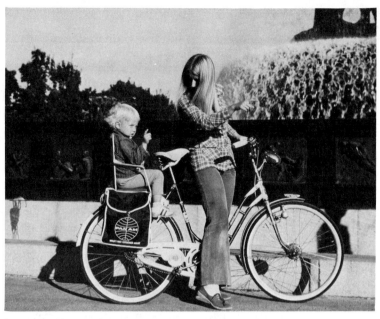

Figure 6. Contemporary parents are judged by much higher standards than were their parents. (Photograph by Brad Powell)

promise with their own beliefs, underscores some of their own doubts and reservations, and is primarily a way of accommodating their children to a society that has not yet wholly caught up with their ideas.

Thus, we see both the New Breed and the Traditionalists transmitting to their children the most basic of American traditional values:

- Duty before pleasure
- My country right or wrong
- Hard works pays off
- People in authority know best
- Sex is wrong without marriage[55]

SOCIOLOGICAL FACTORS AFFECTING CONTEMPORARY PARENTING

Lerner has written that it is evident that in no other culture has there been so pervasive an anxiety about the rearing of children.[57] It might be fair to say that most parents of today are concerned and often confused as to what childrearing technique best fits not only their style but their child. Many of the sociological factors that affect parents have affected parents through the ages, but some of them are new. Davis[58] lists 11 factors, including the rate of social change leaving a considerable gap between parent and child and no models to follow; conflicting norms; competing authorities; sexual tension; and vertical social mobility. Davis argues that in a larger family system, authority and its related feelings are more diffused among several adults than they are in our intense nuclear system![59] Riesman also postulates that the margin for parental error shrinks as the family system grows smaller, and the outcome for each child becomes more crucial.[60] No wonder our modern day parent is anxious.

Today's parent is unquestionably judged by higher standards than were previous generations (Fig. 6), and many people have become critical observers: the children, as well as professionals such as physicians, clinical psychologists, teachers, speech therapists, and social workers.[61] Here we see amateurs judged, not by their peers, but by experts. What is more, parents are expected to attain instant success and 100 percent of the time, at that. There are no learning labs for women or men to practice parenting. At the child's birth they must begin immediately to cope with the problems of childrearing and they are not allowed to make errors for the next 18 to 20 years. There is no way they can quit the job; they must see it through. What is more, they cannot raise their children as they were raised—they must raise them better.

Some of the factors mentioned earlier in discussing changes in the contemporary family also

50

have an impact on parenting: marital instability, new roles for American mothers, urbanization, and the emergence of a youth peer group. Mass media has a powerful influence on children that is difficult for parents to counteract. Some examples are the advertisement of cigarettes, the promotion of free sex, violence, and other moral (or immoral) messages, which vary with the parents beliefs and the goals that they hold for their children.

LeMasters sums it up as follows:

> Parents have been made the bad guy in the drama of modern living, blamed for failures of all other basic institutions in our society—the schools, the church, the government, the mass media, the economic system, the armed forces and so forth. What is more, today's parents are responsible as ever—even more so—for their children but have much less authority over them because of the changes in society.[62]

Parents' confidence in themselves has gone into a steep decline under the thumb of disapproving experts. As health professionals, anything we can do to give mothers back their confidence and permit them to use their common sense in deciding what is appropriate for the child should improve the rearing of America's children.

There are, however, some problems in modern day childrearing. Child neglect and abuse have probably existed for centuries. Only within the past 30 years has the problem penetrated society's consciousness as an appropriate concern for public policy,[63] and for that reason we are now somewhat aware of its pervasiveness. In 1976 alone, 47,167 validated cases of abuse and neglect were reported to the American Humane Association,[64] and that is believed to be only the tip of the iceberg.

Violence within the family is not rare. Many reasons have been given, including the unstable economic system and television. There is also a close association between the amount of violence experienced by the parents as children and the rate of abuse toward their own children. It has been suggested that each generation learns to be violent by growing up in a milieu in which they observe and are victims of violence.

Today's parents, according to a recent study, are as reluctant to discuss sex with their children as were their parents, but perhaps for very different reasons. They seem confused about the accuracy of their information and the relevancy of their own values and life-style for their children. They often retreat in silence when questions about sex are asked by their children, resulting in the children learning not to ask questions and to conduct sexual experiments on their own.

The study entitled *Family Life and Sexual Learning*[65] came out with the following findings:

1. Fathers do not talk about sexuality with their children. When discussion takes place, mothers provide the sex education for both sons and daughters.
2. Parents have more "relaxed" or tolerant attitudes about erotic conduct for their sons than for daughters when they are grown.
3. Parents seem confused and uncertain about sexuality. Most retreat in silence and do not discuss sexual issues with their children.
4. Disapproval of nudity in the home, admonitions against masturbation, and avoidance of in-depth discussions on such issues as anatomy, menstruation, and wet dreams limit the opportunities for growing children to learn about sexual development.
5. Parents say they think their children should learn about erotic sex before they reach adolescence, but this is the very issue that most parents never discuss with them.
6. Parents support sex education for their children; 80 percent believe that sex education should be taught in the schools.

It is ironic that after the so-called sexual revolution of the sixties, many parents approach the eighties perhaps more tongue-tied than ever when it comes to talking honestly with their children about sexuality. We know that teen-agers today are more sexually active, but from the study above, it does not look as though they are much better informed than were their parents.

POSTSCRIPT

No matter how many problems the matrix culture of America is having with the problems of childrearing, think how the problems are increased for the immigrating cultures. They must not only cope with the usual problems of childrearing, but do so in a strange and dynamic culture, which is itself experiencing new and difficult problems in the field of childrearing. Basically, that is the reason for placing this chapter at this place in the book.

REFERENCES

1. Clark, A.L.: *Maternal tenderness—cultural and generational implications.* Clinical Conference Papers, Kansas City, American Nurses Association, 1973, p. 101.
2. Demos, J.: *The American family in the pool.* American Scholar 43: 422, 1974, p. 443.
3. Hechinger, F.M.: *American childhood: the utopian myth.* National Elementary School Principal 55:10, 1975.
4. McClain, S.R., et al.: *Parenting the culturally different.* Paper presented at Annual Conference on Minority Students (La Crosse). April 23, 1977, p. 10.
5. Ibid.
6. Mead, M., and Wolfenstein, M.: *Childhood in Contemporary Cultures.* University of Chicago Press, Chicago, 1955, p. 7.
7. Sears, R.R., MacCoby, E.E., and Levin, H.: *Patterns of Childrearing.* Harper & Row, New York, 1957, p. 11.
8. Mead and Wolfenstein, p. 21.
9. Devereux, E.C., Bronfenbrenner, U., and Rogers, R.R.: *Child-rearing in England and the United States.* J. Marriage and the Family 31:257, 1969, p. 257.
10. Borstelmann, L.J.: *Dr. Locke and Dr. Spock: continuity and change in American conception of child rearing.* Paper presented at the southeastern regional meeting of the Society for Research in Child Development (Chapel Hill, N.C.), March 1974, p. 1.
11. Mead and Wolfenstein, p. 17.
12. Devereux, E.C.: *Authority and moral development among German and American children: a cross-national pilot experiment.* J. Comparative Family Studies 3:99, Spring 1972.
13. Wesley, R., and Karr, C.: *Comparison of opinions and educational attitude between German and American mothers.* Psychologische Rundschau 19:35, 1968.
14. Devereux, *Child-rearing,* p. 257.
15. Ibid., p. 269.
16. Peterson, D.R., and Migiorino, G.: *Pancultural factors of parental behavior in Sicily and the United States.* Child Dev. 38:968, 1967.
17. Ibid., p. 988.
18. Ibid., p. 989.
19. Rebelsky, F., and Abeles, G.: *Infancy in the First Three Months.* Boston University. Headstart Evaluation and Research Center, November 1968.
20. Bronfenbrenner, U.: *Two Worlds of Childhood: U.S. and USSR.* Russell Sage Foundation, New York, 1958.
21. Caudill, W., and Weinstein, H.: *Maternal care and infant behavior in Japan and America.* Psychiatry 32:12, 1969, p. 15.
22. Ibid.
23. Goldberg, S.: *Infant care and growth in urban Zambia.* Hum. Dev. 15:77, 1972, p. 85.
24. Ibid., p. 86.
25. Ibid., p. 84.
26. Munroe, R.L., and Munroe, R.H.: *Levels of obedience among U.S. and East African children on an experimental task.* J. Cross-Cultural Psychology 6:498, December 1975.
27. Bronfenbrenner, p. 143.
28. Whiting, B.B., and Whiting, W.M.: *Children of Six Cultures: A Psycho-Cultural Analysis.* Harvard University Press, Cambridge, 1975.
29. Bronfenbrenner, p. 143.
30. Duval, E.M.: *Family Development.* ed. 4. J.B. Lippincott, Philadelphia, 1971, p. 27.
31. Cavan, R.S.: *Marriage and the Family in the Modern World.* ed. 2. Thomas Y. Crowell, New York, 1965, p. 52.
32. Solnit, A.J.: *Changing psychological perspectives about children and their families.* Children Today 5:6, 1976.
33. Norton, A.J., and Glick, P.C.: *Changes in American family life.* Children Today 5:2, 1976.
34. Solnit, p. 8.
35. Ibid.
36. Chinn, P.E.: *Child Health Maintenance. Concepts of Family Centered Care.* Mosby, St. Louis, 1974, p. 50.
37. Ibid.
38. Demos, p. 443.
39. Ibid.
40. Karson, A., and Karson, M.: *The Influence on American Parenting Styles of Puritanism, Rationalism and Romanticism.* Michigan State University Press, 1976, p. 1.
41. Ibid., p. 2.
42. Ibid., p. 5.
43. Ibid.
44. Mead, p. 146.
45. Stern, H.H.: *Parent Education, an International Survey.* UNESCO Institute for Education, Hamburg, 1960, p. 6.
46. Watson, J.B.: *Psychological Care of the In-*

fant and Child. W.W. Norton, New York, 1928, p. 121.

47. Senn, M.J.: *Speaking Out for America's Children*. Yale University Press, New Haven, 1977, p. 43.
48. Sears, p. 6.
49. Wolfenstein, M.: *Trends in infant care*. Am. J. Orthopsychiatry 23:120, 1953.
50. United States Department Health, Education, and Welfare, Office of Human Development: *Infant Care*. Children's Bureau Publication, Washington, D.C., 1973, pp. 62-63.
51. LeMasters, E.E.: *Parents in Modern America*. ed. 3. Dorsey Press, Homewood, Illinois, 1977, p. 57.
52. United Press news report, *Wisconsin State Journal*, January 23, 1974.
53. General Mills: *Raising Children in a Changing Society, The General Mills American Family Report, 1976–1977*. Minneapolis, 1977.
54. Ibid., p. 27.
55. Ibid., pp. 30-32.
56. Ibid., p. 28.
57. Lerner, M.: *America as a Civilization*. Simon & Schuster, New York, 1957.
58. Davis, K.: *The sociology of parent-youth conflict*. Am. Sociological Review 5:523, 1940.
59. Ibid.
60. Riesman, D., et al. (eds.): *The Lonely Crowd*. Yale University Press, New Haven, 1961.
61. LeMasters, p. 5.
62. Ibid., p. 53.
63. American Humane Association: *National Analysis of Official Child Neglect and Abuse Reporting*. Englewood, Colorado, 1978, p. 1.
64. Ibid., p. 4.
65. Roberts, E., Kline, D., and Gagnon, J.: *Family Life and Sexual Learning*. Project on Human Sexual Development, Cambridge, Massachusetts, 1978.

BIBLIOGRAPHY

Anderson, J.G., and Evans, F.B.: *Family socialization and education achievement in two cultures: Mexican-American and Anglo-American*. Sociometry 39:209, 1976.

Aries, P.: *Centuries of Childhood*. Alfred A. Knopf, New York, 1962.

Bee, H.L., et. al.: *Social class differences in maternal teaching strategies and speech patterns*. Developmental Psychology 1:726, 1969.

Bigner, J.J.: *Parent education in popular literature: 1950–1970*. The Family Coordinator 21:313, 1972.

Brim, O.G.: *Education for Child Rearing*. Russell Sage Foundation, New York, 1959.

Brody, S.: *Patterns of Mothering*. International Universities Press, New York, 1956.

Bronfenbrenner, U.: "The changing American child—a speculative analysis." In Rebelsky, F. (ed.): *Child Development and Behavior*. Alfred A. Knopf, New York, 1970.

Chamberlin, R.W.: *Parenting styles, child behavior, and the pediatrician*. Pediatr. Ann. 6:584, September 1977.

Durret, M.E., Bryant, S.O., and Pennebaker, J.W.: *Child-rearing reports of white, black, and Mexican-American families*. Developmental Psychology 11:871, 1975.

Eiduson, B.T.: *Child development in emergent family style*. Children Today 7:24, 1978.

Erickson, M.L.: "Meeting the needs of parents and children in well-child settings." In Erickson, M.L. (ed.): *Assessment and Management of Developmental Changes in Children*. Mosby, St. Louis, 1976, Chapter 10.

Gesell, A.L., and Ilg, F.L., with G.E. Bullis (rev. ed.): *The Child from Five to Ten*. Harper & Row, New York, 1977.

Ginott, H.: *Between Parent and Child*. MacMillan, New York, 1965.

Instructors special report. Instructor 8:59, 1977.

Lourie, R.S.: *The concern of one generation for the next*. Children 17:234, 1970.

Newman, L.F.: *A bicentennial view of child-rearing; notes of an anthropologist*. R.I. Med. J. 59:221, May 1976.

Ongiri, D.O.: *A comparison of educational and childrearing practices of urban America and British Colonial Africa*. Paper presented at the National Conference on Black Families in America, Black Youth (Louisville, Kentucky), March 6, 1976.

Pearlin, L.I.: *Social class, occupation and parental values. A cross national study*. Am. Sociol. Rev. 31:466, 1966.

Piaget, J.: *Science of Education and Psychology*. Orion Press, New York, 1970.

Raths, L.E.: *Meeting the Needs of Children*. Charles B. Merrill, Columbus, Ohio, 1972.

Rebelsky, F., and Dorman, L.: *Child Development and Behavior*. Alfred A. Knopf, New York, 1970.

Roe, K.U.: *A cross-cultural study of empathy in young children*. Paper presented at the annual conference of the Western Psychological Association (Los Angeles), April 8–11, 1976.

A study of the American family, 1977. Med. Times 105:114, November 1977.

Sands, R.M.: *Toward communal child rearing*. Social Work 18:54, May 1973.

Schiffelbein, D.: *Cross cultural research . . . What makes the differences?* Menninger Perspective 6:10, 1975.

Senn, M., and Hartford, C. (eds.): *The Firstborn Experiences of Eight American Families*. Harvard University Press, Cambridge, 1968.

Spock, B.M.: *Baby and Child Care*. Hawthorn Books, New York, 1968.

Whiting, B.B.: *Folk wisdom and childrearing*. Merrill-Palmer Quarterly 20:9, 1974.

Yarrow, M.R., Campbell, J.D., and Burton, R.V.: *Child Rearing. An Inquiry into Research and Methods*. Jossey-Bass, Inc., San Francisco, 1968.

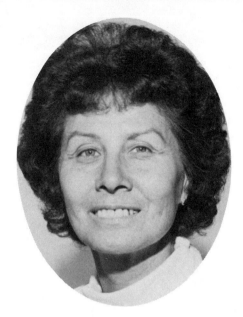

Chapter 3

Charles E. Farris was born near Sallisaw, Oklahoma, where he attended the public schools. He received his bachelor's degree from Northeastern State University, Tahlequah, Oklahoma, and his master's degree in social work from St. Louis University, St. Louis, Missouri. He is an enrolled member of the Cherokee Nation of Oklahoma, and was one of the original members of the Association of American Indian and Alaskan Native Social Workers' organization, for which he is currently the southeastern regional representative. He is actively involved in local, tribal, and national professional organizations, and is a member of the National Association of Social Workers, Academy of Certified Social Workers, Council of Social Work Education, and board member of the Clinical Registry of the National Association of Social Workers. He is an Associate Professor and the Chairman of the Social Welfare Policy and Services curriculum sequence of the Graduate School of Social Work, Barry College, Miami, Florida. He has published articles on the American Indian in professional journals and also teaches Indian courses and is the Project Director for the American Indian Graduate Social Work Student Program at Barry College. He has served as a consultant and participant on professional programs involving the American Indian.

Lorene Sanders Farris was born near Vian, Oklahoma, where she attended Dwight Presbyterian Mission School, Sallisaw City Schools, and completed high school at Sequoyah Indian School, Tahlequah, Oklahoma. She is an enrolled member of the Cherokee Nation of Oklahoma. She received her diploma in nursing from Sibley Memorial Hospital, and her bachelor's and master's degrees in Nursing from Washington University, St. Louis, Missouri. She also has a Master of Science from Barry College, Florida, and is currently a doctoral student at the University of Miami, Coral Gables, Florida. Her nursing experience has encompassed public health, clinical nursing, and nursing education, and she has published articles in nursing and social work journals. She is President of the American Indian/Alaska Native Nurses Association.

The American Indian

*Charles Ed Farris, M.S.W., and
Lorene Sanders Farris, R.N., M.S.*

Major changes affecting the American Indian family came about when destructive forces arrived with non-Indian people and continues today despite treaties, congressional hearings, task forces, reports, conferences, missionaries, legal litigation, and resistance by Indian peoples. The effects of these changes have disrupted the Indian family structure and resulted in a variety of social, health, and developmental problems for the American Indian child.

It is a difficult task to describe childrearing in the American Indian family since there are nearly 300 different tribes, speaking 250 living languages, and each tribe with its own unique cultural orientation. What one says of the Athasbascan of Alaska is not the same as one can say about the Cherokee of Oklahoma. Therefore this chapter does not imply that Indian childrearing practices can be described in generalities, but that there are some relevant similarities and many significant differences. It will attempt to examine some of those similarities and differences and explain that Indian childrearing is person-oriented and stresses personal relationships. Looking only at one specific area of the child's life, such as childrearing and development, will not lead to a definitive or true understanding of the Indian child. A comprehensive search and examination of how the child fits into his total family, tribe, and place of residence would be more productive and accurate, but that is beyond the scope of this chapter.

HISTORICAL OVERVIEW

The American Indian family did most of the teaching and educating of the young and was responsible for childrearing. Only rarely did formal education replace the family and provide this aspect of childrearing. In fact, just the opposite is recorded as early as 1744, when the Virginia legislature offered the Six Nations an opportunity to send six Indian youths for education at the Williamsburg College of William and Mary. Connassatoage spoke for the Six Nations replying:

> We know you highly esteem the kind of learning taught in these Colleges, and the maintenance of our young men, while with you, would be very expensive to you. We are convinced, therefore, that you mean to do us good by your proposal; and we thank you heartily. But you who are so wise must know that different Nations have different conceptions of things; and you will not therefore take it amiss, if our ideas of this kind of education happens not to be the same with yours. We have had some experience of it. Several of our young people were formerly brought up in the colleges of the Northern Provinces; they were instructed in all your sciences; but, when they came back to us, they were bad runners, ignorant of

every means of living in the woods, unable to bear either cold or hunger, knew neither how to build a cabin, take a deer, or kill an enemy, spoke our language imperfectly, were therefore neither fit for hunters, warriors, nor counselors, they were totally good for nothing. We are however not the less obliged for your kind offer, tho' we decline accepting it; and to show our grateful sense of it, if the gentlemen of Virginia shall send us a dozen of their sons, we will take great care of their education, instruct them in all we know, and make men of them.[1]

There is no evidence to indicate that the Virginians took advantage of the counteroffer.

Indian families were the responsible institutionalized tribal force for helping children learn to talk, to behave in approved ways, and to utilize the family and tribe as a socializing agent as they grew into adulthood. Families in the Indian community were not just biological families, they were what is now termed "nuclear" families, consisting of the husband, wife, and children. Perhaps more importantly they also had the familial relationship defined as the "extended family," which included sisters and brothers of the parents, their husbands and wives, their children, and the grandparents. A recent legal definition of the extended Indian family says that "the extended family member shall be defined by the law or custom of the Indian child's tribe or, in the absence of such a law or custom, shall be a person who has reached the age of 18 and who is the Indian child's grandparent, aunt or uncle, brother or sister, brother-in-law or sister-in-law, niece or nephew, first or second cousin or stepparent."[2] An interesting phenomenon of the extended Indian family is that all people in the extended family, including the Indian child, are considered equals and have only one horizontal class of relationships.

An example of the Indian's strong feelings and deep love for his children is illustrated by the simple fact that no Indian language has words for orphan, illegitimate, or adoption as defined by the non-Indian culture. Children who have no parents simply find a home in the extended family, usually with the grandparents, uncles, or aunts. Informal adoption was usual rather than the exception. In many families, children called the wife of the family "Mother," even when she may be the grandmother, aunt, sister, or cousin. The physical relationship was close, with all family members living in one large shelter, for example, the Iroquoian longhouses, or nearby in several shelters known as a camp. This arrangement is still evident today on many reservations and in the Pueblos.

The Indian child was always welcome in all Indian homes. If he was visiting a distance away from his home and it became night, there was no question about his spending the night as a welcome guest. This was the expected and accepted Indian way. If the visit was with a family where there were older Indians, they would often entertain the children with tribal legends, and traditional Indian foods would be served.

The extended Indian family is an important component in tribal life, not only in child care planning and development, but also as a primary resource to be utilized when assistance is needed. Compton's study found that when the extended family and other tribal institutions are strong, developmental and disciplinary problems can usually be effectively handled, but when the extended family and other traditional social institutional controls have been weakened or have broken down, the problems become particularly acute.[3] Owing to past injustices and rejections, Indian peoples tend to turn within and to the extended family during times of adversity and crisis. This often results in the under-utilization by the contemporary Indian of non-Indian community resources, and unemployment and poverty continue as major problems. Per capita mean income for individual Indians was $3377 in 1973. Unemployment rates of 40 to 75 percent are not uncommon.[4]

Culturebearers

With certain exceptions, until recent times most Indian tribes did not have written histories. Tribal legends were orally passed from generation to generation. Some Plains tribes used pictographic records by painting significant chronological tribal events on their tepees. The child in the American Indian family has traditionally been the one to maintain the customs and traditions of the tribe. Indian people have always felt that any Indian child was a child of nature and therefore a very special person. Locke reports an example of this tribal love for children in the Dakota people, who have a tribal concept of the "Beloved Child." The Beloved Child is one born after a time of particularly deep tribal travail. He is considered a gift from God and is treated in a very special way. Even the soles of his moccasins are beaded and many people are invited to a special feast and celebration to see this child.[5] The Beloved Child is a symbol in a real sense of all Indian children, because all Indian people have been through many travails and have a special feeling for their children.

It is not only tragic but true that many of the massacres of Indian people by White people involved not just Indian adults, but also the indiscriminate murder of many childbearing aged women and children. Two incidents come readily to mind. The first relates to the Southern Cheyenne who were wintered at Sand Creek, Colorado. Their chief, Black Kettle, had been promised and naively believed that if his people remained at peace, they would be protected by United States soldiers. When attacked during a chill morning in November 1864, Chief Black Kettle held the United States flag as instructed, to indicate he was friendly, and made no move for protection or hostility. The troops moved in and massacred a total of 300 Indians, most of whom were women and children (only 75 were men).[6] The second tragic incident, so eloquently written about by Dee Brown, is the massacre of Wounded Knee. Sioux Indians camped near Wounded Knee Creek were surrounded by United States troops, and a fatal shot was fired, history does not say by whom. The troops immediately overwhelmed the partially disarmed Indians. The Indian loss was total, including many women and children. No medical aid was allowed into the area for 3 days, although it was available.[7]

It is the feeling of these authors that military extermination was only one of the more obvious genocidal methods that the invading White immigrants used to exterminate Indian people in order to conquer and ultimately to take the Indians' land for their own. It is an amazing thing that any Indian culture survived. Since the beginning of the United States government, there has been war between it and one tribe of Indians or another. The Seminole Tribe of Florida have never signed a peace treaty with the government and still consider themselves "the Unconquered Seminoles."

EARLY CHILDHOOD

The importance for the individual Indian of being in harmony with nature and having basic and close spiritual relationships with the environment (e.g., earth, water, mountains, and trees) is initiated in the early years and emphasized and practiced in Indian child care standards by the family. One might wonder how this emphasis occurs. To the Indian, the world is regarded as interrelated, and all forms of life are sacred and to

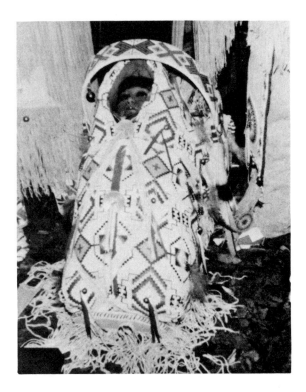

Figure 1. An ornate cradle board for the Indian infant.

be revered. This is a common spiritual truth that is taught to children in all Indian families. The emphasis is upon being as close to nature as possible. It is demonstrated by the Indian practicing a certain life-style with appropriate ceremonies and rites, which are often alien and not understood by the non-Indian (Fig. 1).

Food

Indian families are noted for their traditional hospitality. They are generous with their possessions, and this includes food, even with strangers. The women of the family always set food before any visitors. To not do so would be considered a serious social breach and an affront, inviting tribal censure. If hungry, the guest eats, if not, politeness requires that he taste the food and offer thanks to his host.

Regional foods were the main staple of the Indian child's diet. In the Northeast, berries, fowl, roots, and fresh greens were used. They were supplemented in the winter by dried meat, fruits, and vegetables. In the Dakota area, foods were made from wild rice strained and mixed with the broth of venison. Venison and maize were the mainstay diet of the child until he grew teeth, and then he ate from the table. In the Northwest, fish, often salmon, was the main tribal staple food. Salmon was also used in religious ceremonies. Maize (corn), berries, roots, beans, and squash were almost universal staple foods for most of the Indian families. The buffalo provided vital meat for the Plains tribes. Many tribes were horticulturally oriented and never moved until their forced removal to reservations. Other tribes made seasonal migrations following and searching for certain foods and medicinal herbs. Today, corn still is a major food staple for many tribes. Dried corn is either home-grown or purchased in the grocery stores. The Seminoles of Florida make a popular dish called Sofkee, a gruel type food dish with a corn base, which may be either drunk or eaten with a spoon. Cherokees from North Carolina and Oklahoma make Conutchee, a corn dish mixed with nutmeats and often served at Indian dinners and powwows.

Studies have shown that when Indian foods are consumed in their natural state, they are nutritionally adequate. It is when they are commercialized into modern convenience foods that the nutritional values are lost and health suffers.

Indian time in relation to food is interesting. Indian families eat when they are hungry, and of course this also applies to the Indian child. Early Indians were oblivious to time as non-Indians record it. The day was not artificially measured in hours and minutes, but rather by when the sun rose and set. That is the span of time for a person to do what he wants and needs to do. Even today, Indians can conform to non-Indian time if it means job security, but the value of time is not perceived by the Indian person in the non-Indian's materialistic frame of reference.

Toys and Play

Indian children were encouraged to play. Dolls for the girls have been found in almost every tribe. They were fashioned out of stone, ivory, clay, corncobs, shells, skins, or doughbread. Other toys found were miniature bows and arrows, dog sleds, blow guns, tepees, and cradle boards. Excavation of pre-Columbian tribes has found toys with wheels, although it is not known if the wheel was ever utilized by the adult Indians as a labor-saving tool. Kachina dolls were fashioned after living men who dress in Kachina costumes as symbolic representations of the spirits of their ancestors. The dolls are given to the Hopi girls on the last day of the festival to pass on this part of symbolic and religious ceremonies of the Hopi.

60

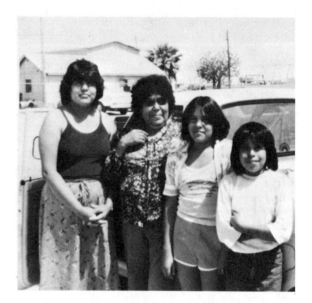

Figure 2. A Pima Indian grandmother with her three granddaughters.

Discipline was and is extraordinarily permissive and mild by non-Indian standards. Shame and ridicule were ordinarily effective in achieving the desired behavior. Traditionally, corporal punishment was rarely used. However, as a last resort, some tribes utilized traditional scratching as a behavior control for especially obstreperous youth. This was done by painfully raking a sharp toothed object on the arm or upper body and was administered by a maternal male relative, usually the child's uncle. As part of discipline, Indian children were taught to not cry out at night. This was a precautionary protective measure for the welfare and benefit of the tribe, especially if they were being hunted and a child's cry would reveal their hiding place. Many Indian families feel their children are competent to care for themselves at an early age and older children are often given supervisory responsibilities for younger children. Some non-Indians label this as objectionable neglect and child abuse, and it may conflict with the non-Indian society's child care standards and laws, resulting in removal of the child from his family.

Story-telling by grandparents often was educational and had a moral of what one should do (Fig. 2). The constant repetition of the right way to do things resulted in producing tribally acceptable social behavior. Indian children are well behaved but are often described by non-Indians as overly shy and withdrawn because of the way that they conduct themselves in public or away from their family. This is not shyness, but the result of both Indian children and adults having conditioned themselves to wait and assess any new situation before they commit themselves and become involved. This type of tactically withholding behavior by the individual Indian reinforces the non-Indian's stereotype of the passive Indian.

CULTURE AND RELIGION

One cannot critically examine cultural and religious influences on Indian childrearing practices without being aware of the many different tribal cultures and religions. Now for the first time since their removal to the reservations, there are more non-reservation Indians than reservation Indians. Although each tribe developed its own cosmology and relationships with the supernatural and spiritual world, there are many common practices and beliefs that cut across tribal boundaries.

Lewis describes "spirit power" as a belief in the presence that is said to sustain the Salish Indian individual, to direct occupational pursuits, and to furnish unique passions, which he could display in ceremonies and in which he could find release for himself and strength in the eyes of his people.[8] This concept of the supernatural is a common belief in Indian families. It is supported by the resurgence and maintenance of the status of the medicine man/woman, holy man, shaman, conjurer, and other traditional specialists in Indian communities all over the nation.

When one considers the Indian's religion, one must recognize the delicate and positive interbalance between it and the tribal social mores and customs. Indian religions, like all religions, reflect a formalized system for institutional moral controls and planned manipulation of desired individual and group behavior. The Indian's traditional religions uniquely reflected a special eclectic relationship with his Mother Earth and Nature. Indian languages do not contain words of sacrilege or profanity. His deity is a part of his total life experiences and not compartmentalized into certain rituals and days of the week, although there are days of fasting, sexual abstinence, sweat baths, vision seeking, and seasonal ceremonies, such as the Green Corn celebration, in which he rejoices in a full harvest.

The total life of the Indian child from birth onward is affected directly and indirectly in numerous ways by his religion. After puberty, as a part of their developmental growth process, Indian youths are active participants in tribal religious rites and ceremonies. They receive special training in their responsibilities from their extended family and tribal spiritual leaders and medicine men/women. The rituals of purification, sacrifice, and the vision quest are a special means for the young Indian as an individual to purposefully reach out to his supernatural surroundings for meaningful spiritual contact.

There have been few Pan-Indian religions, but an example of one is the "Ghost Dance." This movement began about 1880 when a Paiute from Nevada known as Wovoka experienced a vision that incorporated a better world for Indian peoples. There would be a new world with no White people, who would be engulfed by a flood. Dead Indians would return to life and the buffalo would come back. Wevoka urged Indians to be nonviolent, to be faithful to family life, pray, dance a unique happy circular dance, stop intertribal differences, and become Indian brothers. Somehow, the idea developed that the Ghost Dance shirt would protect the Indian from the White man's bullets. Unfortunately, for the Indian, that this was not true was tragically demonstrated in the 1890 massacre at Wounded Knee.[9]

Modern Indian religious freedom was not achieved until 1978, when the Federal government enacted legislation that made the religious use of feathers, peyote, and sacred sites inviolate legally.[10]

PSYCHOSEXUAL DEVELOPMENT

Indian societies, like all societies, have formal and informal sex mores and taboos. In most tribes there were few inhibitions or restrictions regarding the intermingling of the sexes up to the age of puberty. Bodily functions were accepted as a normal everyday part of living and sex play and body curiosity by children were not subjected to shaming or disciplinary punishment. When an Indian child reached puberty, ceremonial recognition was and is still given in many tribes. The individual boy in many tribes would go on a specially planned vision quest to an isolated place in the woods or upon a mountain that had special significance for his tribe. There he would fast and wait for a vision or dream that would have special meaning and give spiritual direction to his future life. The vision might convey a special name or a guardian spirit, or give him some supernatural power related to his future destiny. It was a part of an expected maturing process that tested and reinforced his tribal identity.

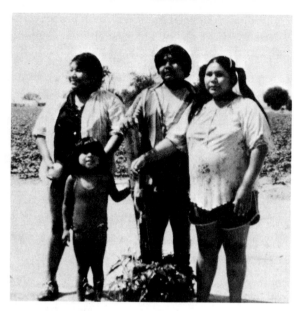

Figure 3. Older girls learn about child care by assuming early responsibility for their siblings.

Unfortunately modern Indian life has failed to develop a satisfactory maturational substitute for today's Indian youth, and this is often reflected tragically in a lack of purpose and direction, high incidence of alcoholism, drug abuse, school under-achievement and dropping-out, and suicide. Current suicide rates among Indian youth have reached epidemic proportions. The seriousness of this is demonstrated by the 1974-1976 age-adjusted suicide rate among Indians, which is 2.1 times as high as the overall United States.

Prior to the onset of puberty, Indian girls were instructed by the older women of the tribe in their responsibilities as a wife and mother (Fig. 3). At puberty there usually were symbolic ceremonies in which she played a leading role signifying her attainment of adulthood with its attendant rights and responsibilities. One example of such a ceremony is the Apache "Gahns" (sometimes called "Mountain Spirits"). It is an event sponsored by the girl's family, with many sacred and social meanings. Today, such ceremonies are becoming rare, primarily because of the prohibitive expense of feeding the many friends and spectators, plus the fees for the medicine men/women and singers. Many Apache families feel they can no longer afford such an expensive ceremony that may no longer be appropriate or necessary in a modern Indian society. Many Indians today feel

that the abandonment of such tribal ceremonies will ultimately destroy tribal identity and true "Indianness." They feel that the traditional uniqueness and strength of Indian culture have always been a strong tribal identity as reflected through tribal rites and ceremonies. However, today if one asks an Indian his identity, he will invariably answer first that he is a Cherokee, Apache, and so on. "Pan-Indianness" is still of apparent secondary importance.

In traditional Indian life, a different and stricter set of moral values took over in adulthood. Chastity and sexual loyalty were highly valued. Punishment for adultery or alienation of affections was swift and sure. In some tribes, an unfaithful wife's nose could be cut off, and she and her paramour permanently banished. Indians in most tribes observed forms of strict incest taboos; for example, subject to severe social censure, husbands avoided direct contact with their mothers-in-law and certain female relatives, neither looking at nor speaking to them except through acceptable intermediaries. Most tribes viewed homosexuality positively, and it was not considered a tribal threat. To the contrary, it was believed that such persons were a special spiritual asset to the tribe.

DATING AND MARRIAGE
Dating was generally unrestricted among Indian youth, but was primarily within one's own tribe. There were usually no tribal class distinctions and one could date and marry anyone except for the incest prohibitions relating to members of one's own clan.

A modern phenomenon regarding dating has developed as a result of the intertribal mix found in the student bodies of the Bureau of Indian Affairs (BIA) boarding schools. It is not unusual to find not only intertribal friendships but marriages resulting when students from different tribes meet (Fig. 4). Today, there is apparently little concern by young Indians for observing the traditional incest prohibitions for taboos regarding intertribal dating and marriage within the same clan. However, such intertribal marriages do present some unique legal and social problems for the husband, wife, and their off-spring. Tribal membership requirements usually allow individual membership in only one tribe, that is, an Indian can only be a voting member and receive benefits from one tribe. Unfortunately, the quantum of "Indianness" of the children from

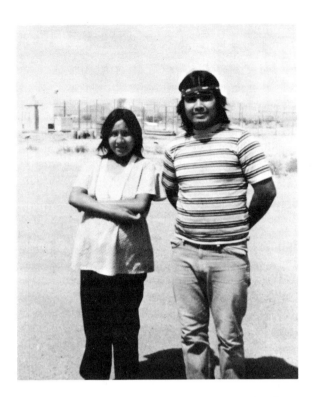

Figure 4. An Apache expectant father with his Pima wife.

the intertribal marriage may become diluted to such an extent as to make them ineligible for membership in either one or both of their parents' tribes. It may in effect make them non-Indians. This tribal membership restriction may also create familial divisiveness with serious problems relating to tribal loyalty and family allegiance in a family that may already have serious adjustment problems.

Another problem of family relationships results from the fact that traditionally many tribes were matriarchal and the children belonged to their mother's clan and took their mother's surname. All tribal rights emanated from this maternal relationship. Today, this may create friction in estate settlements and parental and sibling relationships. The most important man in matriarchal tribes for an Indian child may not be his natural father but his mother's oldest brother. Not only was this uncle responsible for parental training and discipline, but he introduced the child to the clan and sponsored his initiation into important tribal societies. He was an effective father surrogate and role model, but one without legal sanction from the non-Indian society.

It is expected that the Indian youth will be different, and he is encouraged to be independent. In particular, Indian boys are reared to be physically daring and impetuous. If he does not perform an occasional controversially defiant act, he will be less acceptable as a son, brother, friend, or sweetheart. Indian boys are reared to be proud and are expected to a degree to resist outside behavior controls. They have certain familial obligations, but their primary behavior models often come from peers. A major problem with this adolescent peer emulation is that with extra time on their hands, in a relatively unsupervised setting away from the family, such as boarding schools, adolescent acting out and testing may lead to dangerous antisocial experimentation in prohibited areas such as truancy, drugs, alcohol, and premarital sex. This behavior is usually nonviolent. In many Indian communities this type of behavior is abetted by poverty, isolation, alcoholism, and in many cases the apparent permissiveness found in traditional family controls of the extended Indian family.

HEALTH

The tragic tolls of neglect are paid by contemporary American Indians in the nation's highest rates of health problems. One must deduce that, if the child is the father of the man, then many of the problems faced by the Indian have their origin in poor health and a deprived childhood. Treaty commitments by the Federal government to the Indian have always included provisions for health care. Since 1955, the Division of Indian Health Service (IHS) of the United States Public Health Service has assumed the major responsibility for providing Indian health programming.

There is no doubt that poverty and substandard living conditions directly contribute to the lack of well-being and poor health of the Indian child. Leading causes of death among Indian infants continue to be respiratory, digestive, infective, and parasitic diseases, and congenital malformations. All are directly related to the lack of proper nutrition and generally inadequate living standards. Despite concern reflected in corrective and preventive programming, a major health problem continues to be otitis media, the inflammation of the middle ear that results in chronic drainage and possible permanent hearing loss, which in turn directly affects the school and social performance of the child. Periodontal diseases continue as a major reason for tooth decay and loss.

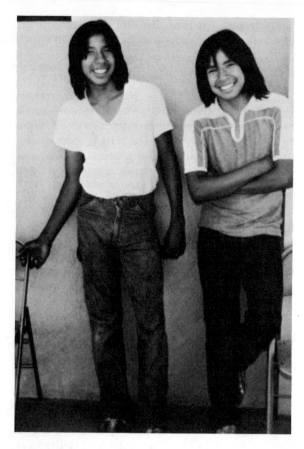

Figure 5. Teen-age brothers at an Indian reservation in Phoenix, Arizona.

Traditionally, the care of the Indian's body was an individual responsibility. Bathing and other health practices were common among Indian peoples. The use of hot springs and of the sweat house was not only for cleansing but also had extra significance for medicinal and religious rituals.

If an Indian youth became ill, treatment included the readily available medicinal herbs, rituals, and baths. Tribal medicine men/women were consulted and healing rites and ceremonies could be administered if indicated. If there was no improvement after treatment, it might be felt that inadvertently a taboo had been violated, and appropriate countermeasures would be instituted.

Physical stamina and endurance were important and admired traits. Tribal and intertribal athletic events were an important part of tribal life. Jim Thorpe, the great Sac and Fox Olympic decathlon winner, is a good example of how Indian people strive for athletic excellence.

FAMILY RELATIONSHIPS

Social erosion in Indian cultures has resulted in Indian family relationships changing significantly in recent years. One major change has been in the role and function of the extended family. Instead of being an available viable resource of support and self-sufficiency, it has become an anomalous, impermanent structure for retreat and withdrawal for those individuals who are insecure. Another important change in Indian family life has been in the weakening of the relationship and role of the Indian father to his children. He no longer has marketable skills and knowledge to teach and is not a positive role model for his children to emulate. Male youths tend to turn to their brothers and peers for support and role models (Fig. 5). There are also new roles and relationships between females, with only token gestures toward traditionally important relationships. Special importance and status are given to the obtaining of a non-Indian education and successful and well-paid employment.

EDUCATION

The academic under-achievement and dropping-out of school of Indian students are major concerns of tribal leaders and educators. Dropout rates range from 25 to 75 percent, and in 1976, 11,000 reservation Indian children were not attending any school.[12] Over 40 percent of all Indians over 25 years of age have an elementary school education or less, and only 3.8 percent have completed 4 years of college.[13]

Historically the Indian child's developmental education and vocational training were largely a matter of imitating the skills and roles of his extended family, especially his mother and father. Young girls played with dolls and made miniature tepees and clothing and eventually learned appropriate home-making skills (e.g., to cook, make clothing, and construct the tepee). Boys were given miniature bows and arrows and encouraged to hunt small birds and game and participate with other boys in games of skill, such as war games, hoop and javelin, and target shooting. As the boys grew older, they were progressively given adult responsibilities. In Plains tribes they became expert horsemen at an early age and spent much time developing skills of hunting and war-making from horseback.

For the contemporary Indian child, primary

formalized education is through the BIA education programs, which are the result of his tribe's relationship by treaty with the Federal government. In 1974, the BIA was operating 75 boarding schools with an enrollment of over 30,000 students.[14] Critics of the BIA school programs have maintained that placements in their boarding schools are often made for social behavioral reasons rather than educational reasons. This is because of the lack of adequate resources, such as group homes, foster homes, and professional counseling services at the tribal level for Indian children and their families. This is unfortunate because boarding schools also lack adequate professional counseling programs to properly help the children with adjustment and guidance problems.

On the reservation level there is need to develop group programs such as Scouting and 4-H Clubs, with a major thrust toward Indian-oriented activities focused upon individual and group needs of Indian youth. An important part of any such projected program should be the teaching of culture, language, and tribal history by interested and qualified elders.

PROFESSIONAL IMPLICATIONS

In spite of the alleged commonalities between professional services and the American Indian, there has not been widespread acceptance or use of their services by Indian peoples. A critical examination will quickly reveal the major reasons. Although those professions are apparently effective with many of the problems of the dominant society, their probing, clinically oriented methodologies are incompatible with traditional Indian values and life-styles, which respect an individual's rights of privacy, confidentiality, and self-determination. Yet these professions myopically persist in using treatment methods that invade and violate those Indian values. Consideration should be given by health workers to developing programs with treatment methods that truly reflect and respect the Indian's values and cultures. There is need to systematically and critically examine and research the various social and economic forces and pressures impinging upon the individual Indian and his life. The professional must recognize and seek to alleviate the negative forces and conflicting value pressures on the Indian and his family.[15]

Professional health workers who implement programs and take actions that are contrary to tribal interests will alienate Indians and further weaken Indian family life by depriving these families of needed services. The lack of recognition of the extended family and the enforcement of non-Indian norms and patterns of licensing and recruitment standards, which reflect only White middle-class values, cause problems. These racist policies exclude many fine Indian foster and adoptive homes, both on and off reservations, and result in the unnecessary and cruel removal and placement of Indian children. There is concern that Indian children are removed from their natural homes at a disproportionate rate and are placed in non-Indian foster and adoptive homes. Even though the non-Indian foster and adoptive parents may be dedicated and well-motivated in their desire to help the Indian child, there is a strong probability that the Indian child will develop negative feelings of racial confusion and abandonment when he enters adolescence and adulthood. Questionable agency practices were in the unfortunate national adoption program that placed Indian children with non-Indian families without clear prior consultation and approval from the involved Indian people. Even conceding there may have been some neglect by non-Indian standards, the failure to recognize and utilize the child's extended family is uncalled for and unprofessional.[16] To help correct this problem, Congress passed the Indian Child Welfare Act, which gives proper recognition to the Indian's culture and life-styles and allows individual tribes to become directly involved in the placement needs of their own children.[17]

Compton's study found a critical need for more tribal group and foster homes, emergency shelter care, and other facilities for delinquent and predelinquent Indian children. Because reservations rarely have adequate emergency facilities, children are often placed in jails, many of which are old and overcrowded, or in a group home, if one is available, or they are simply released. In addition to being professionally questionable, the detaining of juveniles in group homes on an emergency basis can disrupt the services being offered to other residents of the facility.[18]

Comprehensive programs should be developed to help individual Indians and families with personal and family relationship problems. Services such as individual and group counseling, advocacy, and self-help groups should be encouraged.[19] Since many professional counseling methodologies and techniques are apparently incompatible with Indian life-styles, new and in-

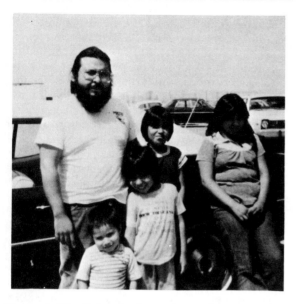

Figure 6. The father is the authority figure for this four-child family.

novative approaches must be researched and jointly developed by professionals and sensitive tribal leaders. The collaborative utilization of the Indian medicine men/women should be integrated into all programs that serve Indian clientele.

The importance of childrearing practices in any society has long been an established fact. However, there continues to be an unfortunate lack of relevant information and programs about the American Indian child. This is a serious indictment against the helping professions. Fortunately, it is one the professionals can correct by providing appropriate leadership to help the American Indian people in developing needed programs for Indian children.

A large number of American Indians live off the reservation and seek health care in facilities where nurses are a part of the staff. These nurses could better meet the health needs of the Indian child and his family if they would initially approach the family in a quiet and unobtrusive manner. The nature of Indians in general is one of being quiet, unassuming, and assessing the situation before speaking or making any commitment. The health provider must first allow time for the Indian person, parent or child, to make his assessment and to ask questions, and then the health provider may prepare to intervene. This is in opposition to the usual approach to the nursing process in which the nurse does the initial assessment immediately.

At this time in most tribes over the United States there is a revival of tribal rituals and Indian medicine, which in some way may establish a pattern of family disorganization, depending on degrees of previous acculturation. This produces a conflict between belief and current reality for the Indian child, so that he may be in the middle of a cultural conflict that affects the health of both child and family. For example, an Indian family may invest money and time to seek relief for the child's illness from an Indian medicine man, but to no avail. The time and money spent in seeking this relief should be anticipated by the nurse and accepted as part of the family's response to an illness.

For effective follow-through of a prescribed plan of care in the home, it is necessary to identify which adult is the authority figure and who is the one that will care for the child (Fig. 6). The involvement of the significant adults in the child's care cannot be overlooked. We think it is different in the Indian family than in the White family (more adults may be involved).

Physical facilities where care is administered is often white and sterile looking. This is seen as an affront to Indians, who are more comfortable with natural or earth tones in furniture, walls, and other equipment.

In Indian communities where there are parents who are more comfortable in the use of native language, efforts to obtain native interpreters will encourage and improve compliance with the plan of care. Even one native nurse would help, as all Indians have a sense of relatedness with one another that is not seen in the White culture.

REFERENCES

1. Armstrong, V.I.: *I Have Spoken: American History Through the Voices of Indians.* Pocket Books, New York, 1972, p. 19.
2. Indian Child Welfare Act. (P.L. 95–608) November 8, 1978.
3. United States Department of Health, Education and Welfare. Office of Human Development, Office of Child Development, Children's Bureau: *Indian Child Welfare: A State of the Field Study.* Washington, D.C., 1976, p. 20.
4. United States Department of Commerce, Bureau of the Census. United States Gov-

ernment Printing Office. Washington, D.C. 1970. P.C. (2)-1F. June 1973, p. 120.

5. Locke, P.: "Supportive care, custody, placement and adoption of American Indian children." A National Conference Sponsored by the American Academy of Child Psychiatry. April 19–22, 1977, Bottle Hollow, Utah, p. 18.

6. Longstreet, S.: *War Cries on Horseback.* Curtis Books, New York, 1970, pp. 186-187.

7. Brown, D.: *Bury My Heart at Wounded Knee.* Holt, Rinehart and Winston, New York, 1970.

8. Lewis, C.: *Indian Families of the Northwest Coast: The Impact of Change.* University of Chicago Press, Chicago, 1970, p. 2.

9. Marriott, A., and Rachlin, C.K.: *Peyote.* Mentor Books, New York, 1971, pp. 25,26, and 32.

10. American Indian Religious Freedom Act. Public Law No. 95–341. August 11, 1978.

11. United States Department of Health, Education & Welfare. *The Indian Health Program.* U.S.P.H.S. 1978, p. 9.

12. American Indian Policy Review Commission: "Report on Indian Education." Task Force Five: Indian Education. United States Government Printing Office, Washington, D.C., 1976, p. 8.

13. United States Congress, Senate Committee on Interior and Insular Affairs, Subcommittee on Indian Affairs: *Hearings, Indian Child Welfare Programs.* 93rd Congress, 2nd Session, April 9, 1974, p. 380.

14. American Indian Policy Review Commission, p. 8.

15. Edwards, E.D., and Edwards, M.E.: "Minorities: American Indians." In Turner, J. (ed.): *Encyclopedia of Social Work.* National Association of Social Workers, New York, 1977, p. 952.

16. Fanshel, D.: *Far from the Reservation.* Scarecrow Press, New York, 1972.

17. Indian Child Welfare Act.

18. United States Department of Health, Education and Welfare, Office of Human Development, p. 26.

19. Farris, C.E.: *American Indian social worker advocates.* Social Casework. 10:10, October 1976.

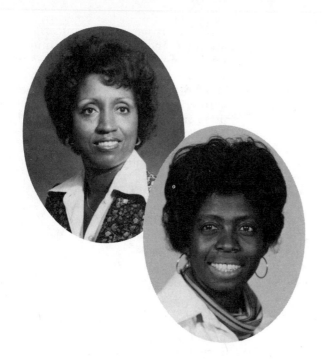

Chapter 4

I, Betty Greathouse, am a Black American woman, wife, mother, friend, and university professor. Yes, I am a very diverse, complex, and yet simple human being. This is so because of the myriad of people, places, and things that have touched me.

My parents, Oliver and Mae Lizzie Harris, had the greatest impact on my life. Without them, I would not be! Dad and Mama made quite a team. I was never quite sure which of them was the head of the family. Mama was hardly a castrating quarterback, nor was she the water-girl; sometimes decisions were made by my father and on other occasions Mama had the last word. They just seemed to know when it was their turn to carry the ball.

My appreciation for education, work, flexibility of roles, and religion was acquired from my parents. Dad worked two jobs and my mother worked outside of the home, also. He worked as a truck driver and yard man; she worked as a domestic worker, cleaning motels and houses. My parents wanted to provide a good home and education for their seven children.

Dad, who had a fourth-grade education, not only talked about the importance of a Black person getting an education; he would sit down with me and a big old 5-cent tablet with primary grade spacing and go over my "times," as he called them. In other words, he didn't just tell me to do my homework; sometimes he worked with me. He was so concerned about getting us educated that he would not allow us to work as teen-agers. In fact, I had very few friends because he felt peers would deter me from that primary goal—an education.

My childhood and early adolescent weekdays were filled with education in segregated schools. Up to the mid fifties Blacks, Anglos, Indians, and Mexican-Americans attended separate elementary schools in Arizona. But the schools weren't equal and buses weren't provided. Each day I walked a mile to get to a "Black school," which was exactly eight blocks further from my house than a nearby "Mexican-American school." Reading, swimming, and religious activities consumed my weekends, evenings, and summers. Oops—I forgot that I also went to the movies most Sundays, after church, that is. Perhaps I wanted to forget about sitting in "Niggers' Heaven." "Niggers' Heaven" was the place designated for "Negroes" in the theater. By the way, we were called Negroes before we discovered Black was beautiful. As a child I detested the word "colored," and as a woman, I detest the term Negro.

Mom stressed the importance of religion. She took us to church at least two times a week. Her kids knew more scriptures, religious songs, and

The Black American

Betty Greathouse, Ph.D., and
Velvet G. Miller, R.N., B.S.N., M.Ed.

prayers than most of the youngsters in Pilgrim Rest Baptist Church. And when we stood up to recite, we were "clean." As a child, mom took me to the beauty shop every 2 weeks to have my hair straightened and recurled. She, a mother with a ninth-grade education, encouraged me to draw the dresses I wanted our seamstress to make. That was quite an experience. Mrs. Allen, a loving, sweet, Black lady, could make any dress I could draw. She didn't need a pattern. As a child, I wondered why she cleaned house rather than designed and constructed clothes full time. But now I know. Now I think of it, via subtle encouragement to do many different things, Mama conveyed to me that she thought I was capable. Hence, I learned to view myself as a capable person.

As a family we made weekly trips to Mesa to visit my father's mother and a host of aunts, uncles, and cousins. I always enjoyed the visits, especially the figs, oranges, grapefruits, and apricots that followed the hugs and "nosey" questions.

When I was growing up my friends told me I was supposed to hate school. But I never did. I liked it because I performed well and this earned me the praise of my parents and teachers. I never missed playing with and pleasing my peers, so I guess my need for adult approval was stronger than my peer affiliation motive.

I married George Greathouse, a high school football player, and promptly had two boys within a 2-year period. However, this did not prevent me from reaching that much desired goal. After marriage, George and I, with a lot of family support and encouragement, completed high school and went on to college (thanks to our extended families and Black solidarity).

During the subsequent years, while parenting, teaching, and working in the community, I earned an M.A. and a Ph.D. in Education. My present work at Arizona State University, Tempe, Arizona, involves teaching preservice and in-service teachers and parents from different ethnic and linguistic backgrounds about child development and the role adults can play in facilitating children's growth and development.

Therefore, it is with pleasure that I write from a Black perspective, utilizing the theories and methods learned from social science and modifying these contributions and methods based on my experience.

I, Velvet G. Miller, remember: the trips to Mississippi when we drove non-stop because there was no safe place to stay; the cotton fields and watermelon patches and grandmother dipping sweet Garrett snuff. One granddaddy was an AME preacher; the other was an agricultural consultant for the government. I remember the time my mom shook her finger in old man Johnny O'Reilly's face for threatening my older brother and calling him a nigger, and Dad's disappointment, perseverance, and final success when he got his real estate broker's license after seven attempts. My brother had me convinced I was named after a horse until I was old enough to read the book National Velvet. I remember how he laughed when I told him Velvet was the girl, not the horse!

I often wonder how they did it! I was born in Reading, Pennsylvania, to two very special people. My brother and I were raised to be proud of who and what we are, with no less respect for anyone who may be different. Mom and Dad taught us to be absolutely and irrevocably conscious of our dignity and worth and everyone else's. It was not uncommon for our home to have Yellow, Brown, Black and/or White, Jew, Hindu, Catholic, or Muslim folk visiting, calling, or sharing tears and laughter. I grew up knowing lots of different cultures and most of the time I felt good about my "differentness." For a Black child in America that's not easy. Now that I am a parent, I wonder how my parents did that.

I earned a B.S.N. from Wagner College in New York City in the sixties. I took advantage of the cultural opportunities of the city and the Black social revolution opportunities of the times. My Black self-consciousness was heightened and deepened. It was during the sixties and the early seventies that may career goals and direction crystalized. I have worked as a community health nurse, acute care staff nurse, medical surgical supervisor, staff development instructor, and director. Following the completion of a Master of Education degree from Temple University, I joined the faculty at Arizona State University College of Nursing in the Continuing Education Program. I am currently the Associate Director, Nursing Division, at Scottsdale Memorial Hospital in Scottsdale, Arizona.

My professional goal is to in some way influence and enhance the quality of nursing and health care for all people with special emphasis for ethnic people of colors. To effect a change in the educational preparation of health care providers, particularly professional nurses, through formal and continuing education is one means of achieving this goal. Facilitating consumer health education classes is another

means to which I remain committed. Contributing to this book is another route to actualizing my professional goal.

Langston Hughes once wrote a poem that said, in part, "beautiful are the souls of my people." Mom and Dad, Sonny, Bigmom and Bryant, Littlemom and Bigdaddy, and others like them are very strong, proud, beautiful, soulful people. I often wonder how, through all the struggles, they remained that way. As I face the responsibility of rearing my son, Toby, I wonder how I can foster the same.

70

Our people have been talked about, written about, and studied largely by White social scientists. It would seem, then, that so "much ado" has been made about us, that the dominant society would be accurately and well informed. However, much of the information has been in the same vein as the now famous (or infamous) Moynihan Report. The Moynihan Report plays the game of "blaming the victim." Utilizing data from the United States Census Bureau, the author contends that the problems in the Black community are due to the structure of Black families.[1] His report imputes a cause-and-effect relationship between family and society, ignoring the effects of institutional racism and the existence of a Black culture that has evolved as an adaptive mechanism.[2] Given this treatment of Black families in American scholarship, it is not surprising that the larger society continues to harbor gross misconceptions about Black family life.[3]

However, a few authorities on the Black community, Black and White, have written about the vast strengths and adaptability of the Black family. They marvel at the ways our people have adapted to poverty and racism, and yet emerged relatively unscarred.[4] We hope this chapter will show that Dr. Martin Luther King's words about the significance of Black family life were not just rhetoric: ". . . for no other group in American life is the matter of family life more important than to the Negro. Our very survival is bound up in it . . . no one in all history had to fight against so many physical and psychological horrors to have a family life."[5]

Since their involuntary arrival in this country, various labels and names have been used to describe our people. We have chosen to use the term Black Americans throughout this chapter. We are no longer colored or "cullud" people. The term Negro no longer reflects the increasing pride in our heritage and ethnicity. Nor are we simply Africans living in America. While we proudly acknowledge our African heritage and cultural links, we have evolved as a distinct and unique ethnic group. The negativism associated with the color black and blackness has in recent years been turned into a statement of cultural and self-pride. We are Black Americans.

HISTORICAL BACKGROUND
The family life and childrearing practices of Black Americans are greatly influenced by history. Because of our uncharacteristic arrival and history in this country, four specific factors distinguish the Black population from other immigrant groups: (1) the Blacks' country of origin had norms and values that were dissimilar to the Anglo-Saxon American way of life; (2) they represented a wide variety of tribes, each with its own traditions, language, and culture; (3) initially, they came without women; and most importantly, (4) they came in bondage.[6]

Consequently, the American Black family—its characteristics, form, and function—is not solely the result of American experience of slavery. Many aspects of our African cultural heritage transcended the atrocities of enslavement and continue to be reflected in the basic structure and functions of Black American family life.[7] The next section will describe the family life and childrearing practices in the preslavery, slavery, and postslavery periods.

Preslavery Period
The bases of African family life were (1) the kinship group and tribal survival and (2) oneness of being and union with nature. The ethos or guiding principles included humanitarianism and interdependence of the members of the group.[7] Kinship groups were bound by common interests of corporate functions and blood ties.[8] Every member of the tribe had been included in the family prior to Europe's intrusion into the continent.[9] Each tribe had its own code of conduct and systems that governed marital and family behavior.

Marriage in most African communities concerned and united all the family members and not just the two individuals. A woman was the wife of the family and not simply the man's wife. As a result of the extensive involvement and commitment of many persons within the community, dissolution was an action of last resort. Payment by the husband's family was made to the bride's family for compensation of their lost services and as a guarantee of good treatment. This was not intended as a purchase of a woman who subsequently became her husband's property.[8]

Central to the patriarchal authority pattern of the family was the reverence attached to the man's role as protector and provider for the family.[8] However, emphasis was placed upon the flexibility and interchangeability of the familial relationships. Family elements were not seen as separate and distinct, but as inclusive, integral, supportive, and interdependent.[7]

Children were seen in African families as the symbols of continuity of life.[10] In West Africa, the most revered relationship in the tribal society was between the grandparents and a child. Grandmothers were the most honored of all relatives. Believed to be and valued as the living links with the past, grandparents were the source of family history, folklore, proverbs, and other traditional lore.[11]

Children were the recipients of much love and attention. Responsibilities to the family were taught early in the developing years. As the children matured and proceeded through the various rites of passage, role requirements and responsibilities to the family were more specifically delineated. The cycle continued until the era of European colonialism and slave trade.

Health was viewed as being in harmony and union with nature. A long life was a sign of proper habits of living. Death after a fruitful life was seen as a natural process. Illness was a result of disharmony or disease. It was believed that illness was caused by evil spirits or demons acting on their own or on behalf of a living or dead soul. Conjure men and women, or voodoo doctors, were curers who specialized in magico-religious powers and the restoration of balance and harmony.[12]

Slavery Period

According to some authorities, the first Black to arrive in this country was Pedro Alonza Nino, who accompanied Columbus as the navigator of the Niña. Although this is disputed, it is known for certain that several members of the French and Spanish expeditions were Black, including Jean Baptiste de Sable, founder of Chicago.[13] Regardless of when the earliest Black arrived, they did not come as slaves. Between 1619 and 1860, however, over 4 million Black people were unwillingly transported to America as slaves.

Numerous historical documentaries, novels, and a mix of both, or "faction," have been written describing the inhumanities and atrocities of the slave trade. Universal comprehension of the tremendous hardships the captured people experienced has been greatly expedited by the novel and televised version of Alex Haley's Roots. According to the many accounts, the strongest and healthiest were captured primarily from West Africa, frequently from the Gold Coast (modern day Ghana) and the Congo.[13] More men arrived initially; it was not until the 1800s that the female slave population equalled that of the males.[14]

The slaves were chained and packed, loosely or tightly and often in spoon fashion in the hold of the ships en route to America. In most instances the slaves were not cared for. Many died or were permanently injured from disease or injuries they received on the way. Upon arrival in the West Indies, the slaves were "seasoned" or taught their new work roles under the whips of overseers. From the West Indies they were transported to the American colonies, with a rapid increase following the invention of the cotton gin in 1792.[15] Families and kinship groups were separated because it was economically advantageous and it minimized the potential of resistance and uprising. Slaves were considered subhuman and treated as chattel and investment properties. An 1809 South Carolina court held that "young slaves . . . stand on the same footing as other animals."[16] Relations between mothers and children were viewed solely on their property value by the slave owner. When children were considered marketable, they were frequently taken from their parents and sold. Historians continue to debate the question of how many slave families were involuntarily separated by their owners.[17] Records indicate that some family units, parents and children, remained together for years. Economics, and not humanity, remained the keystone to that decision.

Many slaves were used primarily as breeders. Native African languages were prohibited. Religious and other customs and practices were forbidden. Slaves could not by law be taught to read or write.[18] They were completely cut off from their past with no hope for the future. It can be stated without much debate that no other immigrant ethnic group faced such treatment upon arrival in America.

A new sense of family evolved during this period. The community of slaves became the kinship group from which the slave found his identity. Slave marriages did exist and, although not legally recognized, were highly valued and regarded by the slave community as the symbol of a lasting, meaningful bond. Many times the system did not permit the individual families to remain together for long periods of time, but the institution of the family was an essential asset in the age of slavery. It was one of the most significant survival mechanisms for the descendants of Africa, despite the prevalent theories of slavery causing the destruction of the family.[17]

During the slavery period, Black children were usually put to work at very early ages as field workers or house slaves. The children who served as helpmates and personal servants to White children were often expected to be available 24 hours a day. The slave parents had minimal time and opportunity to rear their own children. Often the slaves were expected to rear the slave master's children, providing special attention to the physical and emotional needs of these children while their own children were denied the benefits of such parenting.[19]

Because of the constraints of the system, slave parents put great emphasis on the psychosocial development of the children. Socialization of the slave child became the most important facet of slave childrearing practices. As a matter of survival, they cushioned the shock of bondage, provided another frame of reference for self-concept other than that of the slave owner, and taught them ways to avoid pain, suffering, and death.[20] Childrearing practices in today's Black families include elements of this same socialization process. For example, the doggerel, "if you're white, you're right; if you're brown, stick around; if you're black, get back," is a remnant of the historical experiences of the Black child.

The love, support, and struggle of the Black family enabled most of the children to survive. However, many did not. Many slaves and their children suffered serious illnesses and injuries because of the poor health care provided. Often the illnesses and injuries resulted in physical and emotional impairments for life.[21] Health care during this period was learned as a method of survival. A slave was only allowed to be sick or ill when he was unable to function. Otherwise, he was simply "ailing" or "out of sorts." Cost effectiveness was the primary concern of the slave owner. Therefore, to give care to a slave who was too old or too sick to be productive and work was not efficient business.[22] Health care was provided most consistently to the pregnant female slaves and their newborn. This was considered cost effective. For the most part, however, slaves who were ailing were self-treated or were administered to by other slaves. The health care was a combination of knowledge brought to this country from Africa, observation of what transpired in the White household when someone was ill, and trial and error.[22]

Postslavery Period

Following the Emancipation Proclamation in 1863, several laws were passed, culminating in the 14th Constitutional Amendment which ended the formal institution of slavery for Blacks. However, a new system of oppression quickly replaced the old institution. Extensive and pervasive codes that clearly cemented the second-class citizenship of Black Americans were established.[23] The sharecropping system created a form of economic slavery. In many ways the chains of slavery had not been unshackled. Freedom remained a dream.

Children were valued even more during this era, as newly freed slaves relived memories of their offspring being sold away. Those parents born during slavery cherished their children and committed themselves to providing for and protecting the family.

During the late nineteenth century, a strong female role emerged. Many men preferred that their wives remain at home, because working women reminded them too much of slavery times. However, Black men had difficulty obtaining stable work. Consequently, Black women had to work if the family was to survive. Teaching female children not to avoid work became an integral part of the socialization process.[25]

The systematic deprivation of educational and work opportunities fostered a high level of role integration within the Black family. Males shared equally in childrearing and women helped to defend the family. Role flexibility enabled the family to survive incredible odds.[26]

Most Blacks could not afford the expense of health care of the prepared and recognized providers during this era. In addition to cost, facilities were often unavailable or inaccessible to Black Americans. Home remedies, however, from persons known to be successful healers, were available. Missionary societies from community churches also visited and tended to the community or extended family. Help to orphans and widows was considered an inherent responsibility of the group. In Puritanical jargon, it was *Christian duty* to render such care.

The family life of the African, with its high value on kinship, unity, collective worth, and children as the continuity of life, was intentionally and systematically disrupted. Yet in spite of this overwhelming inhuman and inhumane treatment, the Black family survived.

Although Black Americans are viewed as a group, and our culture is distinct and unique, we are a diverse group. It must be recognized that "the" Black family does not exist. Variations within our group behavior are dependent upon the part of the country in which one lives, the

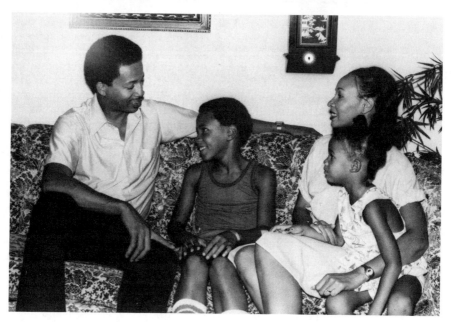

Figure 1. The nuclear family.

education and social exposure one has had, and one's economic level. Therefore, the following influences mediate the same general culture: whether we live in the urban South, the rural South, or the urban or suburban North; and economically, whether we fall in the upper class, the middle class, or the lower class.[27] Childrearing and health-seeking behaviors are also influenced by these factors. Diversification exists; nevertheless, we are bound together by a sense of peoplehood, common historical heritage, and universal definition and treatment by the larger American population.

The cultural values of Black Americans reflect the African heritage and adaptive mechanisms from the American experience. These values include interdependence, mutual aid, compassion, adaptability, flexibility, kinship and group survival, and racial pride and loyalty. There is no question of the impact of the Black Revolution of the sixties on the crystallization and group acknowledgment of the ethos of today's Black Americans.

The survival of Black people is largely due to not only their willingness to help their brothers and sisters, but also their concern for their fellow man, regardless of race and other differences. Compassion is usually widespread among a group that has a history of oppression and poverty. Hence, Blacks are noted for their compas-

sionate behavior. Adaptability is readily discernible when one considers the many masks Blacks wear when dealing with Whites and the number of roles they play in the family and in the larger society.[28] Evidence of interdependence is apparent in the large extended families and strong extensive bonds within the Black community. Although some Blacks still reflect the results of systematic planned separation within our group, there is a growing call for Black unity. Assimilation, which has been interpreted as "becoming white," is no longer a primary goal of the Black American family. The Black family, through all of its tribulations, has been existent, consistent, and strong.

FAMILY STRUCTURE

Nuclear Family

In 1975, there were 5.5 million Black families. Sixty-one percent of those families lived with both a father and a mother.[29] Yes, most Black families adhere to the nuclear family model (Fig. 1). Some of those households have no children. These are often families of young married couples who have not had time or economic security to start their family, older couples who have not been able or willing either to have their own children or to adopt others, and still older couples whose children have grown up and left the home.

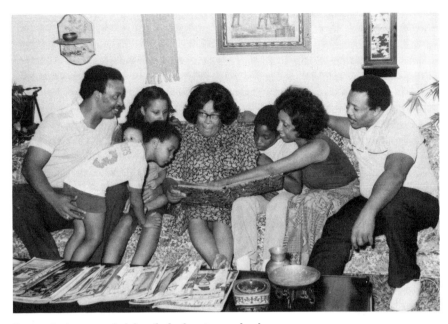

Figure 2. An extended family looks at scrapbook.

Contrary to widely spread myths, some Black families have no children. A few Black homes are childless because their children have been placed in foster homes owing to illness or other factors incapacitating one or both parents. Childless Black homes are an important and complex aspect of Black family life, yet they are almost completely ignored in studies of Black families. Homes of this family structure offer an important potential for the care of Black children in the Black family. Other couples have their natural or adopted children living together in their own household with no other members present.[30]

Extended Family

Out of the sense of peoplehood and the need to survive, some Blacks live in extended families (Fig. 2). The simple extended family includes other relatives or in-laws of the family head. Relatives who can and often do come to live with Black families are not always minors such a grandchildren, nieces, nephews, cousins, and young siblings. Sometimes adults related to either family head move in—parents of husband or wife, aunts, uncles, or grandparents.[31] The incipient extended family, composed of a husband and wife who are childless and take in other relatives, helps sustain Black folk also.[32]

Extended family members provide mutual psychological, social, and economic support for each other. For example, a young couple may marry early, and because of unexpected pregnancy have to move in with parents until the couple becomes economically sound. While pregnant, the daughter-in-law may cook and babysit for her mother-in-law, who may have younger children. Father and son may share a car so that both will have transportation—one buying the gas one week, another the next week. Sometimes a mother who can no longer survive alone economically moves in with her daughter. The grandmother may become the primary authority in the house and take responsibility for child-rearing and maintaining the house. Often, if the grandmother is ill or unable to care for herself, her children or grandchildren will take care of her.[33-37]

Augmented Family

In the face of oppression and sharply restricted economic and social support, Black people often live in augmented families. These families have unrelated individuals living with them as roomers, boarders, or other relatively long-term guests. This family structure is known as the "augmented" family because these unrelated persons often exert a major influence on the availability of resources, such as food, clothing, privacy, transportation, books, and toys.[38]

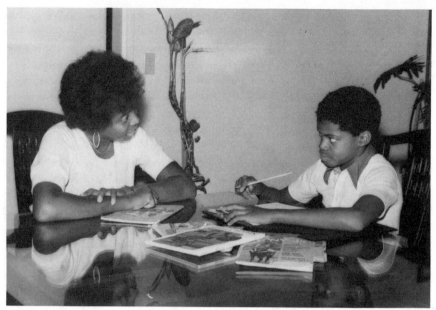

Figure 3. Single parent talks with son. Single parenthood is common in the Black American culture.

Single Parent Family

The attenuated nuclear family, more commonly known as the one parent family, is a viable structure within the Black culture. This important family structure's most frequent form is mother and children living together (Fig. 3).[39] Single parent households exist within the Black community for many of the same reasons they exist among Anglos. However, there are some factors that affect Blacks that have little or no impact on Anglos. The sex ratio between Black men and women also contributes to the large number of female-headed households. In the age range of greatest marriageability, 25 to 64, there are about 45 Black males for every 100 Black females.[40] The abnormally high mortality rate for Black males of a marriageable age or younger, owing to the effects of ghetto living, contributes to the number of single parent households. The economic factor is a major reason for single parent families among low income Blacks. Some men must leave so their wives and children can receive financial support.

Owing to poverty and racism, an unusually high percentage of Black males are in prison, which removes them from the family scene.[41] Black families also lost an unusually high number of Black males during the Vietnam War. According to the United States National Advisory Commission on Selective Service, Black casualties accounted for 23 percent of all deaths related to the war. This raises serious questions when one recalls that Blacks constitute 11 to 12 percent of the total American population.[42]

Births out of wedlock account for a number of single parent Black families; however, it is significant that recently there has been a steady decline in the out-of-wedlock births to Black women, while the rate among Whites has shown a steady increase.[43] Joyce Ladner cites many reasons for child birth before marriage among low income Blacks. She contends that Black females reported that premarital sex provides a substitute for other areas of gratification that could not be fulfilled through other channels: a sense of belonging, feeling needed, a system of exchange (sex-gifts), and a strong indication of being a woman. Also, the moral stigma of premarital sex is not nearly so strong, because sex is considered a very human act among many Blacks.[44] However, most Blacks strongly disapprove of pregnancy before marriage.

The greatest problem for parent and children living in female-headed homes is one of economics. Although it is commonly believed that dependency is characteristic of most of these families, only half of them receive welfare assistance. Thus, the majority are not completely dependent on welfare. Recent census data indicate that three fifths of the women heading Black families work (most of them work full time), although 60 percent of them are poor.[45] In spite of their determination to work and support their families, economics remain a crucial concern to single parents.

Whether born into a nuclear, extended, or single parent family, children are highly valued in the Black American culture. Children, especially males, are seen as a special contribution to the family's existence. This is closely tied with the African view of continuity of life.[46]

FAMILY SIZE

Historically, Black families have been large. To our ancestors, having many children was God's will and consequently unavoidable. In the past, although they were emotionally valued, children were also seen as economic necessities. The children could contribute additional economic support to the family and provide care and protection to aging parents. Most families today, however, are more conscious of the economic burden of childbearing and many Black adults make decisions and choices with this in mind.

The average Black household was 3.3 persons in 1975.[29] Although Black women have the highest birthrate, our family size has been on the decline. Few people are aware that childlessness is higher among Black couples than White couples.[47] Also, Black middle-class women have the lowest birth rate among all women.[48,49] Middle-class women perceive a direct link between large families and low income. These women have to stay in the labor force to maintain their middle-class status; moreover, higher education makes them more aware of and effective in using birth control.[50] However, becoming a mother in America today is still of great importance to Black women, especially women of low socioeconomic status. Black families who live in the South or have a recent southern background account for the highest birth rate among Blacks.[51]

FAMILY PLANNING

In spite of the value placed on children and motherhood, and the high birthrate among Blacks, national surveys, studies, and our own experiences demonstrate that most Black parents in general prefer fewer children. Many believe that family planning services should be made available to the poor.[52] The lack of avail-

ability and accesibility of family planning services to Blacks minimizes effective family planning.

In 1976, 50 percent of Black couples were using the pill or the IUD or had been surgically sterilized. Use of the two most effective methods, the pill and the IUD, had declined from 75 percent in 1963 to 62 percent in 1976. There is a significant increase in the use of non-medical and folk methods (condoms, foam, rhythm, withdrawal, and douche) among both high-income and low-income Black women.[53]

Ms. Wattledon, National President of the Planned Parenthood Federation of America, says: "I believe it is genocidal for black women to have children they don't want, the future and strength of the race is for women to be able to have kids when they want them and to love and provide them with the tools they'll need to get through a hostile world. . . ."[54] According to Joyce Ladner, however, some Blacks may not utilize such services because they believe planned parenthood services are an attempt to "wipe out" the Black population.[55,56] Black genocide has been a fear of many Blacks and has been specifically addressed by many leaders. There is some evidence that these fears are based on reality. Many county, state, and federal attempts have been made to include abortion and sterilization as part of a program of recommended punitive action that may include loss of welfare benefits, the imprisonment and/or fining of the mother, loss of custody of children, and various combinations of these.[57] Consequently, a September 1979 court decision specifically ruled against such actions.[58]

The practices of birth control can apply to both men and women. However, in the Black community women are expected to assume primary responsibility for preventing pregnancy. Although an increasing number of Black males have been sterilized, most refuse to have this done. Many Blacks believe vasectomies will affect the man's sexual performance. Therefore, the woman is usually responsible for selecting a contraceptive method.[59] For many, childbearing is believed to be a natural process and should not be interfered with by employing birth control methods or abortions. Folkloric beliefs held by some Black women cause them to fear contraceptives. They believe that deformity, stillbirth, prolonged illness, and sometimes death to the female are largely due to contraceptives. The use of birth control conflicts with the religious beliefs of some Blacks. Some feel that contraceptives are synonymous with abortion, which is considered murder.[55]

Abortion is also perceived by many to be a means of Black genocide. According to Dr. Mildred Jefferson, a Black physician who is president of the National Right to Life Committee, Inc., abortion is another method of annihilating Black Americans.[60] Supporters of abortion contend that ethnic women of color are denied the right to safe health care as well as the right to choose to have or not have an abortion. Because of the high value placed on life, children, and group survival, the issue remains highly controversial to the Black community. Economics are a major influencing factor for each family confronting this decision.

FAMILY STRENGTHS

In spite of racism and poverty, the Black family—the institution that is primarily responsible for the socialization of Black children—has been able to not only survive, but has indeed moved to a higher level of existence and humanity. This survival, this progress, is due largely to the strengths of the Black family.[61] Our experiences and review of the literature on Black families reveal that at least five major strengths of the Black family have been functional for our survival, development, and stability, namely, strong kinship bonds, strong work orientation, adaptability of family roles, strong achievement orientation, and religious orientation.[62]

Strong Kinship Bonds

These are demonstrated among Blacks by the absorption of individuals—minors and the elderly—into the family: the number of blacks that maintain the extended family structure, and the practice of informal adoption of relative babies and children.[62] Black family solidarity has definitely been a key to our survival. Families help one another with financial aid, child care, and other forms of mutual aid.[36, 63, 65] Hence, the strong kinship network within Black families has proven itself to be an effective mechanism for providing extra emotional and economic support in the lives of Black children.[66]

Work Orientation

Black families place a strong emphasis on work and ambition. Poor Blacks are more likely to work than the White poor. More Black women work (although at lower paying jobs) than White women. Black youth enter the labor market at an earlier age than non-Black youths. However, in the overwhelming majority of Black families, whether poor or not, the husband assumes the primary responsibility of bread winner.[67] Robert Hill has written that "despite this perseverance, the economic picture of blacks is still a national tragedy. The median family income of Blacks is less than two-thirds that of Whites. Blacks are three times as likely as Whites to be poor. The Black unemployment rates remain at recessional levels, even during periods of prosperity."[45]

Adaptability of Family Roles

Another source of strength and stability for Black family members is the flexibility of family roles. Because of the high proportion of working wives in Black families, it is not uncommon for older siblings to serve as parents of younger siblings. In many two parent Black families, especially those with working wives, occasions often arise that require the wife to act as the father, or the husband to assume the traditional role of the wife. Such role flexibility helps maintain the family in the event of separation (because of a sustained illness, divorce, separation, or death) of the husband, wife, or key family member. Contrary to the opinions of Frazier and Moynihan, there is much sharing of decisions and tasks in most Black families.[68–71]

Achievement Orientation

Despite the inauspicious circumstances under which many Black families must conduct the socialization process, they have a very high level of aspiration for their children.[72] High achievement orientation among Black families has contributed significantly to the upward mobility of Blacks. Most Black parents pressure their children to get an education. Also, contrary to popular belief, the overwhelming majority of Black college students come from low-income families in which a few parents have little high school education and most have no college experience.[73] Thanks to sheer determination, Black parents have sent their youngsters to college and on to great achievement.[74]

Religious Orientation

Religion plays a central role in the lives of Black families. Not only does it provide a means for worshipping God and obtaining instruction in religious ideology, it has been used as a mechanism for survival and advancement throughout our

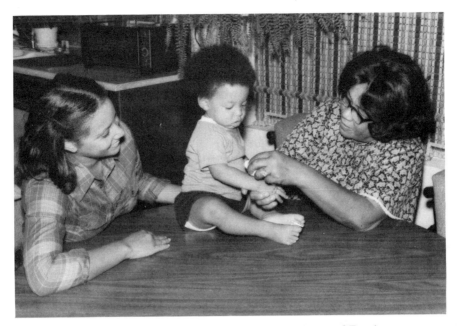

Figure 4. Great-grandmother and mother discuss child care of Faraja.

history.[75] The following statement succinctly reveals the importance of its role: "the fact is that it's the most organized thing in the Negro's life. Whatever you want to do in the Negro Community, whether it's selling Easter Seals or organizing a non-violent campaign, you've got to do it through the church, or it doesn't get done."[76]

Religion meets a variety of Black needs. The Black church usually stands as a conserver of morals, a strengthener of family life, and final authority on right and wrong. Through the church, Blacks are able to obtain a sense of recognition, develop leadership abilities, organize Black protest activities, release emotional tension, socialize, and amuse themselves.[77]

The Black family, because of and perhaps in spite of its long history, is the most effective instrument Blacks have had in their precarious struggle to survive in American society.[78] Primary socialization of the Black child takes place within the context of this institution. Specific childrearing practices for the Black child will be addressed in the next section for each developmental stage.

CHILDREARING
Early Infancy

Although there is a slight edge of preference for a son, the newborn child, boy or girl, is received into a household of warmth, humor, and love.[79] The infant is the center of attention as the parents pride themselves on the evidence of their contribution to life, and measure of their sexuality and maturity.

Early in the newborn's life the mother often will check for any birthmarks and the coloring of the baby's finger joints, toe joints, and knees, or any other area of heavy melanin deposit to assess the final coloring the infant will have as an adult. With the decreased negativism regarding dark coloring there is less worry expressed by the parents for the future of the child. The operating assumption has been that the lighter in color the better the chances for less discrimination and better job and social opportunities. Now, however, color is not as important. There is less worry and emphasis by parents and society on the high yellow, coffee brown, and jet black colors as determinants of the infant's future status and success in life. Any unusual marking on the baby, usually an encapsulated macular area of hyperpigmentation, may be considered a birthmark. Such markings, especially if they resemble food items, are said to be results of food cravings during pregnancy. The mother of a neonate might say, "I wanted steak so badly when I was pregnant, my son was born with a 'steak' on his left thigh!"

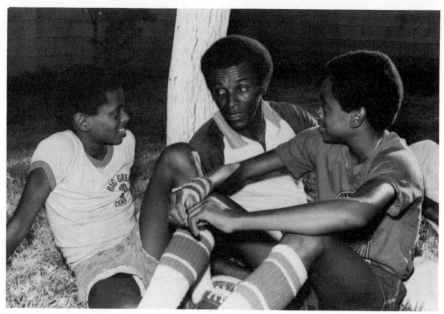

Figure 5. Black middle-class fathers spend significant amounts of time with their families.

The grandmother is often an important figure in the life of a Black child. In many instances a Black child is more likely to have a grandmother in the same household. Frequently the grandmother is likely to take the child into her own home. However, if the grandmother lives with one of her children, it will most likely be her daughter. This family member—grandmother—often plays very significant roles in the family and especially in childrearing. Grandmothers often assist the working parents as babysitters for the infant, providing warmth, affection, and a link to the past. The classic description by E. Franklin Frazier remains valid: "Black grandmothers are the guardian of the generations"[80] (Fig. 4).

One of the many preventive measures handed down from generation to generation in our families is for the mother to tie a black silk string around the wrist of a baby who is prone to constipation. This was to prevent straining of the abdominal muscles and discomfort for the baby. The string is to remain on the wrist for several weeks following the return of normal bowel movements. Because of the concern for preventing umbilical hernias, "belly bands," white linen or muslin cloth, are frequently pinned around the abdomen of the infant. The bands are cleaned and changed frequently.

Older siblings or other kinfolk share in the re-

sponsibilities of caring for the infant. It is understood that everyone is interested in helping the mother and doing the best for the newborn; therefore, child care during infancy may be provided by several members of the extended family. For young couples living away from extended families, fathers, especially middle-class fathers, do more than they normally would with the infant in an attempt to fill the void of minimal or no kinfolk.

There are many Black fathers in all economic strata who have a very significant role in the life of the infant and throughout the child's life. Most frequently they are representative of the middle-class image of the ideal father, with their major interests in the home and the family. They are very attentive to their children and strive to have excellent relations with them.[81] There is increasing evidence that Black middle-class fathers participate more in the lives of their children than do low-income Black fathers or White middle-class fathers (Fig. 5).[82]

However, some child development experts contend that some Black babies are understimulated. Although there is no evidence of lack of love, there seems to be limited interaction between some Black parents and children during infancy. Many Black families dealing with economic and other kinds of stress have difficulty sustaining prolonged feelings of warmth and finding time to play with or adequately stimulate their children. Social and economic conditions in America cause a greater percentage of the Black population to experience a wider range of stress, which impacts childrearing practices.[83]

Another explanation related to this issue is the perceived risk of spoiling the infant with too much attention. Comer and Poussaint, two Black male psychiatrists, state:

> If baby cries, avoid removing him from his crib or bed or picking him up for as long as possible. You are asking for trouble if you place him in your bed. Be confident in your ability as a "sandman." Your anxiety and fear that baby will not go to sleep may cause you to hug and squeeze too much. . . . The baby will wake up and demand to be held again. Eventually, you'll get tired and angry and you and yours will soon be in a "sho' nuff" struggle.[84]

Many Black parents believe that too much attention and show of affection will not adequately prepare the infant to cope with the harsh realities and frustrations of life. One of the authors vividly remembers the night her 2-week-old son began to cry after being fed and cleaned at 2 A.M. After checking all safety and comfort measures, she repositioned him in his cradle and cried with him. He fell asleep quickly. She continued to cry. The critical lessons of coping and survival begin in infancy.

So do the lessons in self-image and identity. Early infant care greatly influences the child's primary core and identity. The infant's first concepts of himself as a person depend upon the responses of others. Although infants become aware of color and other differences, these things have little significance to them. Black parents, however, are beginning very early in the child's life to introduce Black dolls and toys. Unfortunately, all Black parents are not aware that whatever self-image, sense of identity, or rage the family and caretakers have, the infant will begin to model.

Naming the infant is another means of bestowing the child with his own identity. The names given infants in Black families as in other cultures frequently are chosen from significant others in the extended family. Since the Black revolution in the sixties, many young parents are selecting names with African origins. Two examples from our families are Faraja, meaning *leader of the way,* and Turmani, meaning *our trust and hope.* The process of naming a child is another means through which ethnic pride is expressed. Nicknames are not only a substitute or additional name for Blacks, but also very often reflect characteristics and events in the life of the child.[85] Bill Cosby's Fat Albert and friends reflect this pattern. Many of these names are acquired later in life. Another example is the nickname "doodie gal," short for "my doodoo girl." One of the authors has been affectionately called this since infancy by her father.

Emphasis is placed upon feeding the infant. In fact the quality of parenting is often related to how well the child eats. Infant feeding practices, however, are varied. Breastfeeding seems to be dependent upon income, locale, and religion. Muslim women are encouraged by their religious principles and teachings to breastfeed.[86] Often because the mother must return to work early, breastfeeding, if selected, is only done for a brief period of time. In general, Black mothers are more permissive than Anglo mothers in the feeding and weaning of their children.[87]

Eating habits are developed early in childhood. For some families there is more concern about feeding the child with whatever is affordable and available. Black families may begin an earlier introduction to solids than what is customarily suggested by health professionals. Often the concern is to make certain the infant is "full" and happy.

Black mothers are quite rigorous in their efforts to toilet train their children.[87] It has been our experience that we do not adhere to the calm, patient, non-pressure approaches advocated by many childrearing authorities. Frequently, having a child toilet trained makes the difference for the working mother in obtaining child care. Therefore, there is a great sense of urgency for the child to do his share of helping and contributing to the family by becoming toilet trained as soon as possible. Love and caring are not denied the child. However, there is minimal time or patience for "foolishness," that is, uncooperativeness. Out of necessity the children are potty trained early.

Growth and development patterns of Black infants have been studied by many. It has been reported that Blacks tend to be lighter and shorter than Whites at birth. The weight difference may be as much as 200 grams and the length variation as much as 2 centimeters.[88] Robson and colleagues further indicate that in the second year of life, Blacks tend to exceed Whites in height and weight achievement up to the age of 18 months, when growth equalizes. They concluded that race- and sex-specific standards are necessary before growth achievements in infants and children can be properly evaluated.[89] An Anglo nursing colleague recently commented on how often she felt Black children appeared physically and emotionally mature at an early age. In fact, she said, "they look like little men." Many factors in addition to growth and development patterns may contribute to this appearance.

Preschool

Although Black children are affected by other agents, parental attitudes and practices are usually most influential. Black mothers who have more leisure, education, and income are less authoritarian in their interactions with their preschoolers than parents who have less of the aforementioned. Middle-class mothers are more likely to provide explanations about why they are expected to behave in a certain way. The motivation for obedience among low-income children is derived from the authority of the role of the parent.[90] Subsequently, these same parents view disobedience as the most unacceptable behavior.[91] Emphasis is placed on wanting the children to behave. Low-income parents use physical punishment to discipline their children more frequently than their middle-class peers. While Black parents tend to use physical punishment, rather than verbal punishment, to enforce rules, this technique is often buttressed by the love expressed for the children. Confining a child to his room or stripping him of his play privileges is more common to middle-class Black families.[92]

A unique problem of the lower-class Black family is that the children are subject to discipline, but the parents often cannot give rewards except in love and devotion. Parents are not able to offer status rewards. Because the educational and social opportunities are circumscribed by an exclusive, hostile social order, there are few available rewards in the society that the lower class can enjoy.[93] Hence, obedience, which is expected, often goes unrewarded because of a greater sense of hopelessness and futility.

Respect for adults is expected by Black parents. Many feel their children must be taught to fear adults for their own good. While many Black parents report it is desirable "to get children out of the helpless stage of infancy as early as possible," these same parents contend that children should be protected from disappointments, difficult situations, and life's little problems. Of course, this is a difficult task, especially for the economically poor. Low-income Black parents feel that children must not be encouraged to talk about their problems, because the more they are allowed to complain the more they will complain.[94] Some Black parents may feel that since they have such little control over their environment, time should not be wasted talking about things they cannot change. This attitude and practice is often misinterpreted by some as an unwillingness for Black parents to listen and communicate verbally with their children.

The Black child tends to be an integral part of the total family structure more than his White counterpart. Black children are allowed to view and participate in most adult-centered activities, especially those of the family, at an early age. Children are encouraged to join the adult in dancing and sometimes drinking, on special occasions. What is often called the natural rhythm of Blacks actually derives from the Black child's early dancing experience.[95]

Within the family the preschoolers acquire communication patterns. The mode of communication is culturally determined. In the Black family, the use of touch as a means of establishing trust and confidence, and Ebonics, or Black English, are frequently used.[96] Ebonics is different from American English, not inferior. Black English is a dialect characterized by intonation, diction, inflection, structure, and form. It has proven to be functional and advantageous within the Black community. However, there is a wide range of use of the dialect by Black Americans.[97] As preschoolers further develop their language patterns, they exhibit the same patterns as their parents, siblings, and kin.[98] Black parents generally want their young children to learn "standard" English. However, many Blacks feel that their children should be able to use both modes of communication. Black parents know that children who take on Anglo speech are considered suspect in the Black community. Therefore, we view bidialectism as being advantageous.

What many parents call aggressive behavior, Black parents may call defensive behavior. Some fear that passivity or non-aggressiveness in our children has or can lead to acceptance of and adjustment to an unjust society.[99,100] However, some Black parents, especially mothers, feel that aggression in the form of boxing, wrestling, and hitting another child must be suppressed.[94] They believe these behaviors lead to trouble for their children. However, most Blacks feel that youngsters must be taught to protect themselves at an early age.

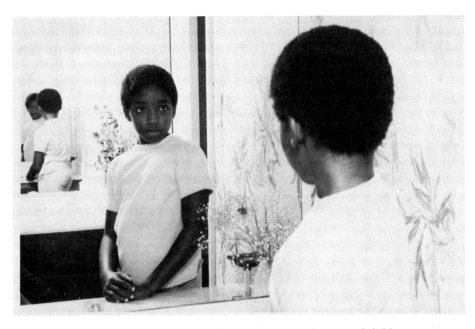

Figure 6. Development of a positive self-image is a crucial aspect of childrearing in Black families.

Childrearing/socialization in America has always presented a double challenge for Black parents as they must teach their young not only how to be human, but how to be Black in a White society.[101] Consequently, basic behavioral patterns have developed. The first was one of reserve: because they believed no White person could be completely trusted or taken into the Black society, no genuine intimacy was viewed as possible. The second pattern set the limits of approved, or even permitted, behavior toward Whites.[102] For example, young Black children, especially males, were taught the rituals of servitude and docility from the time they could talk.[103] Although the negative experience that many Black children and their parents encounter today continues to foster and perpetuate some suspicion and distrust, behavioral patterns of passivity and subservience are seldom taught.

Most parents who have an extreme dislike and distrust of Whites usually do not move to neighborhoods comprised of a large number of Whites. If they do relocate in a predominantly White neighborhood, they seldom discourage their children from playing with White children. However, they are warned not to trust them completely and to protect themselves at all times. If the children have a "spat," these Black parents may often assume that racism on the part of the other youngster is the cause.

It is during the preschool period that Black children become more keenly aware that they are different. Each of us can share numerous stories of our own and our children's discovery of their Blackness. One of the most unique experiences, however, was when one of our sons, at age 4, came running into the house crying. When asked what the problem was, he said one of his Anglo playmates called him "honky." Racism can be confusing to preschoolers!

Most Black parents are aware of the need to bring their children up to be comfortable with their blackness, to be secure, to be proud, and to be able to love. But many Black parents themselves have mixed feelings about being Black. Some have negative self-concepts they acquired as children.[104, 105] Hence, they tend to convey, verbally or non-verbally, the message that Black is inferior, or less. They may communicate this by giving preferential treatment to their light-skinned child, or making negative comments about the darkest child in the family. Other parents ignore their children's concerns about blackness until the children ask.

Since the civil rights movement of the sixties, more and more Black parents see Black as being positive, beautiful, and equal, if not better than (Fig. 6). Most parents acquaint children with the facts of blackness.[106] They teach their children to have pride in their race and culture and defiance

83

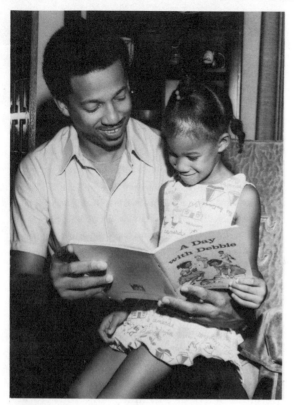

Figure 7. Angela reads to her father from a book with stories about Black children.

toward racism.[95] No longer is the White doll the most common toy in the children's bedrooms. Not only are parents buying Black dolls, but also, books and magazines for and about Black children, such as *Ebony, Jr.* (Fig. 7). Black parents who are aware of the damaging effects of negative modeling and have time to monitor activities, discourage their children from watching programs that portray Blacks in a derogatory manner, and some serve on book selection committees to ensure that Blacks are represented in a realistic manner. These recent changes and others in Black life have elevated Black children's self-esteem.[107, 110]

Many studies have revealed more advanced and rapid skeletal and motor development in Black infants and preschoolers than in Anglo children. During the first 2 to 3 years, Black children are reported to sit up and crawl earlier. They also seem to show greater manual skills through 4 years of age. When using standard charts for growth and development, a Black child that may be assessed as developing normally may actually be underdeveloped by Black norms. Skinfold thickness is thinner in Blacks than in Anglo children. Since this has been a measure for assessing nutritional status, skinfold thickness could be misleading when assessing Black children.[111]

The Middle Years

Between the ages of 6 and 12, children gradually leave the center of parental attention. Black girls from low-income families, at a fairly young age, assume heavy household responsibilities, such as cooking, cleaning, and child care. Many of them by the age of 9 are given the task of taking care of their young siblings. The sharing of household responsibilities tends to build a positive relationship between mother and daughter. The close relationship Black mothers have with their daughters has led to the claim that Black mothers express preference for the female over the son.[112] Our experience and review of the literature does not support this contention.

The young lower-class Black girl usually becomes consciously socialized into the role of womanhood by her immediate and extended family. Although she spends more time with her nuclear family, it is often members of the extended family who serve the vital function as well.[113] Another important agent of socialization for the young Black girl is the peer group. However, during the middle years, the peer group seems to impact on the male child more than the female, because of the amount of time the female spends in the house. Also, many Black mothers do not expect nor want their boys to do housework. However, we have noted that all mothers do not socialize their children to fulfill the traditional male-female roles.

Depending upon the family's socioeconomic level and geographical residence, some young children, especially males, have odd jobs outside of the home, as newsboys, shoeshine boys, and fieldhands. Often parents encourage them to earn their own money for candy and other childhood pleasures; for some it is a matter of family survival. In many southern towns, the children of sharecroppers are exploited as a source of cheap or free labor. However, the primary responsibility of most Black youngsters is to attend school.

In the past, Black elementary school schedules were so arranged that Black children could be released to pick cotton and other crops during the harvest seasons. Their education was secondary to meeting the labor needs of the planta-

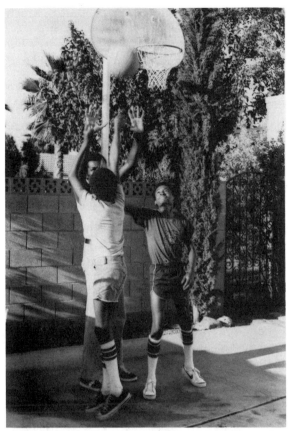
Figure 8. Peers and sports are frequently major influences in children's lives.

tion bosses. Similar patterns exist in certain parts of the country today.[103]

Suburban Black parents, some who do and also some who do not necessarily harbor animosity towards Whites, often take their youngsters to all-Black organized and informal activities, such as *Jack & Jill.* Hence, extra effort is made to ensure that their Black children will be able to relate to other Black children and understand Black cultural elements that may be absent from predominantly White suburbia. We have found that many Black middle-class children's lives are over-organized by their parents.

Although a number of Black youngsters continue to identify with both their parents during the middle school-age period, the peer group has a significant influence on the children (Fig. 8).[114,115] In the context of the peer group, the cultural content is often communicated and created. The Black child's language, skills, roles, moral standards, and code of conduct are partial products of this interaction.

Realizing the potential impact of the peer group, many Black parents make some effort to control the kind of youngsters their children play with. Low-income urban parents seem to exert the least amount of control. They are sometimes unavailable to supervise their children adequately themselves and can not afford to pay for regular baby sitting or organized children's activities. So often the children have great freedom to do as they please. Sometimes relatives or neighbors check on them periodically. Upon leaving for work, usually the parents' final remarks are something like "and stay away from those no good Jones on 160th Street." We have known some parents to forbid their children to leave the apartment while they are away. Because there are so many possibilities for trouble, these parents rank their children more by what they do not do rather than what they do.[116]

If the friends give evidence of being an impediment to their children's success, especially in school, middle-class Black parents recommend that their youngsters discontinue seeing those children.[116,117] Some Black parents who hold high aspirations for their children will even move out of an area in order to prevent their children from playing with children from "bad families."[117,118] Supposedly, this move enables Black middle-class parents to exert a powerful and continuous pressure on their children to study, to repress aggression at school, to inhibit sexual impulses, and to avoid lower-class playmates.[119]

In the urban Black community, children grow up learning a variety of verbal games. During the middle years they practice playing the dozens—a game most common to the Black adolescent male. The dozens is a verbal contest in which the emphasis is placed on exchanging insults most often directed at your opponent's mother or other kinsmen. I recall the following verbal exchange from my childhood days: Charles says, "Yo family is so po that yo moma have to wear combat boots." Roy's response, "U's so po yo moma ain't got no boots." During a verbal contest such as this the responses become progressively more negative. The above exchange is more typical of the middle school-age male child than the male adolescent.[120,121] The middle school-age child also spends time preparing for adolescence by learning to rap. Rapping is described as a fluent and lively way of talking, characterized by a high degree of personal style through which the speaker intends to draw attention to himself or some aspect of himself that he feels is attractive or carries weight with his crowd.[120] Rapping is a verbal skill that is of great value in heterosexual relationships in the Black community. Rapping appears to be more widespread among Blacks of various socioeconomic levels and geographical regions than playing the dozens. Urban Black youngsters enjoy imitating the slang of "street talk" of older siblings or friends and adults. This verbal skill is largely concerned with vocabulary—assigning different meanings to otherwise established word meanings (e.g., bad=good).[3]

Black middle school-age youngsters are not only verbally adept, they are also creative. Out of economic necessity, urban children have created play items that youngsters have enjoyed for days and days non-stop. We recall using old fruit crates to make doll houses, stores, and go-carts. Small pebbles were excellent substitutes for jacks. Pop bottle tops made non-sliding checkers. The best swings were made from an old rope and a tire. Sometimes, nothing was nicer than just rolling a tire down the sidewalk. We could go on and on.

When low-income youngsters receive gifts, they are for very special occasions and are usually functional, such as clothes for one's birthday. Unfortunately, the middle-class child is often robbed of the opportunity to be creative. They receive many toys and gifts, often more than their White counterparts because Blacks want their children to have more than they had when they were growing up. However, some middle-class children continue to receive functional gifts as well as educational toys.

Adolescence

In the Black world, adolescence starts early. Many of these youngsters do not enjoy the luxury of a period of playtime and learning that extends into their teens. Most have had to assume the responsibility and burdens of adulthood at an early age.[74] Thus, an early central concern of the Black youth, like all other Americans, is what Erikson has called the search for identity: coming to know who one is, what one believes in and values, and what one wants to accomplish and get out of life.[123] The task is to come to terms with a new kind of body, with new potentials for feeling and acting, and to rearrange his or her image accordingly.

During adolescence, girls growing up in the inner cities, in many ways, share the same concerns, fears, joys, and questing ventures as other young girls.[124] Often, it is the peer group in which the young girl can share her joys, fears, surprises, and disappointments. Therefore, the peer group can be viewed by the preadolescent and adolescent girl as having many integrative functions that help her to survive and understand life from day to day.[125] Many Black girls first discuss menstruation, sexual intercourse, boy friends, kissing, and so on, with their girlfriends before these topics are discussed with their mothers or other adult females.[126] Often they are never discussed with parents. Almost every facet of a girl's sexual ideas is verbally tested with her friends.[127] The sharing of information and counsel on pregnancy, abortion, and contraception is common. The peer group has a definite influence on the definition of womanhood for Black girls. However, some middle-class Black girls discuss many of the aforementioned topics with their mothers. It has been our experience that some mothers will initiate such interactions rather than wait until the teen-ager brings up the subject.

Parents vary in the extent they will allow their daughter to experiment with such valued items in their identity kits as lipstick, hosiery, tight sweaters, padded bras, and hair styles. In spite of the quality of the mother-daughter relationship, Black girls place strong value on having sincere friends who can be depended on to share secrets, offer sound advice, and provide companionship when needed.

Feminine identity is expressed in a number of ways. From preadolescence to adulthood, there is a preoccupation with making oneself physically attractive, which includes wearing fashionable clothes, jewelry, makeup, and hair styles. Girls who come from the more financially secure homes are usually allowed to secure the proper clothes and shoes and go to the beauty shop without a problem.[128] Other Black teen-agers borrow pretty clothes, purchase stolen goods at reduced rates, steal clothing, or go without. Low-income Black parents usually can not afford to buy clothes their daughters desire.[129] This preoccupation with buying pretty clothes is fulfilling a basic need as well as providing aesthetic satisfaction. In a minor way this preoccupation might be viewed as a compensation for all those things that they cannot afford. It can be viewed as a positive approach because it enables them to indicate worth and possibly also increase their level of self-esteem. It is, perhaps, a part of the Black cultural tradition to "look clean" and "in style," or perhaps it is a reflection of the strong influence the dominant society has had upon them.[130]

Hair care is a primary concern for male and female children. Much time, energy, and often expense is expended toward hair grooming by adolescents. There is an increased ethnic pride for the thick, extra-curly hair characteristic of Black folk. During the 1960s when the drive for identity among Blacks was intense, the natural or Afro hair style was adopted. The popularity of the Afro has waned. Ethnic pride is expressed in a greater sense of peoplehood and feeling and not just in appearance. Current hair styles, including cornrowing and mild relaxers, reflect the individual's creativity and expression of pride and freedom. Because most Anglo nurses are unfamiliar with hair grooming techniques for Blacks, attention to this aspect of restorative health care is often neglected when Blacks are hospitalized. The patient's identity and integrity may be threatened.

Black girls' conceptions of what kind of women they eventually are to become are influenced also by their associations with older sisters, mothers, grandmothers, aunts, and a variety of other role models. They frequently select a model who has been successful. Success is measured among lower-class Black females by the degree to which one can take care of oneself and assist others in the family.[131] Black middle-class girls are socialized to define a successful model as one who has a college education and a professional job—such as teaching. In fact, to insure that their young Black girls continue to value a college education and professional job, many Black parents send them to the "best" Black college in the South.

The start of menstruation for any adolescent female is a major developmental event. Many traditional "preventive" health care practices to be carried out during the cycle are taught to young girls by their mothers, grandmothers, and significant others. Girls are strongly admonished not to wash their hair, take tub baths, go swimming, or submerge their feet in water. Cleanliness is stressed, however.

The anticipation of womanhood is symbolized by certain acquired characteristics that are felt to result in independence. One of these characteristics of independence is shown in the belief of some lower-class Black adolescents that having a baby will help them to achieve a certain kind of responsibility, and consequently womanhood, that they could not otherwise enjoy. Many, however, do not want to have children and see having

children as the road to trouble.[132] Working outside the home is one means of acquiring some semblance of independence. Owing to the historically high unemployment rate among Black youth, this route often does not provide the desired payoff.

The strongest concept of womanhood for the young Black female is that of how she has to play a strong role in the family. Another major conception is that she will probably have to work to help her mate support a family. Few Black girls grow up expecting to stay home and care for the children, but anticipate that they will work outside the home.[133] Indeed, they are socialized to be strong because they more than likely will have to use their resourcefulness.[134]

Learning how to relate to members of the opposite sex is also part of the preparation for womanhood. Relating to boys appropriately is a skill learned within the same-sex peer group early in life. Boys become sexual persons at an earlier age for the lower-class Black girl than for the middle-class Black girl and her White counterparts.[132] Also, heterosexual relationships, such as dating, develop at an early age in the communal setting of Black social relationships (Fig. 9).[135-137]

While young Black male adolescents are becoming more adept at the technique of rapping, the female is learning to discriminate between a guy who is "for real" and one who has a "weak rap." When the male makes a play to develop a relationship of varying degrees of sexual intimacy, she may agree to participate or decline.[138] Her decision will be influenced by her peer group, degree of internalization of parental values, religion, and her self-selected goals. Black girls who engage in premarital sex tend to be more critical of parental control and to feel that their parents do not understand the needs and problems of adolescents. Some young Black females told Joyce Ladner that some reasons for participating in premarital sex are that they perceive it as (1) a substitute for other areas of gratification that could not be fulfilled through ordinary channels, (2) an attainment of a sense of belonging and feeling needed, (3) a system of exchange (sex for gifts), and (4) an indication of being a woman.[139]

Most Black parents urge their daughter to remain chaste until adulthood. However, more emphasis is placed on the practical consequences of premarital sex (pregnancy), rather than on the religious stance—sex relations before marriage are sinful. Girls who decide to have

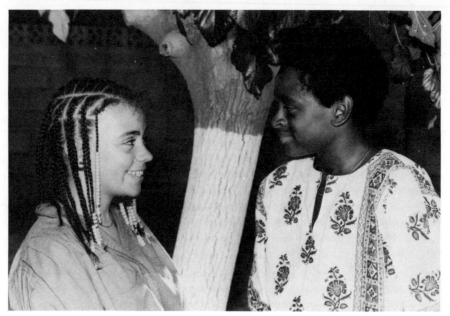

Figure 9. Adolescent dating.

intercourse are rarely condemned by their peers, nor are those who decide to refrain.[140] Most Black parents, especially lower income, like their White counterparts, do not begin to have an impact equal to that of the peer group on their children, especially in the area of sex education. Many are unable to discuss this topic freely and seldom provide adequate information. For example, Joyce Ladner, in her excellent study of the Black female, recorded the following folklorish approach to the description of menstruation:

> Mother told me that the monkey was going to "split his tongue" one of these days and he was going to bleed. . . . So, I started looking for my monkey . . . I was about fifteen. At first I was kind of scared because I thought she was talking about a real monkey that had cut his tongue out. I didn't really know what she was talking about at first. . . .[141]

Another of Ladner's subjects gave the following account of her sex education experience:

> My mother told me . . . not to let a boy touch me or I would have a baby. And I always thought if a boy touched my hand I was pregnant. . . . One day a boy bumped against me. I was scared. I went home and laid in bed and I said, "Oh, Lord, I'm pregnant."[142]

While many parents provide little or no information about sex, a few are providing adequate in-

formation early in life.[143] *What's Happening to Me?* by Peter Mayle[144] and other books are used by some middle/class parents of young adolescent children.

It has been the authors' experience that an increasing number of middle-class Black parents, who discover that their adolescent females are participating in premarital sex, will suggest or see that their daughter obtains some form of contraception from their family doctor. If the middle-class Black female becomes pregnant before marriage, her parents are more likely to see that she gets an abortion than parents of her lower-class counterpart.[140] However, abortion is not a likely alternative for the majority of young Black females, nor is adoption. Although there is much ambivalence over the birth of children outside marriage, the first pregnancy is perceived as more of a "mistake" than a sin.[145]

In spite of the "mistake" attitude, parents usually react negatively at first to the pregnancy of their daughters with hurt, shame, and sometimes shock. Later there is an acceptance of the fact. Some teen-agers are mistreated by their parents because of pregnancy. Subsequently, they become very strict with them and younger siblings. However, most parents feel that the child has the right to live and should not be punished for his mother's mistake. Regardless of how dire circumstances become, and no matter how upset the girl and her parents are over the impending birth, the mother and her family usually keep the child and rear it.[146]

One of the most salient differences between the socialization of young Black males and the females is in their sex education.[147] Females seem to receive a more thorough orientation to sex within the family and at an earlier age than the males. Also, often when parents are giving advice to males, it is limited to their double standard attitude. Boys are advised not to "mess around with girls," but at the same time it is emphasized that messing around is natural for boys.[148]

The same-sex peer group's influence on the Black male peaks during the adolescent period. Within this group he obtains the bulk of his sex education and sex-role behaviors. Among his friends he hones his verbal skills—rapping, jiving, and playing the dozens to a fine art. Jiving, playing the dozens, and the use of slang are techniques utilized for a variety of purposes, such as maintaining one's status in "the group," reaffirming one's identity as being Black, isolating non-Blacks, having fun, or putting down a brother. He can now use his linguistic ability—rapping to convince the female that he is worthy of her interest and as a verbal prelude to more intimate activity—more effectively. His success is dependent to a large degree upon his ability to use such words as "cool" and "baby" in the proper context. This demonstrates you are "together" and worth her attention. The tone and the quality of his words are significant. He must remember to use a different rap for lower-class females than middle-class females.[149,150]

One of the most difficult problems facing Black parents is assisting the adolescent deal with his or her sexuality. While all parents must contend with this problem, the myths and stereotypes associated with Black sexuality make the task more difficult. Both boys and girls can be entrapped in trying to live up to the image of sexual prowess. However, the Black male occupies a very special sexual role in the American society.

The young male adolescent becomes acutely aware that Black men are seen as the "super studs," the ultimate in virility and masculine vigor. He is also regarded, however, as socially, economically, and politically castrated.[151] Identity, self-worth, and position and function in the society also come into question at this stage. The conflict, testing, questioning, and experimentation of adolescent sexuality is compounded by racist attitudes in the American society. Parent-

ing and growing up Black are not easy tasks.

It is purported that Black girls were often socialized to be independent, disciplined, and puritanical. In contrast to Black boys, there seems to be some evidence that there are fewer social conformists among Black females at an early age.[147] On the other hand, Black boys have frequently been socialized to be obedient and compliant, not to be too ambitious or aggressive. Historically, parents have been fearful for the safety of the son. Today there is emphasis on survival and ethnic pride. Racism is seldom tolerated and more apt to be confronted.

Today, within the Black community, males are socialized to be strong, aggressive, and independent. A boy who seems "weak" is often reprimanded and ridiculed by his father and other adults, including his mother and older sisters and peers.[148] While Black males and females are encouraged to get an education, the Black male frequently emulates professional athletes and is subtly encouraged by parents and the community to develop athletic and physical prowess. They view sports as a vehicle to a successful future and physical prowess as an indication of "maleness."

A high degree of independence is acquired by the young Black male at an early age. Many work part-time jobs during high school and college, if they are fortunate enough to get a job. Usually they contribute a portion of their salary to support their family.[152] In 1950, two out of three Black male teen-agers were in the labor force; that figure has dropped to less than two out of five. In some large cities, Black teen-age unemployment approaches 65 percent. Consequently, many Black teen-agers are jobless, which prevents them from helping their family and causes them to withdraw from college.[153] The high unemployment and limited opportunities for Black adolescent males have a negative effect on their ability to gain independence, to have access to higher education, and to even subsist. Hence, a young Black male's identity is often in jeopardy.

The conditions under which many young Black males live are largely responsible for an increase in the use of drugs and the kind of crime rate that goes with it. "It's all built into the kind of despair and lack of projection—who gives a damn?"[154] Fortunately, a number of Black youths are able to find jobs, complete their education, and establish successful careers. This success is largely due to the Black child's high resilience and survival skills. Halpern attributes this to (1) the love and security he enjoys early in life; (2) his inclusion in most family activities;

(3) his early opportunities for the assumption of physical independence and responsibility; (4) the security provided by many mothering figures at his disposal.[155] Thus, in spite of racism and other difficulties, Black parents, for the most part, have traditionally helped Black children develop a positive inner core.[156]

HEALTH CARE IMPLICATIONS

Everyone is a cultural being. Values and practices, including childrearing, socialization, and health response behaviors, are culturally determined. The contents of this chapter have attempted to provide you with information regarding the Black family, the children, childrearing considerations, and some related aspects of health care unique to our ethnic group. Although bound together by common values and a sense of peoplehood, diversity in behavior exists. Many factors influence these variations, including the degree to which the family and/or the child identify with the ethnic group. The higher the sense of group identity, the more apparent are the cultural/ethnic influences in behavior.

Stemming from the traditional African belief about life and the nature of being, Black Americans' perception of health is related to the degree of harmony or discord in one's body, mind, and spirit.[157] These three facets of existence are not considered separate entities. Being ill is when one is at odds with nature—out of sorts. Emphasis is placed on health promotion. Preventive measures, such as three nutritious meals a day, especially a hot breakfast, occasional laxatives to "clean" the system, and cod liver oil to prevent colds, are introduced early in the life of a child. The childhood memories of routine doses of castor oil, Phillips 666, or Black Draught bring sour tastes and smiles to our mouths!

Self-care and folk medicine are very prevalent among Blacks. Emphasis is placed on health prevention through the use of tried and proven traditions. If an illness does occur, parents may use home remedies and the prescribed medical treatment. It is important for the health care worker to know what methods have been tried and to work in support of and with respect for the patient, the family, and their cultural beliefs. As long as the folk medicine is not contraindicated for the mutually derived plan, the combining of the folk or traditional methods with the Western modality should not be problematic.[158]

The belief that serious illness can be avoided is so strong that an individual is not viewed as ill as long as the person can function—walk, talk, work, and eat. Consequently, many Black Americans may not consider early signs and symptoms of disease processes as a state of illness. The perception of illness as well as other factors influences when Western medical intervention is sought. The health care provider must be careful not to be critical of what may be at variance with her own culture's perception of health and illness.

The state of health is also closely related to the religious beliefs of Blacks. The laying on of hands and rooting, a practice derived from the practice of voodoo, are healing practices for some Blacks. Prayer is also a common means of preventing and treating illness.[159] The Black clergyman is considered a significant spiritual support by many Black families. Because of their understanding of the folkways, rituals, and mores of the culture, clergymen are frequently sought by family members to help them cope with sickness and suffering.[160] Visitation by the family minister is sought, expected, and valued. He is frequently considered a significant and vital other at a time of family crisis.

In addition to clergy and parents at the bedside of a hospitalized child, aunts, uncles, cousins, and distant relatives may be in attendance at the bedside.[161] Owing to the close social network and Black solidarity, it is important to include kin and significant others in the planning and implementation of care. Decisions regarding care of a child may require consultation with several members of the extended family. The parents usually assume responsibility for signing appropriate forms. However, respect for the process rather than impatience by the care provider will facilitate matters.

Keeping the family and patient informed of the plan of care is good nursing care for any patient. However, because of the deep-seated distrust and suspicion by Blacks of the health care system, it becomes even more important. Fear of experimentation or mistreatment of a sick child will lead to conflict and miscommunication. The treatment plan and the reasons for a given treatment must be shared with the patient and family.[158]

Health care workers must be careful not to erroneously interpret the use of Black dialect as evidence of perversity, stupidity, or uncooperativeness.[162] A sensitive and thoughtful understanding of the culture and the language may expedite effective communications. Any suggestions of cultural imposition, condescension, imitation, or encouragement to "speak English" may be interpreted by the patient or family as evidence of covert racism. Such perceptions may further hinder any future effort of therapeutic intervention. Black children are reared to recognize and respond to racism. Many of the problems Black children and parents have in dealing with the health care system are evident in problems faced in other systems as well. However, the inherent and pervasive racism within the health care system cannot be denied.[163] Coping responses to the health care system include testing, suspicion, and avoidance. Testing is an attempt to assess the degree of racism that exists in a new situation and with any ethnically different, especially Anglo, person.[164] It is assumed that racism exists. The question to be answered is "how much?"

Testing is done in numerous ways. Examples of this behavior include (1) going to a clinic or health care facility, sitting or standing, and simply observing for a period of time without registering, then abruptly leaving; or (2) sending an older child to the clinic for one-time treatment. Both of these examples are methods to measure the friendliness and concern of the staff, preferential treatment of anyone, and the potential risk of being made to feel inferior and without worth. If testing results are unfavorable, family and friends are warned.[164]

Suspicion is another response closely related to testing. Because of the history of exploitation and deceit, Blacks are very distrustful and suspicious of being used as guinea pigs or being involved in a "beneficial" program for Blacks which may be and has been used to perpetuate stereotypes and myths. Numerous accounts of mistreatment and explorative activities by health providers are documented and reinforce suspicion and negativism. One of the most inhumane was the Tuskeegee experiment study conducted by the United States Public Health Service over a 40-year period. Four hundred Black patients infected with syphilis were denied proper treatment so that scientists could observe the "natural history" of the disease. Over 100 of these Black people died as a result of this federally funded health research project.[165] Suspicion of Black genocide, mistreatment, and second-rate care are nutured by such incidents.

For many Blacks, the push for sickle cell anemia testing is also suspect. While acknowledging the value of knowing if one has the disease or the trait, Blacks are often in conflict regarding screening for fear of becoming labeled and discriminated against in jobs and insurance once the diagnosis is confirmed. The politics of disease and treatment, as well as the current emphasis on ethnic inclusion in health care, are met with seasoned caution by Blacks.

Avoidance is also used as a coping mechanism by Blacks to preserve self-esteem and dignity. We may simply stay away from situations that may result in rejection or harm in confronting Whites. Unfortunately, there are times when use of this defense is to our detriment. This defense may also contribute to postponement of early treatment and result in a longer, more serious illness and a less complete cure.[166]

Great concern is expressed regarding the risk of being in a vulnerable situation, stripped of any independence, identity, and knowledge. The Black experience in America has indicated the cruelty of such treatment. In addition to these common problems of most patients entering a health care facility, it is acknowledged that most Anglo health care providers know very little about Black hair care, skin care, or shaving problems of Black men.

Assumptions on the part of some health care providers also breed caution and distrust in Blacks. An example is that upon admission to the hospital, all Blacks were asked for their medical assistance cards.[167] Or if a Black teen-age girl comes to the emergency room for acute abdominal pain, it is assumed to be pelvic inflammatory disease. Or the assertive Black parent is perceived to be a radical, belligerent person and about to start a riot in pediatrics. The potential humiliation fosters avoidance.

A major health concern of Blacks is the importance of survival in a hostile society. The mental anguish is severe. Grier and Cobbs in their book, *Black Rage*, discuss at length the psychological impact of parenting and growing up Black in America.[151] A culturally relevant psychological assessment is critical. What may be interpreted as aggressiveness in a child may actually be a healthy defense to a situation. What may be diagnosed as paranoia may be an accurate assessment by a Black of a situation. The realities are that if you are poor and Black you are more likely to be institutionalized for emotional illness than a member of any other ethnic group.

In a study by Hammonds, the health status of urban Black preschool children revealed physical, mental, and emotional problems resulting from circumstances affecting the family (i.e., survival) and communication failures. Since the majority of Blacks are urban residents, comprehensive health care systems with culturally sensitive providers are needed if we are to impact the future health of today's Black child.[168] The health professional must keep in mind the value Blacks place on children and the responses to the health care system. Communication will be facilitated if done in a manner that shows respect for the family and their beliefs. Whenever this is not present, barriers to therapeutic communication will exist.

A critical evaluation of one's self and peers for racist attitudes and behaviors is essential. Actions do speak louder and are interpreted more quickly and sometimes erroneously by those who have experienced prior negativism.

Other Black family health issues, such as drug abuse, Black professional education, specific disease propensity, and health promotion have not been addressed in this chapter. Excellent resources are available for such content. However, Black family strengths and childrearing practices have been addressed. While there remain several other aspects of this topic not included in this chapter, we hope it will foster a better understanding to the health care provider of the unique aspects of the Black family and the role it plays in the socialization of a great resource—our Black children.

REFERENCES

1. Moynihan, D.P.: *The Negro Family: The Case for National Action.* U.S. Department of Labor, Washington, D.C., March 1965.
2. Billingsley, A.: "Black families and white social science." In Ladner, J. (ed.): *The Death of White Sociology.* Vintage Books, New York, 1973, pp. 431-450.
3. McClain, S.R., et al.: *Parenting the culturally different.* Paper presented to the Annual Conference on Minority Studies. La Crosse, Wisconsin, April 23, 1977.
4. Ladner, J.: *Tomorrow's Tomorrow: The Black Woman.* Doubleday, Garden City, New York, 1971, pp. 4-5.
5. King, Martin Luther. Address delivered at Abbott House, Westchester County, New York, October 29, 1965.
6. Staples, R.: *Introduction to Black Sociology.* McGraw-Hill, New York, 1976, p. 113.
7. Nobles, W.W., and Nobles, G.M.: "African roots in black families: the social-psychological dynamics of black family life and the implications for nursing care." In Luckoft, D. (ed.): *Black Awareness: Implications for Black Patient Care.* American Journal of Nursing Company, New York, 1976, p. 7.
8. Staples, *Black Sociology*, p. 114.
9. Nobles and Nobles, p. 8.
10. Staples, *Black Sociology*, p. 115.
11. Staples, R.: *The Black Woman in America: Sex, Marriage, and the Family.* Nelson-Hall Publishers, Chicago, 1973.
12. Jacques, G.: "Cultural health traditions: a Black perspective." In Branch, M.F., and Paxton, P.P. (eds.) *Providing Safe Nursing Care for Ethnic People of Color.* Appleton-Century-Crofts, New York, 1976, p. 116.
13. Bullough, B. and Bullough, V.: *Poverty, Ethnic Identity, and Health.* Appleton-Century-Crofts, New York, 1972, p. 39.
14. Staples, *Black Sociology*, p. 116.
15. Bullough and Bullough, p. 40.
16. Harrison, I.E., and Harrison, D.S.: "The Black family experience and health behavior." In Crawford, C.O. (ed.): *Health and the Family.* MacMillan, New York, 1971, p. 178.
17. Staples, *Black Sociology*, p. 117.
18. Sharpley, R.H.: "A psychohistorical perspective of the Negro." In Reinhardt, A.M., and Quinn, M.D. (eds.): *Family-Centered Community Nursing.* C.V. Mosby Company, St. Louis, 1973, p. 78.
19. Comer, J.P., and Poussaint, A.F.: *Black Child Care: How to Bring Up a Healthy Black Child in America: A Guide to Emotional and Psychological Development.* Simon & Schuster, New York, 1975, p. 16.
20. Staples, *Black Sociology*, p. 118.
21. Comer and Poussaint, p. 17.
22. Jacques, p. 118.
23. Harrison and Harrison, p. 180.
24. Staples, *Black Sociology*, p. 120.
25. Absug, R.H.: "The Black family during reconstruction." In Huggins, N., et al. (eds.): *Key Issues in the Afro-American Experience.* Harcourt, Brace, Jovanovich, New York, 1971, pp. 26-39.
26. Staples, *Black Sociology*, p. 121.
27. Carrington, B.W.: "The Afro-American." In Clark, A.L. (ed.): *Culture, Childbearing, Health Professionals.* F. A. Davis Company, Philadelphia, 1978, p. 36.
28. Staples, *Black Sociology*, pp. 76-77.

29. U.S. Department of Commerce, Bureau of the Census: *The Social and Economic Status of the Black Population in the United States: A Historical View, 1790–1978. Current Population Reports. Special Studies, Series P-23, No. 8.* Washington, D.C., 1979, p. 100.

30. Billingsley, A.: *Black Families in White America.* Prentice-Hall, Inc., Engelwood Cliffs, New Jersey, 1968, pp. 18-21.

31. Ibid., p. 20.

32. Staples, *Black Sociology*, p. 124.

33. Stack, C.B.: *All Our Kin.* Harper & Row Publishers, New York, 1970.

34. Hays, W.C., and Mindel, C.H.: *Extended kinship patterns in Black and White families.* Journal of Marriage and the Family 34(1):51-57, 1973.

35. Cohen, A., and Hodges, H.M., Jr.: *Characteristics of the lower-blue collar class.* Social Problems (Spring) pp. 303-334, 1963.

36. Feagin, J., et al.: *Extended kinship relations in Black and White families.* Journal of Marriage and the Family 33 (Feb.): 51-57, 1973.

37. Bott, E.: *Family and Social Network.* Tavistock, London, 1957.

38. Billingsley, *Black Families in White America*, p. 10.

39. Ibid., p. 18.

40. U.S. Department of Commerce, Bureau of the Census: *1970 Census of Population, Advance Report, Series PC (V2)-1.* Washington, D.C., 1971.

41. Chrisman, R.: *Black prisoners—White law.* Black Scholar (April-May) 1971, pp. 44-46.

42. U.S. National Advisory Commission on Selective Service: *Who Serves When Not All Serve.* U.S. Government Printing Office, Washington, D.C., 1967, p. 26.

43. Staples, *Black Sociology*, p. 123.

44. Ladner, pp. 211-212.

45. Hill, R.B.: *The Strengths of Black Families.* National Urban League, New York, 1971, p. 9.

46. Staples, *Black Sociology*, p. 133.

47. Kunz, P.R., and Brinkerhoff, M.B.: *Differential childlessness by color: the destruction of a cultural belief.* Journal of Marriage and the Family 31(4):717-719, 1969.

48. Kiser, C., and Frank, M.: *Factors associated with low fertility of nonWhite women of college attainment.* Millbank Memorial Fund Quarterly (October) 1967, p. 427.

49. U.S. Department of Commerce, Bureau of the Census: *1960, Census of Population: Women by Number of Children Ever Born, PC (2) - 3A.* Washington, D.C., 1964, Table B.

50. Staples, *Black Sociology*, p. 127.

51. Hill, A.C., and Jaffee, F.S.: "Negro fertility and family size preferences—implications for programming of health and social services." In Staples, R.: (ed.): *The Black Family: Essays and Studies.* Wadsworth, Belmont, California, 1971, p. 129.

52. Ibid., 204.

53. Ford, K.: *Contraceptive use in the United States, 1973–1976.* Perspective 10(5):269, 1978.

54. Lewis, S.D.: *Family planning's top advocate.* Ebony 33(11):86, 1978.

55. Ladner, p. 250.

56. Reid, I.S.: *"Together" Black Women.* Joseph Okpaku Publishing Company, New York, 1975, p. 99.

57. Slater, J.: *Sterilization: newest threat to the poor.* Ebony 28(12):150-152, 154, 156, 1973.

58. Foor, M.: *Abortion as condition for aid ruled illegal.* Phoenix Gazette, September 5, 1979, p. A-17.

59. Staples, *Black Woman in America*, p. 144.

60. *A fight for right to life.* Ebony Magazine 33(6):79, 1978.

61. Hill, R.B., p. XI.

62. Ibid., pp. 5-8.

63. Harper, D.W., and Barza, J.M.: *Ethnicity, family, generational structure, and intergenerational solidarity.* Sociological Symposium 2:75-82, 1969.

64. Stack, pp. 32-44.

65. Shimkin, D.B., et al. (eds.): *The Extended Family in Black Societies.* Mouton Publishers, Chicago, 1978.

66. Hill, R.B., p. 8.

67. Ibid., p. 15.

68. Bott, E.: "Conjugal roles and social network." In Coser, R. (ed.): *The Family: Its Structure and Functions.* St. Martin's Press, New York, 1964, pp. 331-350.

69. King, K.B.: *Adolescent perception of power structure in the Negro family.* Journal of Marriage and the Family 31(4):751-755, 1969.

70. Parker, S., and Kleiner, R.J.: *Social and psychological dimensions of the family role performance of the Negro male.* Journal of Marriage and the Family 31 (Au-

gust): 500-506, 1969.

71. Ten Houten, W.: *The Black family: myth and reality.* Psychiatry 33(2):145-173, 1970.

72. Broom, L., and Glenn, N.: *Transformation of the Negro America.* Harper & Row, New York, 1965, pp. 23, 61, 152, 153.

73. U.S. Department of Commerce, Census Bureau, 1970: *School Enrollment.* October 1970.

74. Comer and Poussaint, p. 20.

75. Hill, R.B., p. 33.

76. Brink, W., and Harris, L.: *The Negro Revolution in America.* Simon & Schuster, New York, 1964, p. 103.

77. Staples, *Black Sociology,* pp. 166-169.

78. Thompson, D.: *Sociology of the Black Experience.* Greenwood Press, Westport, Connecticut, 1974, pp. 79-80.

79. Staples, *Black Woman in America,* p. 153.

80. Ibid., p. 154.

81. Ibid., p. 151.

82. Gillete, T.L.: *Maternal Employment and Family Structure as Influenced by Social Class and Role.* Unpublished doctoral dissertation, University of North Carolina, 1961.

83. Comer and Poussaint, p. 42.

84. Ibid., p. 51.

85. Ebony 32(8):6, June 1977.

86. Carrington, p. 47.

87. David, A., and Havighurst, R.: *Social class and color differences in childrearing.* American Sociological Review II:698-714, 1946.

88. Lythcott, G.I., et al.: "Pediatrics." In Williams, R.A. (ed.): *Textbook of Black-Related Diseases.* McGraw-Hill, New York, 1975, p. 134.

89. Robson, J.R.K., et al.: *Growth standards for infants and children: a cross sectional study.* Pediatrics 56(6):1014-1020, 1975.

90. Hess, R.D., and Shipman, V.C.: *Early experience and socialization of cognitive modes in children.* Child Development 36:869-886, December 1966.

91. Stewart, I.S., and Normak, S.: *The identification of Texas Anglo, Black and Chicano childrearing and childcare practices in relation to childcare competencies.* Paper presented at the annual meeting of the American Educational Research Association, New York, New York, April 1977, p. 6.

92. Davis, A., and Dollard, J.: *Children of*

93. Staples, *Black Woman in America,* p. 150.

94. Radin, N., and Kamii, C.: *The childrearing attitudes of disadvantaged Negro mothers and some educational implications.* Journal of Negro Education 34(Spring):138-146, 1965.

95. Staples, *Black Woman in America,* p. 155.

96. La France, M., and Mayo, C.: *Gaze direction in interrational dyadic communication.* Paper presented at the Eastern Sociological Association, Washington, D.C., May 1973.

97. Taylor, C.: "Soul talk: a key to Black cultural attitudes." In Luckraft, D.: *Black Awareness: Implications for Black Patient Care.* American Journal Company, New York, 1976, p. 2.

98. Seymour, D.: "Black children, Black speech." In *Readings in Human Development, 1973-1974.* Annual Editions, Duskin Publishing Group, Guilford, Connecticut, 1973, pp. 144-147.

99. Comer and Poussaint, p. 23.

100. Watts, L.G.: *The Middle-Income Negro Family Faces Urban Renewal.* Brandeis University Press, Waltham, Massachusetts, 1964.

101. Billingsley, *Black Families in White America,* pp. 28, 30.

102. Lewis, H.: *Blackways of Kent.* University of North Carolina Press, Chapel Hill, North Carolina, 1955, p. 109.

103. Comer and Poussaint, p. 19.

104. Clark, K.B.: *Prejudice and Your Child.* Beacon, Boston, 1963, pp. 22-24.

105. Harrison-Ross, P., and Wyden, B.: *The Black Child: A Parent's Guide.* Peter H. Wyden, Inc., New York, 1973.

106. Ibid., p. 9.

107. Staples, *Black Sociology,* p. 79.

108. Gaughman, E.E., and Dahlstrom, G.W.: *Negro and White Children.* Academic Press, New York, 1968, p. 77.

109. Ward, S.H., and Brown, J.: *Self-esteem and racial preference in Black children.* American Journal of Orthopsychiatry 42(4):644-647, 1972.

110. Barnes, E.J.: "The Black community as the source of positive self-concept for Black children: a theoretical perspective." In Jones, R.L. (ed.): *Black Psychology.* Harper & Row, New York, 1972, pp. 113-123.

111. Block, B.: "Nursing intervention in Black

patient care." In Luckraft, D. (ed.): *Black Awareness: Implications for Black Patient Care.* American Journal of Nursing Company, 1976, p. 29.

112. Staples, *Black Woman in America*, p. 156.
113. Ladner, p. 60.
114. Ladner, pp. 60-61.
115. Scanzoni, J.H.: *The Black Family in Modern Society.* Allyn and Bacon, Inc., Boston, 1971, pp. 145-146.
116. Rainwater, L.: *Behind Ghetto Walls: Negro Families in a Federal Slum.* Aldine Publishing Company, Chicago, 1970, p. 65.
117. Scanzoni, p. 284.
118. Jeffers, C.: *Some perspectives on child rearing practices among urban low income families.* A paper prepared for the Regional Training Institute, Project Enable, Miami, Florida, July 11, 1966.
119. Staples, *Black Woman in America*, p. 52.
120. Kochman, T.: "Black English in the classroom." In Cazden, C. (ed.): *The Function of Language in the Classroom.* New York Teachers College, New York, 1972, p. 32.
121. Foster, H.L.: *Ribbin', Jivin' and Playin' the Dozens.* Ballinger, Cambridge, Massachusetts, 1974.
122. Frazier, E.F.: *Black Bourgeoisie.* Crowell-Collier, New York, 1962, p. 184.
123. Erikson, E.H.: *Childhood and Society.* Norton, New York, 1963, pp. 261-263.
124. Ladner, pp. 68-69.
125. Ibid., p. 72.
126. Ibid., p. 113.
127. Ibid., p. 114.
128. Ibid., p. 115.
129. Ibid., p. 120.
130. Ibid., p. 123.
131. Ladner, pp. 125, 126.
132. Ibid., p. 126.
133. Ibid., p. 131.
134. Ibid., p. 135.
135. Rainwater, L.: *The crucible of identity: the lower-class Negro family.* Daedalus 95(Winter):258-264, 1966.
136. Zelnik, M., and Kauter, J.: *Sexuality, contraception and pregnancy among unwed females in the United States.* Paper prepared for the Commission on Population Growth and the American Future, May 1972.
137. Broderick, C.: *Social heterosexual development among urban Negros and Whites.* Journal of Marriage and the Family 27:200-203, May 1966.
138. Staples, *Black Sociology,* p. 129.
139. Ladner, pp. 211-213.
140. Ibid., p. 202.
141. Ibid., p. 178.
142. Ibid., p. 179.
143. Dollard, J.: *Caste and Class in a Southern Town.* Doubleday Anchor Books, New York, 1957, p. 159.
144. Mayle, P.: *What's Happening to Me?* Lyle Stuart, Inc., Secaucus, New Jersey, 1975.
145. Ladner, p. 214.
146. Ibid., p. 220.
147. Staples, *Black Woman in America,* p. 154.
148. Hannerz, U.: "What ghetto males are like: another look." In Whitten, N.E., and Szwed, J.F. (eds.): *Afro-American Anthropology.* Free Press Collier-MacMillan Limited, London, 1970, pp. 313-323.
149. Staples, *Black Woman in America,* p. 60.
150. Rainwater, *Behind Ghetto Walls,* p. 284.
151. Grier, W.H., and Cobbs, P.H.: *Black Rage.* Bantam Books, New York, 1968, p. 73.
152. Coles, R.: *Children of Crisis.* Little, Brown, New York, 1964.
153. Jordon, V.: *Black youth: the endangered generation.* Ebony August 1978, p. 86.
154. Smith, V.E.: *The drug scene.* Ebony 33(10): 144-46, August 1978.
155. Halpern, F.: *Survival: Black/White.* New York, Pergamon, 1973.
156. Comer and Poussaint, p. 25.
157. Spector, R.E.: *Cultural Diversity in Health and Illness.* Appleton-Century-Crofts, New York, 1979, p. 231.
158. Ibid., p. 243.
159. Ibid., p. 234.
160. Smith, A.J.: "The role of the Black clergy as allied health care professionals in working with Black patients." In Luckraft, D. (ed.): *Black Awareness: Implications for Black Patient Care.* American Journal of Nursing Company, New York, 1976, p. 14.
161. Ibid., p. 12.
162. Taylor, p. 4.
163. Spector, p. 241.
164. Harrison and Harrison, p. 194.
165. Williams, R.A. (ed.): *Textbook of Black-Related Diseases.* McGraw-Hill, New York, 1975, p. XXI.
166. Harrison and Harrison, p. 195.
167. Block, p. 30.
168. Hammonds, K.E.: *The health status of urban Black preschool children.* Journal of National Medical Association 67(1):36-40, 1975.

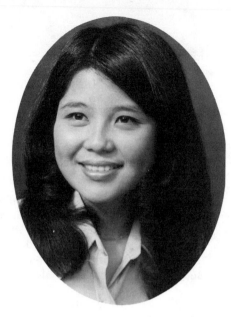

Chapter 5

I am a Sansei, born to Nisei parents—Douglas Ryozo and Clara Sumie (Ueoka) Sodetani. The initial thoughts when writing this chapter brought memories of many cherished moments of my childhood days with my grandparents, parents, and three older siblings—Joyce Reiko, Lloyd Kazuya, and Faith Sachiko—on Maui, Hawaii, where both of my parents, my siblings, and I were born and reared.

My maternal and paternal grandparents migrated to Hawaii during the early 1900s. My maternal grandfather was a Buddhist minister and my paternal grandfather was a carpenter.

From early infancy through high school, much of our time was spent with our grandparents, either in day care or family gatherings. Each set of grandparents lived in their own separate homes. My grandparents spoke very little English, most of which was Pidgin. I can recall my grandparents dramatically telling us samurai and childhood stories from their past, each of which seemed to contain some moral ending regarding one's behavior. The moral teachings seemed always to extend beyond the stories and relate to ourselves, whether they related to manners or etiquette, sibling love, being humble and polite to others, the need to reciprocate a thoughtful gesture, respect for elders, or being a good Japanese child.

Both of my parents were very active in the Buddhist church and community affairs and

encouraged us to participate in them. Everyone had to attend Japanese language school and church on Sundays, which included church related activities such as Girl and Boy Scouts and the Young Buddhist Association functions. My sisters and I also enrolled in piano, 4-H, and Hula or Japanese dance classes, while my brother took martial arts.

Our family celebrated the traditional Japanese festivals of New Years, Girl's and Boy's Day; traditional events of the church (e.g., Buddha or Bodhi Day, O-Bon); and many of the local and Western festivals and holidays, according to the Hawaiian or American tradition.

Throughout our lives there was a great emphasis on education, achievement, ethnicity, and preservation of the family name. My parents worked hard and made many great sacrifices so we could have the advantages of a comfortable living, opportunities for education, and other extracurricular activities. One of the greatest moments in my parents' lives was when I (the last among the four children) completed my college education.

There was always a feeling of love and security at home. My parents were quite affectionate and it always gave me a pleasant feeling to be hugged by them. Even with the atmosphere of achievement orientation, there was still support when one failed and encouragement to try

The Japanese American
Aimee Emiko Sodetani-Shibata, R.N., M.N.

again. My parents have now taken on the role of grandparents, and there is still an environment of love and security created for my nieces.

The roots of this chapter began while I was teaching at the University of Hawaii School of Nursing. In September 1978, I joined my husband Erwin in Seattle, Washington, where I became Instructor of Nursing at the University of Washington.

Each search through the literature seemed to bring a closer understanding about my cultural heritage and my own behaviors. The process has also helped me to become more sensitive to the people of my own culture and leaves me with a hunger to learn more about the Japanese Americans.

"How do the relatively unique ways of thinking, feeling, and acting that characterize different families and groups get transmitted to their offspring?"[42] It is often accomplished directly and formally, such as in educational programs, but to a considerable extent such transmissions occur through the informal interactions between parents and their children in the course of childrearing. These parent-child interactions include the parents' expressions of traditional cultural attitudes, values, interests, and beliefs, as well as caretaking and training behaviors that have probably been modified as they are passed on from one generation to another.[61] Once the child is beyond infancy, his general personality becomes a product of social experiences influenced not only by his parents but also relatives, neighbors, peers, and school.

This chapter was written for the primary purpose of identifying some of the childrearing practices among Japanese Americans and their implications for health care providers in promoting quality care for such families. Other important considerations include an historical review of the culture in Japan and America and significant events that influenced changes in the traditional Japanese behavior, family life, and childrearing practices in America.

JOURNEY TO A NEW LAND
The initial migration of the Japanese people into

the continental United States and Hawaii occurred during 1542 to 1638, when Japan maintained contact with the Western nations through its interest in international trade and travel. A lack of accurate and consistent records makes it difficult to ascertain the actual number of people that arrived or settled in the continental United States and Hawaii. The migration of these people seems relatively insignificant as the numbers were few and many were transient sea merchant traders or students seeking an education abroad.

The migration out of Japan ceased in 1638 when the country under the reign of the Tokugawas adopted a seclusion policy because they were fearful of damaging and exploitative influences on their culture by foreign powers. Although the exclusion and inclusion policy prohibited any migration into or out of Japan, it made provisions allowing only a limited number of Dutch and Chinese traders into the country. In addition, some history books do indicate that a number of castaway fishermen, shipwrecked sailors, and adventurous people smuggled their way out of Japan and reached the shores of the continental United States and Hawaii.[27,30,31,39,43,48,57,59]

At the beginning of the nineteenth century, with the development of improved means of sea transportation and the rapid expansion of economic activity, the seclusion of Japan became threatened. There were many futile attempts to reopen Japan's doors to foreigners. In 1852, the 214-year-old seclusion policy finally gave way when United States President Fillmore commissioned Commodore Matthew Perry to lead an expedition in a major effort to break Japan's isolation. The mission resulted in the signing of a peace and amity treaty (Treaty of Kanazawa) on March 31, 1854. The arrangement opened two sea ports to American ships for provisioning, guaranteed good treatment for American sailors, and provided for the appointment of an American consul to reside at one of the sea ports.

Four years later, in 1858, Townsend Harris, the first American consul-general to Japan, secured the first Treaty of Commerce. Shortly thereafter, other foreign countries signed similar treaties with Japan. The signing of the treaties guaranteed foreigners as well as the people of Japan the right to reside in any of the treatied nations. Japan, however, did not allow any of its nationals to leave the country.

In 1868 the political power of Japan shifted from the isolationist Tokugawas to the Meiji clan. The new Meiji government was more inclined to accelerate the Westernization of Japan's economic and military systems. Consequently the attitudes toward foreign emigration changed. In 1866 legal provisions were made enabling certain classes of its citizens and students who wished to pursue their education abroad to leave the country.[31,59]

Eighteen years later, in 1884, the Japanese government adopted a policy of unrestricted emigration, thereby allowing all of its citizens, including its labor classes, to migrate to foreign countries. As a result of the policy, the extent and the character of the Japanese emigrants began to change. A large majority were young men seeking opportunities of education or a more prosperous livelihood. Many left with hopes of gaining wealth and eventually returning to Japan once they had made their fortunes.

The period of unrestricted emigration, a period that saw the largest emigration of Japanese people into the continental United States and Hawaii, ended in 1908 when the United States government issued a proclamation called the "Gentlemen's Agreement." The proclamation denied the skilled and unskilled Japanese laborers entrance into any continental territory of the United States. The agreement was not a formal document but was more of a voluntary arrangement between Japan and the United States. Despite the agreement, the Japanese people continued to migrate, but the numbers decreased drastically.

The census of Japanese immigrants entering the continental United States and Hawaii increased once again between 1911 and 1924 as a result of more female immigration. Table 1 cites the increase in female population, which was influenced by both birth and immigration.

Many of the female immigrants who migrated between 1911 and 1924 were wives of laborers or "picture brides" (those married after being selected from pictures). Although women were covered under the Gentlemen's Agreement, their immigration became a focus of attention for the American anti-Japanese agitators and caused the Japanese government to voluntarily stop the issuing of passports to the so-called picture brides on February 25, 1920, with the hopes of maintaining international harmony. Those that secured passports prior to that date continued to migrate until 1924.

The Gentlemen's Agreement was replaced by the Asian Exclusion Law in 1924. The new law,

TABLE 1. Japanese female population in the continental United States and Hawaii, 1900–1920[64]

Year	Total in Continental United States	Percent of Total Japanese Population	Total in Hawaii	Percent of Total Japanese Population
1900	985	4.00	13,603	22.25
1910	9087	12.59	24,891	31.24
1920	38,303*	34.50	46,630	42.67

*Includes 34,216 or 30.82 percent of the total Japanese population who migrated between 1911–1920.

TABLE 2. Japanese in the continental United States and Hawaii, 1870–1970[65]

Year	Total U.S. Population	Total Japanese in Continental U.S. and Hawaii	% of Total Japanese in Total U.S. Population	Japanese in Continental U.S.	% of Continental U.S. Japanese in Total U.S. Population	Japanese in Hawaii	% of Hawaiian Japanese in Total U.S. Population	% of Hawaiian Japanese in Total Japanese Population
1870	38,558,371			55	0.000014			
1880	50,155,783			148	0.003			
1884						116		
1890	62,947,714	14,649		2,039	0.003	12,610		86.0
1900	75,994,574	85,437		24,326	0.030	61,111		71.5
1910	91,972,266	151,832		72,157	0.080	79,675		52.4
1920	105,710,620	220,284		111,010	0.100	109,274		49.6
1930	122,775,046	278,465		138,834	0.110	139,631		50.1
1940	131,669,275	284,853		126,948	0.090	157,905		55.4
1950	159,697,361	353,384		168,773	0.090	184,611		52.2
1960*	179,323,175	463,650	0.25	260,195	0.145	203,455	0.114	43.5
1970	207,211,926	591,290	0.29	374,114	0.184	217,175	0.107	36.7

*Statehood in 1959 arbitrarily included Hawaii in the United States census of 1960.

which was issued by the United States, prohibited any oriental immigration into the United States and its territories. It excluded certain select people, however, who were protected by the treaty, and the so-called non-quota individuals, comprised of professional clergymen, professors with their wives and minor children, and bona fide students over 15 years old. The exceptions held little numerical significance. The law remained in effect until the passage of the McCarran-Walters Bill in 1952, which became effective in 1954.[31,39,58]

It is noteworthy to mention the importance of including Hawaii in the discussion of the Japanese Americans. Although Hawaii was not a territory of the United States until 1900, a significant number of the Japanese immigrants settled there. The granting of statehood in 1959 arbitrarily included the Japanese people of Hawaii into the 1960 United States census, thereby increasing the total number of individuals of Japanese ancestry in the United States.

Recently Harry H.L. Kitano, a sociologist, supported the inclusion of Hawaii by stating:

It is difficult to understand the omission of Hawaii when there is a discussion of the Japanese American, but such practice is common. Perhaps there is a feeling that Hawaii is an exception to many of the generalizations concerning the Japanese American, or that it is so small that it is not worth counting. But a glance at population figures shows how erroneous such impressions are; in 1970, 217,307 or 37 percent of the 591,290 Japanese in the United States were residents of Hawaii. . . . numbers alone do not begin to reflect the importance of the islands. . . . the experiences of Hawaii have been different so they provide another frame for looking at the Japanese.[39]

Table 2 cites the number of individuals of Japanese ancestry in the continental United States and Hawaii from 1870 to 1970.

DEFINING THE GENERATIONS AND THE PEOPLE

Japanese Americans are the only immigrant group in the United States who term each generation (Issei, Nisei, Sansei) of its descendants from the original immigrant group by their geographical and generational distance from Japan. Such terms can also distinguish the native-born from the foreign-born, and when used subjectively can refer to unique character types, behaviors, and stereotypes of each generation.

The first generation of pioneer immigrants who were born in Japan and migrated to the continental United States and Hawaii in the 1890s and early 1900s are referred to as the Issei. They are known to work hard, be group and family oriented, and cling to old values and customs.[32,39,48] Nisei are the second generation born in the continental United States and Hawaii; Sansei are the third generation born in the continental United States and Hawaii (Fig. 1).

A term used to identify a subgroup of the Nisei generation is the Kibei. They were Nisei children who went to Japan with their families or were sent there to live with their grandparents, usually for the purpose of education. The practice of sending at least one child back to Japan to be educated was quite popular between 1920 and 1940, but was never resumed after World War II.

After reaching adulthood, many Kibei returned to the continental United States and Hawaii, only to discover that they were in conflict with their Issei parents and many of their Nisei counterparts. Such tensions arose particularly among their Nisei counterparts as a result of their pro-Japanese values, their different perceptions of Japan, and their inadequacy in speaking the English language fluently.[30,31,39,47] Okamoto suggests that the maintenance of some Japanese traditions may have been influenced by the Kibei.[60] (Children of Kibei parents are considered Sansei.)

Okamoto noted that while the utilization of the terminology may be historically convenient to classify the Japanese Americans by generations, such terms do not illustrate their entire population. Complexities arise with children of mixed generations (e.g., Issei-Nisei, Nisei-Sansei) and racially mixed parentage.[60] Matsumoto and associates noted that a child born to an Issei father and Nisei mother is "officially" a Nisei, but may be reared in an environment similar to that of a Sansei. The child would thus have values, attitudes, and behaviors that were more like a Sansei.[50]

Kitano sights two other factors that have contributed to the insignificance of and confusion with the use of the terminology. He notes that as newer generations are born (Yonsei—fourth generation; Gosei—fifth generation) and become more closely acculturated to the American way of life than were their great-grandparents, and as new Issei arrive from Japan only to add to the complexity of the terminology, such terms will

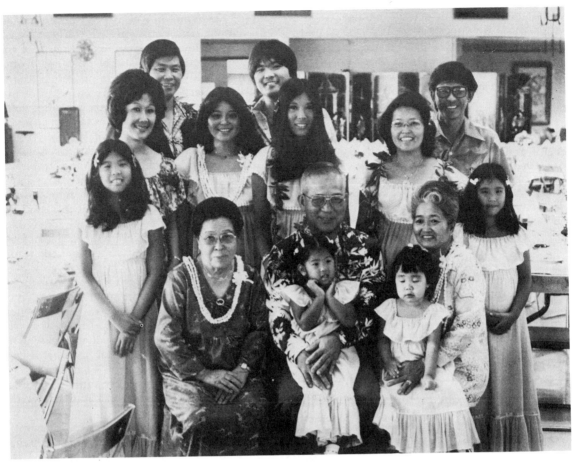

Figure 1. Four generations of Japanese Americans: Issei, Nisei, Sansei, and Yonsei.

eventually become meaningless. The term Nik-kei is now used to include all the generations of Japanese Americans.[39]

Still another factor that is equally important to consider when utilizing these terms, whether objectively or subjectively, is the determination of a person's birthplace and place of rearing. Such distinctions may seem unimportant for those outside of the Japanese-American culture, but for those within the culture and close observers differences do exist, particularly among Japanese Americans born and reared on the mainland and Hawaii.

The Japanese were the first to recognize the differences and created special terms to classify one from the other. The term Kotonk is used for those born in the continental United States and Buddhahead or Pineapple for the Hawaii born.

A popular version of the origin of the term Kotonk occurred during World War II when the mainland and Hawaii Nisei met on a large scale for the first time. There were inevitable arguments, which resulted in fist fights. When the hard hollow head of the mainlander hit the floor it made an audible impression. The term still remains in use today, particularly among the Japanese Americans in Hawaii. Kitano noted that "the mainlander still finds some difficulty in gaining full acceptance into the Japanese American social system, and his island peers will seldom let him forget his Kotonk background."[39]

Kitano indicated that "the general theme is that the mainlander is overly concerned about surface appearances, too materialistic, too careful about impressing the majority group, too acculturated, and in one word, too 'haolefied' (white)."[40] Kitano suggested that the differences between the mainlanders and the islanders were

101

regional and non-specific to the Japanese. He attributes the differences to the islands' casual style of living, dressing, and speaking (Pidgin).[39] He further acknowledged that:

> . . . the Japanese in Hawaii make up a powerful group with a number of alternatives not readily available to most of their peers on the mainland. They are more comfortable in their ethnicity; they are freer to retain their life styles by voluntary choice. Yet, they were also freer to acculturate because the barriers toward Americanization were not as rigid as on the mainland. Even more important, their acculturation was to a more racially tolerant island culture, so many profess surprise when a discussion of racial discrimination, mainland style, is raised. It is the amalgamation of these experiences that has developed the Japanese in Hawaii into something different from their mainland counterparts.

> . . . Japanese in Hawaii were never a small, scattered minority in a vast land but were a large, and sometimes majority group on concentrated islands; they entered into a more racially tolerant society than their peers in California; and they were one of the large number of imported nationality groups. . . . They were geographically close enough to Japan so that homeland influences were much stronger than on the mainland. . . . Japanese in Hawaii offer an opportunity to evaluate the effect of variables like power, a more tolerant social structure, a relative degree of social isolation, and closer ties to the homeland on a Japanese population.

Despite the expressed feelings of differences, the question of differences still remains academic, owing to the lack of research studies. Furthermore, the regional differences could be argued since the large majority of the continental United States incorporates a mixture of life-styles.

It is worth mentioning that all terms should be utilized with care. Okamoto also maintains that while such "historical considerations are significant when reflecting on a client's identification with Japanese cultural beliefs and values . . . care must be taken to avoid using inappropriate stereotypes in an attempt to serve the needs of the people with apparently similar backgrounds but with diverse associations."[60]

MOTIVES FOR LEAVING THEIR HOMELAND

A very large majority of the Japanese people who migrated during the 1890s and early 1900s came from the southwest prefectures of Japan: Hiro-shima, Kumamoto, Wakayama, Fukuoka, and Yamaguchi, which cultivated the largest areas of farmland. They were products of a culture that was undergoing vast social changes from a feudal system (Tokugawa) to an urban and industrial society (Meiji). Many came from individually poor families and were attracted to the widely publicized opportunities to gain economic wealth in a new land. The widely publicized invitations from Hawaii's plantations attracted many of the young, intelligent, and ambitious, seeking opportunities to study or better opportunities to gain a livelihood. Others followed after people returned to Japan with success stories of Japanese people in the continental United States and Hawaii. Such stories made a great many people less passive and less skeptical about journeying to strange lands.[17, 39, 48, 70]

A considerable number were summoned (Yobiyose) by earlier immigrant fathers or uncles.[17] Some utilized Hawaii as a stepping stone to gain entrance into the continental United States. A small number were older men who had failed in business or had found farming or wage labor in Japan unattractive. Whatever the motive, many of the immigrants came with the intention of someday returning to Japan once they had made their fortunes.

Ichihashi sights the Military Conscription Law of Japan as another reason for the Japanese emigration. The Japanese law required that every male citizen at the age of 20 undergo examinations for the military service and provide services for 3 years. Since the law gave privileges of indefinitely postponing the examinations if abroad, an effective means of entirely freeing oneself from the military service was to migrate and remain abroad until one reached the limiting age of 32 years. (In 1910, it was increased to age 37.) For these immigrants, reasons for migration were twofold: to avoid the military law and to obtain economic wealth.[31]

The Japanese ambition of making a fortune proved to be more difficult and took longer than they had anticipated. Therefore, as their families grew and their economic stake in the country became more solid, their hopes of returning to Japan became more difficult to achieve. While the lack of data makes it difficult to ascertain the actual number that returned to Japan, a certain number did return. Many who went back to Japan soon returned with stories that it was even more difficult to start a life there, as things had changed.

THE ETHNIC CULTURE: SOCIAL NORMS AND VALUES

To understand the ethnic culture of the present Japanese Americans, it is essential to understand the circumstances of the Issei's life in Japan. The ethnic culture variables discussed are social norms and values. Kitano defines the variables as follows:

> Norms are shared meanings in a culture that serve to provide the background for communication; values refer to clusters of attitudes that give a sense of direction to behavior. . . . The primary purpose of a social norm is to provide a guide for interpersonal behavior so that an individual has an acceptable way of interacting with others and, conversely, is able to judge the acts of others.[39]

It would be inaccurate to say that all or even most Japanese behave in accordance with the prescribed norms. Nevertheless, knowledge of the traditional norms is important as it provides a background for understanding Japanese American behavior, family life, and childrearing practices.

Ethnic Culture Origin

Strong, in his study of the Nisei, noted that the majority of the Issei had the equivalent of an eighth-grade education and were primarily drawn from an ambitious, intelligent middle class.[63] The Issei have been closely associated with terms such as self-controlled, obedient, patient, diligent, obligated, responsible, loyal, selfless, stoic, and persevering. They are known to be willing to work hard without complaint and consistently strive to improve themselves. They also believe in the hierarchical order of patriarchy and hold a high regard for their parents and elders. The Issei were conditioned with the traditional virtues and felt such qualities, as well as others, were important in a person and therefore emphasized them in the rearing of their children.

The grandparents and parents of the Issei had experienced a direct contact with the feudal culture of the Tokugawa era (1600–1867), which saw a very firm consolidation of culture patterns. The Issei spent their childhood in the Meiji era (1868–1911) that followed. The Meiji era saw many great changes, but in many ways that allowed and encouraged the continuation of the old Tokugawa social order and its supporting values. Many of the sources of identities and behaviors of the Issei and succeeding generations of Japanese Americans can be traced back to the Tokugawa culture.

PRE-TOKUGAWA PERIOD

This was a period of chronic warfare among feudal lords, without a central controlling leadership. The most influential leader of each region maintained a personal residential castle with his familial group and vassals. Defeat meant the total destruction of the fief and family. Under such circumstances, a sense of mutual dependency and responsibility became important. A vassal responded to his lord's generosity with deeds. The samurai (warrior) looked to the peasant for food and labor, while the peasant looked to the samurai for protection.

The samurais, however, soon established their political superiority and forced the peasants into a position of obedience, thereby planting the seed for the authoritarian identity.

TOKUGAWA

After a full century of bloody civil wars, every effort was made to suppress change and to establish a rigid social system for the benefit of the samurai class. To combat social mobility, the Tokugawa Shogunate widened the gaps between each class and within each social position. The Shogunate rigidly defined the social position of each individual and made it virtually impossible for an individual to move into a higher status.

Each individual was responsible to someone higher than himself. He related to "outsiders" by virtue of his overlord's relation to them. An individual soon learned that if he remained in his proper position in life, he was safe and secure. To maintain the enforcement of the codes, the samurais were allowed to behead anyone of a lower status whose behavior was undesirable. The strict structure of the codes resulted in the absence of one's expression, regardless of one's real emotion and enryo (modesty in the presence of one's superior).

Desiring to make the social control more effective, the samurai class sought to make its own moral code (Bushido) the ethics of the nation. To implement this value system, the Tokugawa Shogunate utilized the deeply ingrained ethical and religious systems of Confucianism and Buddhism.

Confucianism

Confucianism was based on two themes: (1) common people or the lower class should be in an entirely subordinate position, and (2) patriarchy and the family are a unit for social action.

Within the family the patriarch, who was the eldest adult male, stood at the head of the family. All family actions centered around the patriarch-heir relationship. "The patriarch was the guardian of ancestry, land, economics, and family unit; his prominence was sanctioned by legal rights and unquestioned obedience."[59] The eldest son was the inheritor of the patriarchal status and was treated with respect. The emphasis on male authority in terms of family inheritance was such that the relationship took precedence over the husband-wife relationship. The bond between husband and wife was secondary to the bond between father and son.

The state was an extension of the family. The final link, which was the only one extending beyond the family, was the association of the ruler with the subject. The ruler in turn was in the position of a son to Heaven. Heaven, the family system, and the state were therefore joined into a single unity. The smooth functioning of the entire system was warranted by each person's adherence to the prescribed rites governing each important action.[48]

As an ethical system, Confucianism taught benevolence, propriety, and wisdom and emphasized obedience to one's parents. Its primary emphasis concerned the problems of behavior and of man's obligations in social and family relations. The system was based on the premise that selfishness hides the true self and keeps one from attaining the state of oneness.

Buddhism

The Buddhist doctrine stresses selflessness, the dissolution of self in infinity, and the destruction of ego. The greatest obstacle to the freedom and liberation of the mind is the self.

The self had two components. (1) Man in his natural state had distinct and unique felt qualities, such as cherished feelings toward his parents or natural objects. But since such things are transitory and mortal, the desire for their immortality was a source of suffering, selfishness, and evil. (2) The aesthetic surrounding component of the self was unchanging and immortal, and if cherished by the self, it would give one a compassionate fellow-feeling for all creatures.

A person's relation to deity as a supreme being was governed by the theory of "on" (ascribed obligation). A supreme being in some form dispensed blessings and it was the obligation of the recipient to repay these blessings. Buddha identified four debts that one owed: to parents, to fellow beings, to sovereign, and to the three holy treasures of Buddhism. Man could not live without the blessings of the supreme being, and since the blessings given were much greater than man's ability to return them, he was always in debt. Therefore, only by devoting himself to the return of the blessing could he be assured of a continuation, and thereby saved from his weakness.

Bushido

The Bushido or the samurai class was seen as the guardian, authority, and protector of morality. It was each samurai's duty to be devoted to his lord or superiors. Self-control was stressed to suppress all desires. As a child, like all other children, he was taught filial piety so that he would fulfill the requirements of loyalty when he reached adulthood. The samurai was instructed to live a frugal and selfless life—to be a person of few words, to leave a festive place when he still had desire to remain, and to know he had more than enough when he was satisfied, for enough was too much. On or off the battlefield, he was expected to control his feelings because his devotion to the lord and warfare came before himself. Showing one's feelings was considered a sign of weakness.[48]

Social Norms and Values

The influence of the rigid centralized authority of the Tokugawa rulers together with Japan's isolation from the outside world for over a period of 260 years contributed greatly to the development of cultural homogeneity. It also led to highly prescribed and predictable behaviors in social interaction, many of which were non-verbal.[21, 26, 33, 44, 55]

The non-verbal communications were very personalized and have come to play an important role in Japanese interpersonal relationships. There are countless expressions and many do not need words for their fluent transmissions. Hearn, in his review of the Japanese non-verbal behavior during the Tokugawa period, stated that:

> Demeanour was most elaborately and mercilessly regulated, not merely as to obediences, of which there were countless grades, varying according to sex as well as class—but even in regard to facial expression, the manner of smiling, the con-

duct of the breath, the way of sitting, standing, walking, rising. Everybody was trained from infancy in this etiquette of expression and deportment. . . . not only that any sense of anger or pain should be denied all outward expression, but that the sufferer's face and manner should indicate the contrary feeling. Sullen submission was an offense; mere impassive obedience inadequate; the proper degree of submission should manifest itself by a pleasant smile, and by a soft and happy tone of voice. The smile, however, was also regulated. One had to be careful about the quality of the smile: it was a mortal offence, for example . . . to smile in addressing a superior, that the back teeth could be seen. In the military class especially this code of demeanour was ruthlessly enforced. Samurai women were required . . . to show signs of joy on hearing that their husbands or sons had fallen in battle: to betray any natural feeling under the circumstances was a grave breach of decorum. . . . In all classes demeanour was regulated so severely that even today the manners of the people everywhere still reveal the nature of the old discipline. . . . Old-fashioned manners appear natural rather than acquired, instinctive rather than made by training.[28]

Similarly, Asch hypothesized that the Japanese people's tendency to smile in adverse situations is due to the major concern with maintenance of control and showing respect to one's superior: "Japanese learn . . . that it is necessary to keep a reserve of strength in the face of crisis in order not to be naked and exposed. The smile in this context has the significance of resisting the shock of pain and sorrow by summoning of inner strength."[7]

Certain expressions were transformed into social norms and values and were incorporated into the Japanese national school curriculum as an ethical doctrine, so the exposure to such techniques was widespread. Some of the more highly stressed were: "enryo," self restraint or modesty in the presence of one's superior; "amae," dependence; "on," ascribed obligation; "giri," contractual or reciprocal obligation; "chu," loyalty to one's superior; and achievement orientation. Through time they have been renewed and changed and given new modes of expression.[39, 48, 59]

ENRYO

Kitano indicates that among the many norms that shape Japanese behavior, enryo appears to be one of the most important. Through the years its meaning and its use expanded to cover a variety of situations—from how one behaves, to

what to do in ambiguous situations and how to cover a moment of confusion, embarrassment, and anxiety. Kitano discusses the enryo syndrome as follows:

Enryo helps to explain much of Japanese-American behavior. As with other norms, it has both a positive and negative effect on Japanese (social interaction). For example, take observations of Japanese in situations as diverse as their hestitancy to speak out at meetings; their refusal of any invitation, especially the first time; their refusal of a second helping; their acceptance of a less desired object when given a free choice; their lack of verbal participation, especially in an integrated group; their refusal to ask questions; and their hesitancy in asking for a raise in salary—these may all be based in enryo. The inscrutable face, the non-commital answer, the behaviorable reserve can often be traced to this norm, so that the stereotype of the shy, reserved Japanese in ambiguous social situations is often an accurate one.[39]

"Ha zu ka shi" (embarrassment, shame, or reservation) is part of enryo. The motive for this feeling is centered on others—how other people will react to you so that there remains a feeling of shame or a feeling that one may have made a fool of oneself in the presence of others. Childhood discipline emphasizes "ha zu ka shi"—"others will laugh at you"—and the norm is used as a means of social control.[39]

The use of "haji" (shame) is a form of "ha zu ka shi" and was one of the most prominent mechanisms to regulate an individual's behavior. The shame orientation of the Japanese individual was highly valued and an effective tool of social conformity. The judgment of your peers and family and what others thought of you was an important determinant in reinforcing bonds of love. If a person failed to perpetuate the open relations of love and trust, then he threatened his position in society and was shamed.[59]

Kitano maintains that "hi-ge" is a part of enryo and is often difficult for many non-Japanese to understand. The Japanese may deny themselves the satisfaction of self-expression and delight in understatements. Thus, when forced to speak about their possessions or a family member, they belittle them as being of no special value. For example, a father in speaking of his bright son may describe him as a "good-for-nothing boy," or when homemade food is served in the presence of guests a Japanese woman may say, "This is not very good, but do have some." Praise, especially in public, is considered to be in poor taste, except in formalized circumstances.[39]

AMAE

Amae is another concept, described by Doi[23],[24] and Meredith,[52] that is important in understanding the basic dependency of the Japanese. The term refers to the need to be loved and cherished, a means of asking for love, and seeking recognition and acceptance. According to Doi, it can lead to serious behavioral consequences such as "ko da wa ru" (to be inwardly disturbed over one's personal relationship) or "sumanai" (to feel guilty or obligated).

Amae was often used by the Issei mother to describe the behavior of her children—sometimes with approval and sometimes with impatience. For example, a mother might indicate that all her children have to have amae, and she will pamper and baby them. Yet, in other situations she might indicate that her children are seeking and behaving with too much amae and refuse their requests or ignore their behavior. For the child, it was a means of interaction, and asking for love, attention, approval, or recognition, and because of his need for amae, he would be less likely to risk being in a position of being scolded or laughed at.

A critical part of amae is the way it is perceived and responded to in the Japanese culture. For example, if a mother sees the behavior of her child as amae, she would not respond with discipline or punishment, since it is understood that amae is an important factor in a relationship. However, if she interprets the behavior in another way, a different response may be elicited. Amae is currently equated among Nikkei with being spoiled and is considered an undesirable action and should be restricted or eliminated. The practice of prohibiting the behavior often deprives the child of a gentle technique for gaining attention or asking for a favor.

The dependency, though different in expression, is carried over into adulthood. For example, today it is not unusual still to find unmarried children in their late twenties or early thirties living with their parents, and who are expected to or expect to continue to live at home or nearby after marriage. In such situations, family problems often arise as a result of conflict between independence and dependence. Its origin stems from the Japanese socialization goal, which stresses the establishment of dependency on the family, the group, the company, and the mutual responsibility that is attached with such a perspective. Conversely, the American goal of socialization stresses the establishment of independence and autonomy as early as possible.

ON

The concept of "on" or obligation to superiors is a passively incurred type of psychological burden and fosters a relationship of interdependence. It covers a child's obligation to his family, status, position, elders, and community. For example, a child is indebted to his parents for having received care and support from them. The child therefore has an obligation to obey his parents (a good child's repayment of parental on does not allow him to question his parents' decisions), show achievement in school and/or community, and care for his parents in their old age.[9],[59]

Recently a Sansei described a family experience that illustrates parental "on," interdependence, and the independence-dependence conflict previously discussed:

After completing my master's degree and being pretty much on my own for about 7 years—with the exception of financial assistance from my parents, I was both happy and relieved, because I had made my parents happy over my achievement and thought finally they wouldn't have to support me.

My decision to return home was mutual . . . I wanted to be near my family and I felt I needed to repay my parents in someway by doing things to make life a little easier or better for them, like helping to care for my grandparents or whatever help they needed . . . and my parents wanted me home too.

Prior to my return, I made plans of getting an apartment and a job nearby—but all plans were shattered when my parents strongly disagreed and decided that I should stay at home because everything that I needed: the family, access to a car, food, a roof over my head, etc. were right at home. The benefits they stressed would be financial as well as emotional. I would incure enough savings in event of marriage and have the companionship of the family.

Similarly, the same Sansei described another family experience that illustrates parental "on" and the resulting interdependence:

When my grandmother suffered a stroke at the age of 86, all of her children and their husbands and wives took turns staying with her on a 24 hour basis during her entire hospital convalescence. When it became apparent that she would make it through the crisis and need care after she left the hospital, all of her children got together on many occasions to discuss where she would live and how care would be given. One mention of putting her in a nursing home almost brought the roof down and it was never again mentioned. After much discussion, my second eldest uncle (since the first had passed away) who was the primary consultant in all major matters that dealt with my grandma prior to her illness, took her into his home. Although the greatest responsibility of her care lay in my uncle and aunt's hands, each child in their own way shared in the responsibility of her care until her death 8 years later.*

GIRI

"Giri" or reciprocal obligation is based on the premise that each individual who has received something, whether material or nonmaterial, from another human being has acquired a debt. The debts are to be repaid with something equivalent to or greater than the original favor, emotion, or gift received, and there are time limits. A person is therefore continually attuned to what he receives and how and when he should repay it. If a person fails to return the energy, he is in danger of losing any future support and assistance.

Ogawa indicated that the reciprocal obligation also had a humanistic dimension, that of dependency between human beings, which reinforced the bonds of affiliation. Therefore, by being obligated one was not only economically involved but was also emotionally linked in mutual help and concern. Friendship became more highly valued than personal sacrifice or selfishness.[59]

CHU

In the traditional Japanese family submission to the father was transferred to the emperor through the institution of "chu" (loyalty to one's superior). Self-effacing obedience was developed to such an extent that a Japanese, when inducted into the imperial military service, was considered as one who was already dead. The utilization of chu was applied in every action or interaction, whether in the family, community, or work force.[46,48]

ACHIEVEMENT ORIENTATION

Throughout Japan's recorded history, high standards of excellence have been sought and

achieved. The strict codes of ethics required the achievement of set standards of excellence by each Japanese citizen. If the standards were unmet, the individual felt shame and guilt.

The standards of excellence grew to emphasize the importance of learning among all classes of citizens during the Tokugawa reign. According to their ideals, ascription alone was not a sufficient claim for status without adequate performance of the prescribed duties.

The Meiji Restoration period, which brought the drive for industrialization and urbanization, left the majority of Japanese relatively unaffected, but expecting more out of life than their fathers. With the abolishment of the samurai class, the new government offered an age of opportunity. It was now possible for the Japanese to achieve status without ascription and believe that courage, energy, initiative, and determination could carry a person anywhere.

The achievement orientation in Japan was derived from one's social self-identity. The extreme form of dedication to a particular social role was originally part of the samurai sense of self. With the abolishment of the samurai class, the models of self-actualization were transferred to the roles of the Meiji government, the educators, and the mother.

The sense of self was acknowledged only through repayment of deeply felt obligations. If the obligations were not repaid, a sense of intolerable guilt would arise. The sense of loyalty to authority and repayment of one's obligation was deeply ingrained from birth. Guilt functioned as the operative superego and was internalized by the individual. Subsequently, the individual feared rejection by those whom he depended upon rather than punishment. Therefore, if a child failed to achieve or to meet the desired societal expectations, the mother would blame herself. As a result, the child felt guilt for the pain he caused his mother and shame for not meeting the set standards. He therefore learned that only by achieving could he rid himself from guilt, make amends for his past misbehavior, and preserve or bring back honor and praise to his family.[48]

LIFE IN THE NEW LAND

The following is a summary of some of the significant life events that the Issei and succeeding generations of Japanese Americans have encountered. The purpose of its inclusion is to il-

---

*Personal interview, Hawaii, 1978.

lustrate some of the external forces that influenced generational changes in the traditional Japanese behavior, family life, and childrearing practices.

Before World War II

From birth, the early "pioneer" immigrant was conditioned and accustomed to put the interests of his family, village, prefecture (ken), nation, and emperor ahead of his personal interests. "His behaviors were dictated by clearly defined rules and obligations. A system of collectivism and ethical interaction provided mutual assistance for group members and proved effective in protecting the individual from cultural shocks of both a rapidly changing Japan and later a new land."[39]

Although the Issei had been born to a social system that may have prepared them for adapting to the difficulties that they encountered in the new land, there were still many barriers that precluded their smooth assimilation into the host society. The major barriers that awaited them were language and differences in custom.

The Japanese that migrated to the continental United States in particular were victims of being in the "wrong country at the wrong time." Those that settled on the west coast of the mainland entered in the midst of an anti-Oriental agitation that was originally directed at the Chinese.[31] Many were forced into agricultural or other manual labor work. But they had little intention of permanently remaining as laborers. Their ambitions quickly carried them from laborers to economic competitors. The upward mobility of the Japanese people disturbed the anti-Oriental agitators, who eventually succeeded in persuading the government to pass the Alien Land Law, School Segregation Law, and Asian Exclusion Law of 1924.

Concurrently, the Japanese that went to Hawaii entered into the plantations as contract laborers and inherited the lowest position in that system. (The theme of the plantation system was to control power by accepting only enough people of one ethnic group to perform the labor, then to switch to another.) They were assigned to the poorest plantation-owned homes and were the lowest paid. Life on the plantations was monotonous and severe. Their lives were controlled by an indifferent and inaccessible Caucasian plantation management in which laborers served as specialized functionaries with little personal or individual identity.

Many of the plantation owners felt that the Japanese were good workers, but were not content to remain on the plantations. To counteract the Japanese ambitions, strategies such as maintaining surplus, playing one race against another, keeping aliens out of the city, restricting government jobs, prohibiting the laborers' movement to the mainland, working through foreign consuls and police officials, and intimidation were instituted.

Consequently, the Japanese people became dissatisfied with plantation life and the working conditions and struck, first in 1909 and again in 1920. The strikes at times split the Japanese community, since values of loyalty and obligation to the employer, hard work, and gratefulness could not be integrated into a militant adversary position.

The strikes proved to be an important factor in building the Japanese people's economic strength, as there was a concerted effort among all Japanese working on various plantations to organize and coordinate their resources. It also resulted in a general improvement of the conditions under which they were to labor, caused some to leave the plantations and engage in other preferred occupations, and above all brought the Japanese community closer together.

Another barrier that the Issei faced was the denial of citizenship. The naturalization laws, which established the criteria for United States citizenship from 1790, limited naturalization to those persons "free, white and twenty-one years of age." It also recognized citizenship for those born in the United States or territories of the United States. The law therefore excluded the Issei from gaining citizenship, but recognized their Nisei children as bona fide American citizens.[59]

Despite the prejudicial attacks and the denial of citizenship, the Issei on the mainland and Hawaii still maintained their racial pride and identity and valued many of their traditional virtues of loyalty, obligation, hard work, and gratefulness. The maintenance of their strong attachments to the Japanese culture was in part due to their infrequent and limited contact with the American culture.

The anti-Oriental sentiments lay relatively dormant through the 1930s. Hosokawa indicated that, during those years, many Nisei on the mainland "were still in search of their identity, seeking to make their reality of the textbook ideal of Americanism."[30] Concurrently, because of their increasing numbers in a smaller community, the Japanese in Hawaii were beginning to draw power in the island economy and Hawaiian politics as more of them reached the voting age.

World War II

The crucial moment for all Japanese came on December 7, 1941, with Japan's attack on Pearl Harbor. The following day President Franklin D. Roosevelt, with the consent of Congress, officially declared war on Japan. Nearly 30 years of anti-Japanese sentiment had preceded the outbreak of the war, a sentiment which cast a shadow on the character, integrity, and adaptability of the Japanese immigrants and their children to the American way of life. Now, dormant impressions of the Japanese awakened and found new means of expression and new aims. For all Japanese, having the face, culture, language, diet, and dress of the enemy during the war necessitated caution, cultural suppression, and superpatriotism to America. The frightened Issei, in particular, were in an awkward predicament—they had lived most of their lives in America, but were still citizens of Japan and were now thought of as enemies of the United States.

In the continental United States, immediately after war was declared, Japanese bank accounts were seized by the United States government, business licenses were revoked, and the Federal Bureau of Investigation began to arrest an increasing number of Japanese people on suspicion of being spies. The chain of actions prompted the mass evacuation of all mainland Japanese to relocation camps on March 2, 1942.

Across the Pacific Ocean, at the actual sight of battle, all surviving residents united to repel Japan's attack. Suspected Japanese enemies, which included Japanese priests, language school teachers, and community leaders, were immediately taken into custody. Once the danger was over, Nisei members of all military forces were disarmed and relieved of their duties.

Simultaneously, top officials in Washington, D.C., deliberated over steps to be taken against the Japanese people in Hawaii. The idea of mass evacuation was unreasonable, since it would require the use of desperately needed ships and additional military men who were not readily available. Because mass evacuation was a matter of manpower and logistics, they proposed that the Japanese people in Hawaii be treated as citizens in an occupied country. Therefore, except for those that were evacuated, the Japanese people in Hawaii were relatively free to live and work within the island community. And in their effort to prove their loyalty, many volunteered for services under the direction of military personnel and campaigned openly for all Japanese to speak English and act American.

Ogawa indicated that the essential differences between the mainland and Hawaiian experiences were a result of how the Japanese community in each respective area stood with the greater community. The Japanese on the mainland were scattered in diverse communities with no cohesive ethnic community, common leader, or common goals. Their manpower, in comparison to what was available from Caucasians or other minority groups, was too insignificant to be in demand. Therefore, the removal of the Japanese would have no absolute impact on the war effort or the stability of the economy of various communities, since they were so few in number compared to the host population.[59]

Ogawa further pointed out that in Hawaii the Issei and Nisei had become socioeconomically interwoven with the greater Hawaiian community. Consequently, the military and humanitarian reasons for relocation seemed irrational in terms of Hawaii's economic state. The removal of Japanese would mean a severe reduction of the working force and a drastic curtailment of the market's buying and selling power, thereby crippling Hawaii and the Pacific war effort. But more important than economics were the ties of friendship that the Japanese community had established with the military, the civil government, and the non-Japanese.[59]

The chain of actions that took place after the attack on Pearl Harbor elicited a wide range of reactions and changes in the lives of people everywhere. On the mainland, many Japanese families were ruined both psychologically and economically by the forced evacuation. Their lands were either lost, stolen, sold, or confiscated and there was little hope for financial recovery. The bleak outlook caused immeasurable damage to the self-respect of the proud and independent group of people.

The war in addition forced many Japanese Americans everywhere to carefully consider their nationality and ethnic identity, something that they had never done prior to the war. The decision was difficult for many Issei and Kibei, as they were torn between a double loyalty. Loyalty in the Japanese tradition is not of one's personal choice; it is predetermined. Therefore, to be Japanese is to be loyal to Japan, and not to be loyal is never to have been a Japanese. The Issei in particular were caught further in the dilema, having lived most of their lives in the new land and having already called it their home; but more important their children were Americans.[39, 48]

In spite of the fact that many Nisei were in the midst of establishing themselves in their life's goals just prior to the war, as a group they remained loyal to the United States. In their effort to prove their loyalty to the United States, many volunteered to fight against fascism when the military service was reopened. The 100th Battalion and the 442nd Combat Team, made up of Nisei and Kibei, became the vehicles for active participation in the war. Those who did not enlist redoubled their efforts in agriculture and engaged in civilian defense work.

Toward the end of the war, when it became apparent that Japan was defeated, the Supreme Court of the United States determined that the confinement of the Japanese people in the relocation camps was a violation of their constitutional rights.

On January 2, 1945, the gates were officially opened after almost 3 years of exile. The evacuees were now free to leave the camps. Hosts of mixed emotions flooded their minds: excitement over their regained freedom, despair over their losses and having to start all over again, fear over the thoughts of returning to their former homes only to reopen the scars of the evacuation and to face hostile neighbors. Their general outlook was gloomy.

This time of rebirth was not easy, particularly for the Issei, who felt the weight of the oncoming years. A new start meant rebuilding clientele and reinvesting savings that had been eroded by the evacuation and devalued by the war. In spite of the bleak outlook, coupled with the anti-Japanese sentiments of the war, the Nisei moved on, determined to achieve a level of security and comfort.

Kitano suggested that the camp life experiences contributed to the Nisei's determination. It provided them with an opportunity to see themselves as Japanese in a new situation—being a Japanese in Chicago was often different from being a Japanese in California—and the experience broadened their awareness. The camps also exposed the Japanese people to an American model of a small community with block votes, community services, community decisions, and schools, giving the Nisei an opportunity to feel what it was like to be a majority.[39]

After World War II

All remembered World War II as a "period of sacrifice, hardship, grief and finally exaltation—a period when generations of Americans would be tempered by war."[59] For one generation of Americans, the Nisei, the war was remembered as a time when they as Japanese Americans had to prove their loyalty to America by cultural suppression and superpatriotism. The Nisei were a generation on trial and their defense during the war helped to facilitate their success after the war.

Kometani suggests that the war may have been a "blessing in disguise."[41] It compelled the Caucasian American soldiers and Japanese American soldiers to live with each other and discover that they had very few differences except for the color of their skin. The awareness, particularly for those who had a misconstrued view of the Japanese people, helped to bridge the gap of racial understanding among "Americans."

Although anti-Japanese sentiments still lingered after the war, the young Nisei, who had proved their loyalty in countless ways during the war, were not discouraged from fulfilling their personal ambitions. Nisei veterans returned with a greater level of confidence and broader horizons from experiences gained during the war—horrors of combat, traveling, meeting with a wide variety of people, seeing racial discrimination in the South. Instilled with aggression and an optimism for success, many veterans took advantage of the G.I. Bill to further their education and training.

For the Nisei evacuees, the war-time evacuation ironically played an important part in changing both the types of employment they expected to obtain and the types that they actually received. In the evacuation centers, a wide variety of occupations were open to them that had never been available before (e.g., teachers were able to teach). For the first time, with their race no longer a factor in competition, Nisei were able to fill every job a community required except for administration, which was reserved for the Caucasians. Japanese competed against Japanese, so that education, training, and ability determined one's success. Camp life therefore instilled the Nisei evacuees with confidence that they took with them after their release.

For most Nisei, the effects and experiences of the war and their cultural background, with the home stressing hard work, education, success, and economic stability, and school teaching democracy and equality of opportunity, helped to build their hope for social mobility, equality, and success.

One by one the barriers—legal (better immigration laws), social (more involvement with the greater American community), occupational—vanished for Japanese Americans. In time the Nisei found that they could live in virtually any area that they could afford and find employment that was more congruent with their qualifications. The rather remarkable story of the Japanese Americans after World War II has prompted some to call them America's most successful minority group.[40]

The 1970 census revealed that the majority of the Japanese people have risen above the lower levels of the American system. Their mobility centered around the areas of education, income, and occupation.[65] Although the Japanese people have risen above the lower-class levels, they as a group (particularly the mainland Japanese) have generally maintained the middleman position. However, some of the recent changes affecting the Japanese in the United States—(1) continued acculturation into American life with each new generation, (2) continued upward social mobility, and (3) rising rates of intermarriage[30]—may mean an eventual decrease in their visibility, indicating a decrease in discrimination and a rise in power, which should diminish their middleman position.[40]

Today the Japanese are as diverse as any American group. Their history in the United States has encompassed in some families as many as five generations (Issei, Nisei, Sansei, Yonsei, Gosei), so that acculturation, multiple experiences, and differentiation have had a chance to be felt over a period of approximately 80 years.

In recent years, the diversity has been complicated with the settlement of newer Issei from Japan. Unlike the "pioneer" Issei who were homogeneous in terms of age, social class, and residential background, the newer Issei are more heterogeneous and reflect the many changes in the Japanese culture in Japan. Kitano stated that the newer Issei in general "have little intimate contact with the local ethnic communities. . . . many appear at least superficially to be more ac-culturated than the Sansei, especially in terms of personality. Where many Sansei still demonstrate reticence and reserve, the new Issei, reflecting changes in modern Japan, often seem more open and receptive to new ideas."[39] Because of their differences, the newer Issei perhaps provide another frame of looking at the Japanese in the United States.

ISSEI

Most of the surviving pioneer Issei today are retired and facing the problems of old age. Many are resigned to the fact that they are aliens, but because they are so deeply rooted in America, they have accepted it as their home. They as a group continue to cultivate their Meiji "Japaneseness." For some, their problems are typical of most of our senior citizens—income maintenance, health care, social isolation, and finding useful family roles. Others, who perhaps are more fortunate, still have a fairly satisfying and productive life within the Japanese community by participating in Japanese-oriented activities through church and community programs developed for senior citizens. Many live near or with their children and are very much a part of the family life.

NISEI

Many Issei, having considered the future of their children more important than the immediate satisfaction of their own wishes, now measure their success in terms of the success of their Nisei children and Sansei grandchildren. The Nisei in general have rewarded their parents' sacrifices, in spite of their traditional position of being faced with the resolutions of two cultural demands that drove them to succeed and achieve.

The Nisei are presently in their middle years, with ages ranging from the thirties to sixties. They, like any group of established, fairly affluent, middle-aged people, find themselves concerned with leisure and community service as well as concerned over the behaviors and successful achievements of their Sansei children and Yonsei grandchildren.[17,39]

SANSEI

The majority of the Sansei are currently between their twenties and forties. Some are in the process of raising their Yonsei children. They have inherited a place that generations before them had struggled to achieve and had given shape and purpose to, creating the status of the

Japanese people as accepted neighbors. Such foundations helped to make the Sansei's assimilation into the American society smoother. Many have also benefited from the relative economic success of their parents, particularly in the area of education. In some families, the Nisei's motivation for success and achievement has exerted a tremendous amount of pressure on the Sansei to excel and become overachievers.

Sociologists have indicated that the Sansei as a group have almost completely acculturated themselves, yet a great number still retain a large part of their ethnic identity and Meiji Japanese ways.[17,32,39,50,52,54] Perhaps more accurately:

> ... the major generalization for the Sansei relates to individual differences. By now the relative homogeneity of the Issei and the Nisei have given way to the Sansei (and the Yonsei, or fourth generation), who are products of a freer and more open world. The boundary maintenance mechanisms entrapping the previous generations in narrow stereotypes are no longer as effective as they once were, nor are the socialization and social-control techniques of parents in shaping their children. Therefore, there has developed a more visible range of individual differences, which has been reflected in a wider span of expectation, life styles, and behavior.[39]

THE TRADITIONAL JAPANESE FAMILY

The traditional social structure and religious values of the feudal fiefs greatly influenced the importance of the family unit and family relations. It emphasized solidarity, mutual assistance, and a patriarchal structure in which the eldest male, usually the father, was the head of the household and maintained a strong authoritarian control over the family.

The concept of family, while stressing Confucian parental authority and filial piety, eventually incorporated the moral duties and authoritarian principles of the lord-vassal relationship, which served as the model conduct in the traditional society. It emphasized hard work, duty, obligation, and responsibility.

The family also incorporated the samurai moral teachings into respect for age and seniority: parent-child, husband-wife, elder-younger sibling, and other familial relationships.

The hierarchical structure concept was eventually incorporated into the inheritance of the family estate, which was passed on to the first-born son. The successor to the estate was treated specially from his early life and siblings were expected to show him respect. The heir, upon the assumption of the headship, also acquired the responsibility of providing and caring for his retiring parents, who frequently lived with his family.

Each individual member of the house was assigned to a definite role in the hierarchical scale, which bound him to others in a network of moral duties and rules for proper conduct. Interaction was therefore based on clearly prescribed roles, duties, and responsibilities rather than on personal affection.

Love, although undoubtedly present in many families, was not the essential element for gaining social control. It was secondary to rules, duty, obligation, and tradition. The Japanese child was more apt to hear "You will obey mother because you have to," rather than the American prescription of "You will obey mother because you love her." Kitano suggests that the early training, emphasizing the more impersonal types of interaction, may have helped the Japanese to fit into the bureaucratic structures with less difficulty.[39]

Another important aspect of family interaction was its emphasis on filial piety (oyakoko). It was a reciprocal obligation between parent and child. For example, the parent(s) may give up the choicer cut of meat for his child or sacrifice his own pleasures in order to send a child to college. The child in return showed respect to his parents, was a "good" child, never questioned his parents' decision, and did not bring shame to the family. Filial piety enjoins all the responsibilities that rest upon the "head of the family to provide for his children, educate his sons and younger brothers, see to the management of the estate, give shelter to relatives who need it and a thousand similar everyday duties."[8]

Benedict noted that the greatest antagonism in the family was between the mother-in-law and daughter-in-law, particularly if the daughter-in-law was married to the family heir. The relationship was built on the premise that the daughter-in-law comes into the home as a stranger. It is her duty to learn how her mother-in-law likes to have things done and then learn to do them. In many instances, the mother-in-law takes the position that the young wife is not quite good enough for her son. The young daughter-in-law is therefore endlessly submissive. It is said, however, that the daughter-in-law eventually becomes a mother-in-law who is as reacting and critical as her own mother-in-law.[8]

One of the most important factors in Japanese life was the "ie" or ancestral clan, or house and its name. In practice, the ie was similar to an extended family. It was a social unit and formed the basis for interaction with the greater social structure. Status, name, lineage, and customs were attached to the ie. Nakane indicated that the ie was a continuum from the past to the future and its members included the present as well as the dead and the unborn.[56]

The ie was one of the strongest reference groups in the Japanese social system and controlled and managed the individuals making up the unit. It was a central factor in the traditional marriages by arranging for meetings between families by the official "go-between" (Nakaodo). The go-between, in arranging the marriage, would be careful to analyze the family lineage to make certain of its proper ranks, background, status, and that it was free from any inferior qualities.

The importance of the ie over the individual can also be seen in the care with which the family members avoid bringing shame to the family. Benedict reported that once a child started school he became a representative of the family. If he engaged in behaviors that brought shame to the family, he could not look to the family for support. The family name had been disgraced.[8]

At the time of the Issei's migration to the continental United States and Hawaii, many left without their parents and grandparents. There was no older generation to serve as a reminder or to fulfill the traditional responsibility of teaching the young roles and rituals of Japanese life, so the culture and the childrearing practices were based on what they had learned and remembered.

THE PIONEER JAPANESE FAMILY

The pioneer families continued many of the traditional Japanese patterns of behavior, particularly in being interdependent with the larger Japanese neighborhood and community units. Many initially lived in rooming houses that were generally maintained and populated by members of the same ken (prefecture).

The early life of the Issei family had many unfavorable aspects to its structure: the arranged marriages, the need to adapt to a new spouse and to a new land, the crowded and inferior housing, poverty, the anti-Japanese sentiments, and little hope for social change. The conditions also made attempts to introduce the traditional village life of their homeland difficult. Though the pioneers were disillusioned, much emphasis was placed on the traditional values of duty, obligation, and "ga-man" (which refers to the internalization of anger and emotion and sticking things out).

The Issei's new life of rapid industrialization and urbanization made it difficult to totally re-create the ie (house) system. But because of the absence of their extended family, since their parents and grandparents remained in Japan, it eventually grew to include other immigrants from the homeland village, ken, and later the entire Japanese community. Although the ie was altered, it still had a significant impact on the family, peer group, and community patterns. It was successful in controlling the behaviors of its members, who in turn were characterized by conformity and little social deviance.

The Issei continued to think of the family as a unit and a foundation of society. When they established homes of their own and children were born, their ideal of family solidarity was used as a basis for training and disciplining their children.

The idea of "family honor" was deeply ingrained within each family member. The family was an important social economic unit and demanded obedience of its individual members, so that their status in the community could be enhanced and protected. The family could not be shamed and each individual member could not do anything that reflected negatively on the image that the family projected to its neighbors and friends. Independence and individualism were secondary to the family image.

The family controlled its members' behaviors by placing emphasis on duty, obligation, responsibility, the use of shame and guilt, and one's ethnic identity. For example, a child quickly learned that his behavior, good or bad, did not end at himself but extended to his family and community. It was his responsibility to be on good behavior, and to be recognized as a good child and a good Japanese because these things reflected on the goodness of his family ("good Japanese family") in the eyes of the community. Bad behavior brought shame to the family and produced feelings of guilt in the member who brought the disgrace. Strong family ties discouraged juvenile delinquency; it was considered a disgrace to the family for a member to be apprehended by the police for breaking the law.

The patriarchal hierarchy continued with the

father as the head of the house and director of the interests of the family group. He was the judge in all matters pertaining to the welfare of the family, was usually central in the disciplinary scheme, and was the official representative in civic affairs.

The position of the female within the family reflected submission and deference more than equality. She usually stayed at home and saw that the father had every possible comfort. She was also responsible for managing the family budget and the everyday domestic affairs of the family. She devoted herself to her family and had very few social activities. In the eyes of the patriarch and the family, a good wife was a woman who, by bringing forth sons, helped to safeguard and perpetuate the family name, and by being obedient, properly humble and diligent, helped to maintain peace and order in the family.

Family meals, particularly dinner, were eaten with all members present. The father is served first, then sons in descending order of age, daughters, and finally the mother.

Non-verbalization was stressed within the family institution. Kitano points out that:

> The most distinctive characteristic of Japanese family interaction was, and still remains, the absence of prolonged verbal exchange. Although some of the common strategies to gain support through manipulation or cajoling were present, very few problems were resolved through open discussion between parent and children. Instead, arguments were one-sided, and most Nisei can remember the phrase da-mat-to-re (keep quiet) that concluded them. Verbalization, talking out, and mutual discussion were actively discouraged.[39]

For some Nisei adolescents, the cultural demands of both the Japanese and the American cultures brought forth familial problems, particularly in the area of language and cultural conflict. Language problems between parent and child arose when the Nisei children picked up English from school and their peers, and since their parents were often too busy to teach them the proper Japanese, spoke neither English nor Japanese correctly. To assist in bridging the gap, Japanese language schools were started to provide a communication medium within the home. The schools also reinforced the traditional norms of proper conduct and behavior as well as the fine arts of the Japanese culture.

Despite the absence of the Issei's parents and grandparents, who usually had the responsibility of teaching the young roles and rituals of Japanese life, the early Issei-Nisei family was intact with prescribed roles, duties, and responsibilities for each family member. Their lives continued in the shared patterns of family respect, obligation, and parental authority, with a sensitive regard for honor, image, and status, and the intense personal identification with the family unit.

WAR AND THE JAPANESE FAMILY

During the war, while the mainland Japanese families were abandoning their homes and possessions for nearly 3 years, the Japanese families in Hawaii, except for those that were evacuated, were generally unaffected by the emotional outrages of the military and public authorities on the mainland. Their family life remained fairly intact and they were relatively free to live and work within the island community.[59]

Kitano reported that the financial losses, together with the camp policies of utilizing American Nisei in positions of camp responsibility, worked to shift power and influences away from the Issei and onto the shoulders of the Nisei. This exerted a definite influence on the structure of the Japanese family and worked to free the Nisei from Issei influences.[39]

The family structure was also affected by the physical conditions of camp life. The lack of privacy, the community mess hall arrangements, the communal duties, and dependency on the government rather than on the head of the household contributed to the reordering, which required certain changes in roles and expectations.

Mealtime ceased to be a family affair: men often ate together, while mothers and younger children shared a table. The older children drifted to other parts of the mess hall with their peers, thus limiting the parents' ability to guide and discipline them. The customary family rituals associated with the mealtime gathering began to disappear.

The changes imposed by the camp life also affected the roles of the husband and wife. Men were no longer the breadwinners; their wives and older children often earned the same amount of wages. This threatened the prestige of the men and they no longer felt as important and necessary to their families, which lead them to loose much of their firm control over their families. These circumstances also forced women into positions of independence.

War also reshaped the Japanese way of life in Hawaii. During the early period of the war, while awaiting news of whether they were to evacuate en masse or not, the Japanese people actively engaged in Americanization efforts in fear and in demonstration of their loyalty. "Speak English" and "Act American" campaigns flooded the islands.

The war and the efforts to exercise a 100 percent Americanism repatterned the roles and relationships within the family. Many of the Nisei were already adults or reaching adulthood and perhaps were better equipped (more American than their Issei parents—they held citizenship and understood the American culture better) to move relatively freely within the society. This forced the Nisei to become the authority in the family, thereby reversing the parent-child roles. Many Nisei children forced their parents to stay at home in fear that they would become the focus of hate and revenge. Children also enforced disciplinary rules on their parents, such as "don't wear kimono," "speak English," and "don't bow like a Japanese."

Ogawa also noted that the war altered the husband-wife relationship, because many Issei and Nisei women joined in the war efforts by volunteering for services at the Salvation Army, Red Cross, and other organizations, and were not able to perform the necessary womanly chores customary in the Japanese home.[59] Women were also freed of the stiff obi bindings and wrappings of the kimono since it was a representation of Japan and had become forsaken. The war imposed new alternatives and life-styles, particularly on the young Nisei women, changes that their Issei parents in previous years would have suppressed. Women were also taken out of the home and put into schools, factories, assembly lines, or professional jobs. The independent employment exposed her to many alternatives outside of the family and the ethnic community. Although accustomed to the role of wife and mother, she found it equally challenging as a co-provider for the family. The working woman soon became a more acceptable role. The pattern of the husband and wife as co-contributors to the family income exposed their Sansei children to a family structure that was more closely associated with the American middle-class family. The passive role of the females in the cultural practices of the Japanese family was even more seriously questioned when Nisei women were recruited into the United States armed services.

Dr. Dennis Ogawa, a sociologist, summarized the familial changes of the war in Hawaii by pointing out that:

> With the changing nature of the Japanese family due to the lessening of Issei parental discipline, the emergence of the Nisei as household authorities, and the liberalization of the female role, the character of the Japanese community was rapidly being transformed. The war was effectively disrupting the rigid boundaries which had separated the Japanese from the non-Japanese. No longer totally restrained by the traditionalism of the Issei culture, many Nisei in defense work, in the military service, and in their daily relations with the broader non-Japanese community expanded their contacts with people of all races. The outcome of these interethnic contacts was an increasing rate of interracial marriages for the second generation. . . . the assimilation of the Japanese community into the Island society was being accelerated.[59]

THE JAPANESE-AMERICAN FAMILY TODAY

Research analysis and studies done by sociologists[1, 17, 25, 32, 39, 59] on the Japanese-American family structure, whether on the mainland or Hawaii, report that "though the family had become structurally attuned to urban society, patterns of relationship stemming from the spirit of ie tenaciously survived."[59] The maintenance of the ie patterns in the family can be seen especially in the development of the Japanese modified extended family pattern. As the family grew and became more nuclear in profile, they were still linked, attitudinally and socially, with an extended kinship pattern. The nuclear family unit was adapted into the entire Japanese-American community in a modified extended network of relational dependence and obligations.

Dr. Colleen Johnson, a sociologist, conducted a study on kinship interactions among a sample of Nisei and Sansei Japanese Americans in Honolulu. The results of her study demonstrated that although urbanization and economic changes resulted in the nuclearization of the family, there was a progressively strong identification of succeeding generations with the extended family network. Her data also indicated that although the ethnic group as a whole had less relevancy to the Sansei lives, the ethnic family composed of parents, grandparents, aunts, uncles, cousins, and so on had a significant impact, particularly in creating cultural and psychological stability in the home. In spite of the fact that the modified extended family did not live under the same roof, they were still involved in relationships of extensive interdependency. Johnson attributes a part of this to the insularity of island living, which has permitted extensive social mobility but limited geographical mobility, resulting in a larger number of accessible kin.[32]

Dr. Dennis Ogawa, in his book entitled *Kodomo no tame ni: For the Sake of the Children—The Japanese American Experience in Hawaii*, maintains that, for the Sansei and their children, the emergence of grandparents as active cultural transmitters also enhanced the ethnic integrity of the evolving Japanese family. "Grandparents, especially in the extended family situation, are 'caretakers' of culture, passing on the cultural continuity of their world view to their grandchildren."[59]

Similarly, Kitano states that although the American styles of the Nisei and Sansei family do not allow the grandparents the same honor and responsibility they would have in Japan, they still have a definite and respected place within the family. Futhermore, since most Issei continue to live with or near their children and are an integral part of the family, the extended family network is allowed to perpetuate.[39]

Significantly, Johnson's study revealed that 75 percent of the Nisei and 58 percent of the Sansei in her study identified respect for elders as an advantage of the Japanese family.[32]

Johnson's study further indicated that the mechanisms that maintained the modified extended family's solidarity were identified as having sources in the value system derived from Japan of the Meiji era. The value system that emphasized sociocentricity (precedence given to the primary group interests over individual group interests), obligation to parents, reciprocity, and dependence was translated into the regulation of kin relationships. For example, she observed that the obligatory nature of the tie between parent and child had laid the ground rules for the binding nature of other forms of reciprocity.

Johnson further reported that the cohesiveness of the family tie has persisted and even increased despite structural changes in the family from a patrilineal to the bilateral American form and despite considerable social mobility. The ef-

fects of the structural change were largely due to a redistribution of indebtedness to parents among the entire sibling group rather than it being centered on the eldest son. She suggests that the sharing of filial obligations contributed to the high kin solidarity.[32]

Similarly, Dr. John Connor, an anthropologist, conducted a study on the retention of characteristics that are associated with the Japanese family system (ie) among three generations of Japanese Americans in Sacramento. The results of his study indicated that while the emphasis on the family and the maintenance of dependency needs among the Sansei were lower than among the Nisei or Issei, the emphasis still remained higher than that found in Caucasian Americans.[17]

In spite of the continuation of the extended family patterns, the male-female relationships continued to undergo structural changes in the 1960s and 1970s, particularly among the Sansei generation. The discrepency between independence and sex-role limitations especially affected the Sansei female. Although the attitudes of the male seemed to be in direct agreement with the dominant male of traditional Japan, there were movements toward a more egalitarian conception of both sexes.[1,5,25]

Finally, it is important to emphasize that while such generalizations about the Japanese-American family may be true for a number of families, each is unique and will reflect variations in attitude and behavior.

THE VALUE OF CHILDREN IN THE FAMILY

The Value of Children—A Cross-National Study, by Dr. Fred Arnold and colleagues, which looked at the psychological, economical, and social satisfactions of having children, as perceived by parents in Korea, Taiwan, Japan, Philippines, Thailand, and Hawaii (this population included the Japanese, Caucasians, and Filipinos), stated the following:

> Children are more than the object of their parents' attention and love; they are also a biological and social necessity. The human species perpetuates itself through children; cultures, religions, and national groups transmit their values and traditions through children; families maintain their lineage through children; and individuals pass on their genetic and social heritage through children. The ultimate value of children is the continuity of humanity.[5]

The findings of the *Value of Children* study illustrated the importance of children for the Japanese in both Japan and Hawaii (Fig. 2). The following includes some of the general results of the study.[5,6]

Psychological Advantages

The majority of the respondents in both rural (Hawaii was excluded in all rural data, because the subsample did not include persons from this socioeconomic group) and urban Japan and Hawaii mentioned various psychological and emotional advantages (e.g., happiness, love, companionship) of having children and frequently mentioned that it was "instinctive" or "natural" to have children.

Socioeconomic Advantages

Differences were seen between rural and urban lower class and urban middle class. The rural and urban lower class showed high expectations for economic assistance from their children when they reached old age. Their responses were further supported by their greater concern over financial costs of raising their children.

Sex Preference

In 1953, the United States Territorial Department of Health in Hawaii conducted a study on cultural beliefs and practices with Issei and Nisei mothers.[66] It was reported that the Issei mothers had a popular saying: "First a girl, then a boy." The family was pleased to have a male child to carry on the family name. (If there were no sons, the oldest daughter married the second son of a family and took her surname to perpetuate the family name.)

The majority of the Nisei mothers did not respond to male sex preference. Those that did stated that it was important to carry on the family name, the husband wanted a companion, and a son could take care of the family.

Similarly, the data from the *Value of Children* study revealed that the majority of respondents in Japan and Hawaii showed a male over female preference. Responses for male preference in Japan were somewhat higher than from their counterparts in Hawaii. In both countries, the major emphasis for the male preference was on the psychological satisfactions provided by the sons while they were children (companionship for the father, positive behavioral and personality traits), and when they were older, continuity of the family name.

Daughters, on the other hand, were still greatly desired in both countries. The most frequently cited reasons were psychological satisfaction, practical help, daughters remained at home with the family, companionship for the mother, positive behavioral and personality traits, and help with the housework. The reasons seem to reflect universal aspects of female sex-role prescription.

Family Size

After the post-war baby boom, the Japanese birth rate in the United States began to stabilize to typical American urban patterns. In 1960, the average size of the Japanese family was 4.0, but dropped to 2.67 in 1970.[65]

The findings of the *Value of Children* study indicated that, in all countries, family size in general was interdependent with the psychosocioeconomic needs of the family. For example, the rural areas saw the greater number of children as a greater burden to educate, but felt that they could afford a larger number of children and had greater expectations of economic help from their children. (The investigators of the study suggested that the conflicting responses on economics may have been due to the respondents' reluctance to say that they could not afford to have children.) The urban middle class felt that they could afford the "desired" number and were able to raise them. They seemed to reflect a desire for children of a higher quality at a greater cost per child.

The study also revealed that the "mean number of children wanted" (number of living children plus number of additional children wanted) by the Japanese in Hawaii living within the urban lower class was 2.7, and in the middle class was 3.0. It was interesting to note that the "mean number of children ideal" (number of children respondents would want to have if they were starting their families again) was 3.1 in both groups. These data also suggest that the respondents seem to have realistic perceptions of the average American family size.

In 1946 Ruth Benedict, in *The Chrysanthemum and the Sword*, reported that Japanese parents, as parents in the United States, want children "because it is a pleasure to have a child."[9] But the Japanese parents also wanted children for other reasons that seem to have much less weight in America.

Japanese parents need children, not only for the emotional satisfaction, but because they have failed in life if they have not carried on the

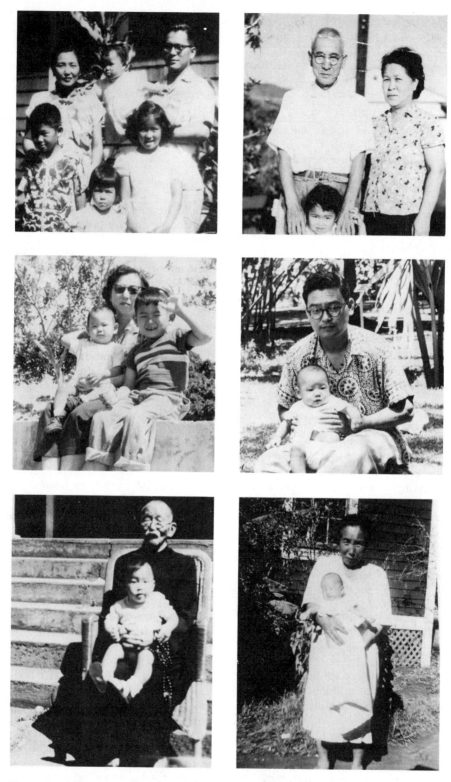

Figure 2. Children are an integral part of the Japanese family life.

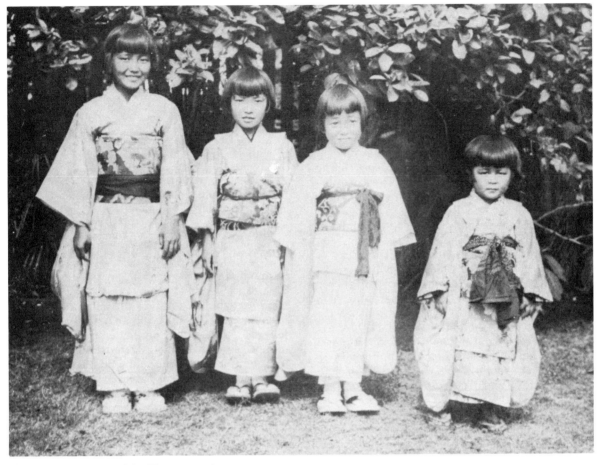

Figure 3. Girls dressed for Hinamatsuri.

family line. The need for children also varies with each parent. As for the male in the traditional Japanese culture:

> Every Japanese man must have a son. He needs him to do daily homage to his memory after his death at the living-room shrine before the miniature gravestone. He needs him to perpetuate the family line down the generations and to preserve the family honor and possessions. For traditional social reasons the father needs his son almost as much as the young son needs his father. For a few years the father is trustee of the "house." Later it will be his son. If the father could not pass trusteeship to his son, his own role would have been played in vain. This deep sense of continuity prevents the dependency of the fully grown son on his father, even when it is continued so much longer than it is the United States, from having the aura of shame and humiliation which it so generally has in Western nations.[9]

And for the female in the traditional Japanese culture:

> A woman too wants children not only for her emotional satisfaction in them but because it is only as a mother that she gains status. A childless wife has a most insecure position in the family, and even if she is not discarded she can never look forward to being a mother-in-law and exercising authority over her son's marriage and over her son's wife. Her husband will adopt a son to carry on his line but according to Japanese ideas the childless woman is still the loser. Japanese women are expected to be good childbearers.[9]

Children have always been an integral part of the Japanese family life. Two practices traditional to the Japanese society that continue to be observed in the United States in the honor of children, though on a smaller scale, are the celebration of special days for girls and boys.

Girls' Day, also known as Hinamatsuri, the Peach Festival, or Festival of Dolls, is held yearly on the third day of the third month (March 3) (Fig. 3). There are many interpretations given for the festival. In traditional Japan, families observe it to encourage filial piety, ancestor worship, loyalty, and above all their love of their children, their joy and pride in them, and their desire to please them.[21]

Families start the collection of display dolls at the birth of a female child. At each succeeding Girls' Day, new dolls are added. They are displayed in the best room of the home and usually consist of at least 15 dolls dressed in the ancient costumes (Emperor and Empress, three ladies-in-waiting, five musicians, two retainers, and three guards), and other artistic productions of miniature household articles. All dolls are displayed on a tier of steps, covered with a bright red cloth. The Imperial couple (Dairi-sama) occupy the top step, followed by the other dolls on the lower steps. Girls quickly learn that they are ceremonial dolls and not to be played with.[20, 21]

Peach blossoms, symbolizing happiness in marriage and feminine characteristics of softness, mildness, and peacefulness, are among the decorations of the stand.

Girls are often dressed in special, bright kimonos and are served hishi-mochi or a diamond-shaped mochi (rice cake) in three colors (white, red, and green) and other special foods. The shape of the mochi is said to have originated from a diamond-shaped medicinal leaf thought to have the property of giving long life to the eater. White represents the snow of winter, red the flowers of spring, and green the fresh vegetation of the summer.

Recently, a Sansei mother of three girls responded to why she celebrates Girls' Day:

> As a parent, I wanted to instill in my children some ideas and acceptance of our traditions, to help them understand and appreciate some of the cultural aspects that are gradually being lost by our modern fast pace of living. So at their early stages of life, I have tried to be that link of information and hope a little will be retained and maybe at least one of the girls will be influenced to carry on what I learned and passed down to them.
>
> Why do I find it necessary to do these little things? Mostly because I believe my role as a parent is to learn and teach my children what I feel is vital to their well-rounded basis or foundation towards live-

lihood. This came about, not instantaneously but because my parents performed their responsibilities to try and lay down a basic foundation that they felt was just as important.

> Reaction of the girls? Even at this early age, they know the Girls' Day dolls are not to be played with but stand for something ceremonious. They also know a little about its history from the information I've read to them. They have helped make certain foods that are eaten on that day. They have been able to share what information I have passed on to them with others, especially at school.
>
> Father's participation and reaction? He being the only child, always helped by building the stands to place the dolls, encouraged me to increase the collection. Enjoyed recording the girls' reaction on photos. Likes to see these things done with our children, having closer relationships with our girls.*

Boys' Day, also known as Boys' Festival, Tango-no-Sekku (the First Day of the Horse) or Shobu-no-Sekku (Iris Festival), is celebrated yearly on the fifth day of the fifth month. One interpretation of tango is that the horses displayed in the festival symbolically represent the manliness, bravery, and strength desired in boys. An interpretation of the shobu (iris) is that its long and narrow leaf represents the sword blade. The boys are bathed in an iris-bath (shobu-ya), which is said to instill a samurai spirit in them. They, too, are dressed in bright kimonos and carry a wooden sword called the iris sword or shobu-katana.[20, 21]

In ancient times, the heirlooms (armor, helmet, leg guard, and weapons) of the samurai ancestor were brought out (today simulated ones are used) and displayed on tiered shelves together with miniature samurai dolls depicting scenes and characters in the well-known heroic stories of Japan. The Boys' Day display like the Girls' Day display was always in the best room of the home.

Koi-noboi (carp streamers) of paper or cloth are flown for each son on the roof of the homes. The symbol of the carp is used because it is believed that the carp has the power to fight its way up the swift streams, and because of its determination to overcome obstacles it is held to be a perfect example for a growing boy, typifying ambition, strength, and the will to overcome difficulties.

Boys are served kashiwa mochi, which is a

---

*Personal interview, Hawaii, 1978.

specially shaped delicacy said to have taken its shape from a samurai helmet, and other special foods.

CHILDREARING

Childrearing is a task that all adults who are responsible for a child face, regardless of cultural identity. The common denominators of the tasks are set by the developmental phases of the newborn and the growing child, but specific ways of handling the child vary widely on the basis of cultural norms and individual variations.

William Caudill, an anthropologist, and his associates compared childrearing patterns among Caucasian American, motherland Japanese, and Japanese-American mothers.[13,15,16] According to Caudill and his associates, a Caucasian American mother was more individual oriented and independent, more self-assertive and aggressive, and would take time to explain what she believed were rational reasons for her actions. She saw her infant from birth as a separate and autonomous individual with his own needs and desires. She therefore helped him to express these needs and desires through her emphasis on vocal communication. She was noted to be more lively and had a more stimulating approach to her baby—positioning baby's body more, looking at and chatting to baby more. Separateness and independence are stressed by having the infant sleep in his own crib shortly after birth and the mother was observed to leave the room once her infant was asleep; early weaning from breast or bottle and teaching self-feeding usually began before the first year. Exploration of the body or environment was welcomed. In general, she seemed to desire a more vocal and active baby.

In contrast, the motherland Japanese mother was observed to be more group oriented and interdependent in her relations with others, more self-effacing and passive, and when matters required a decision she was more likely to rely on her emotional feeling and intuition. The mother appeared to view her infant as an extension of herself. She made a conscious use of many forms of nonverbal communications through gestures and close physical proximity. The mother was observed to rock, lull, soothe, and sleep with her infant and thereby gratify and indulge dependent needs, while independence was less fostered. In general, she was observed to have more physical contact and a more soothing and quieting ap-

proach with her infant and seemed to desire a more quiet and contented baby.

The Japanese-American mothers, on the other hand, appeared to be somewhere in between. They had come to behave like other American mothers, but at the same time retained much of their mothers' behavior.

In 1961 and 1964, Kitano conducted two studies, using the Parental Attitude Research Inventory (PARI). Both studies illustrated changes in parental childrearing attitudes by Japanese generational background.[35,36]

The first study compared childrearing attitudes among a sample of Issei and Nisei in Los Angeles. The data revealed the Issei to have a higher mean score, representing a restrictive way of raising children. The Issei view of childrearing was more traditional; children were recognized as dependent, quiet, unequal, and to be raised with strictness. In contrast, the Nisei view reflected a more contemporary American practice: children were regarded as comrades with whom they could share their experiences, and were encouraged to ask questions and permitted a higher degree of sexual exploration.[35]

The second study by Kitano compared a younger and older Nisei generation with similar age populations in Japan. The findings of the study reflected differences between age groups rather than national groups. Intergroup comparisons of the same age group across national lines revealed similar attitudes. Kitano suggested that childrearing attitudes are a measure of age-generation changes and acculturation.[36]

Higa conducted a similar study using the same PARI scale and comparing three groups of Japanese mother: (1) Nisei Japanese-American mothers reared and residing in Hawaii, (2) Japanese mothers born and educated in Japan and moving to Hawaii with their American husbands after World War II (these women were often referred to as War Brides), and (3) motherland Japanese mothers, born and educated in Japan. According to his results, the Japanese-American mothers were the most restrictive in their maternal attitudes. They were followed by the motherland mothers and lastly by the immigrant mothers. Higa attributed the differences in attitudes to differences in cultural background.[29]

In an attempt to find more meaning in his findings, Higa conducted an unsystematic interview with some Japanese-American and immigrant mothers. His assumption prior to the interview was that Japanese-American mothers acquired their restrictive attitudes from their parents or grandparents who migrated to Hawaii in the early 1900s.

Higa's interview with the Japanese-American mothers revealed that they were extremely conscious of being Japanese Americans, particularly in reference to other ethnic groups in Hawaii. He suggested that the consciousness of the mothers seemed to impel them to become overzealous disciplinarians, instill ideas of not disgracing their race, and drive their children to surpass the children of other ethnic groups.

Although Higa does not support his original assumption, I believe that the data from his interview do reflect a retention of some of the traditional Meiji Japanese values. For example, the mothers' use of ethnic identity, shame, and disgrace can be seen as an attempt to preserve the family's honor and the desire for achievement in their children; this, too, can be related to the pioneer Issei's strong desire for upward mobility—a desire they tried to instill in their Nisei children.

The second part of Higa's interview dealt with the immigrant mothers. He noted that the interview strongly suggested the mothers' tendency toward "hyper-correction or hyper-adjustment," as they seemed to justify their liberal attitude toward their children by asserting that they are in a free, democratic country and that their children are American rather than Japanese. While Higa's assumptions may be true, it is also important to consider the changes in the Japanese culture in Japan at the time of the immigrant mothers' departure, so that appropriate behavioral distinctions (whether they are a result of cultural changes in the motherland or responses to the American culture) can be made.

In addition, Johnson's study on kinship interactions among Japanese Americans notably showed that Nisei maternal attitudes toward children gave precedence to the primary group interest over individual interests. The findings of the study also revealed that a majority of the mothers selected those behaviors related to concern for others, humility, and compassion, while independence as a goal in childrearing was generally rejected.[32]

While the above studies reveal generational changes in the styles of childrearing and reflect a retention of traditional Japanese values in Nisei childrearing attitudes, other studies on the Sansei show an even greater movement toward an American orientation with the retention and alteration of select traditional values.[1,4,10,17,18,25,49,54] The styles of childrearing practices can not help but change from one generation to the next, particularly with the influence of the American media, which actively advertise the availability of the wide variety of resources specific to child care, such as parent education classes, American baby magazines, Dr. Spock's child care books, and other countless resources. Japanese parents in America today are offered a greater number of choices. The selection they make, with individual alterations, and the impact of their own childrearing, which contains a part of their cultural heritage, make each family and child unique yet similar in terms of common cultural norms.

Interviews with a Nisei grandmother and Sansei mother illustrate one example of generational changes in the style of child care with a retention of some traditional ways:

> *Nisei:* When I was raising our children, I read books from the library, did what the doctor recommended, and what my mother and mother-in-law wanted me to do. If there was a problem, I would use what I thought was best. Sometimes it required the utilization of combinations.
> *Sansei:* When our baby was having a period of chronic diarrhea, the doctor recommended that I remove everything from her diet and start with diluted soda pop. I was skeptical about the diet, so I consulted my mom. She agreed with me. I decided to try. But, after a week of no improvement, my mom and I started her on okai (soft rice boiled with a greater amount of water) diet and securely but not tightly bound her abdomen with a soft cloth. [Binding the abdomen is said to prevent the child's stomach from overexertion.] Her diarrhea was cured within the next day or so. My mom learned this from her mom and it worked for us.*

Early Infancy

To the Japanese people, the three most important events in life are birth, marriage, and death. Each are celebrated accordingly.

As it did for their mothers, childbirth for the Issei took place in the home, usually with the assistance of a midwife, although in many instances the father was the primary or only atten-

---

*Personal interview, Hawaii, 1978.

dant. Seeking medical or hospital care was unheard of during those times, as it was usually reserved for the sick. The birth of a child was a family affair and a great event in the Japanese family life.

Unlike their mothers or grandmothers, the Nisei and Sansei experienced childbirth similar to that of the American culture. Nancy Shand-Kovach describes the initial mother-infant interaction as follows:

> . . . a brief glimpse of the infant after birth, perhaps a momentary holding of the infant a quarter of an hour later, then separation for several hours, accompanied by isolation of the mother in recovery and the infant in an incubator. Separation of the mother and infant continues throughout the postpartum hours and days, interrupted only by intermittent feedings during which mother-infant interaction can take place.[62]

Recently, however, there has been an emergence of a reverse trend of mother-infant separation procedures with a return to childbirth as a family affair in a number of American hospitals. There is now family center maternity care, with birthing rooms, active participation of the father in the delivery room (which often includes time for breastfeeding), rooming-in, sibling visitation, and a host of other alternatives offered to childbearing families today. Many young American (Japanese included) families take an active interest and participate in the experiences.

In the traditional Japanese culture, the sex of the child determined the number of days that the mother should convalesce after childbirth: 31 days for a boy, 32 days for a girl. During this time she would take sponge baths and avoid showers, tub baths, and washing her hair. She also needed to avoid doing housework or any strenuous activity. The woman's mother or another relative usually managed the household activities for that period. Today, it is not unusual to find the woman's mother, who if necessary travels a great distance, assisting in the household work after delivery, no matter if it is the first or fourth child. A Nisei mother recently described her experiences:

> I took care of myself with my first two children in the traditional ways: no housework because it was too strenuous, no reading or sewing because it put a strain on one's eyes. We essentially had to avoid anything that put a strain on any part of the body. I had the family support which was nice, but when my

third one arrived, my boss needed me back at work and I needed to keep my job for our family finances. So the working demands made it somewhat difficult to continue such cultural practices.*

Today, the postpartum period varies in length and quality. The usual hospital stay is 2 to 3 days for a normal vaginal delivery. The mother's stay at home is dependent on the variable psychosocioeconomic needs of the mother and the family (e.g., the mother's health, length of time allowed by employer, stability of the family income, her desire to return to work).

CELEBRATIONS

A Japanese tradition that takes place 7 days after the infant's birth is a celebration for its naming. The infant's head is shaved and he then receives a name that has been especially selected by his grandparents. Each name, depending on how it is written, has a special meaning. Names were often selected to help mold the character of the child. Boys were often given samurai names or names with the prefix depicting their birth order. Girls were often given earthy names like "Yukie," meaning snow. After the infant receives its name, the name is written on a piece of paper and placed at the family Buddhist altar. "Chan," meaning honorable child, is often added to the end of the name. Many Issei are known to have carried on this custom in America. A Nisei father reminisces:

> Since many of us were delivered at home by the midwives, and the city didn't have any rules about when a child needed to be registered, there was no real rush to have us named like they do in hospitals today. So, our families could partake in the customs. I was registered with the city 9 days after my birth, so my legal birthday is not accurate.*

The traditional celebration of naming the child was not carried over to today's Japanese-American family life, but the selection of the infant's name is still quite important. Japanese-American children are usually given an English first name and a Japanese middle name, which is often specially selected by their grandparents or great-grandparents, or sometimes taken from a close ancestor.

The next traditional event in the infant's life is "Miyamairi," meaning shrine visit. If the infant

---

*Personal interview, Hawaii, 1978.

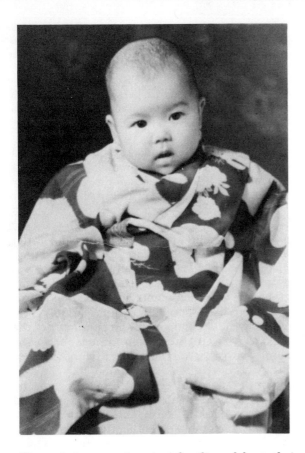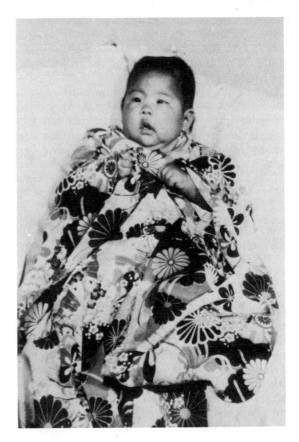

Figure 4. Japanese-American families celebrate their children's 100th day of life.

is a boy, it takes place on the thirty-second day, and if it is a girl, the ceremony is held on the thirty-third day. On the occasion, the infant is taken to the shrine of the local deity to give thanks and to pray for the child's welfare—that he grow up strong and healthy. The infant is dressed in his best clothing and is carried in the arms or on the back of his grandmother or nurse. The mother is not allowed to attend because she is considered impure and cannot yet approach the presence of the Kami or god. The party, consisting of relatives and friends, forms a procession to the shrine, each carrying one of the baby's beautiful kimonos.[21]

Arriving at the shrine, the priest performs a ceremony of purifying and blessing the infant. The infant is thereby freed from all evil that it may have brought from the other world and the child enters this life clean, pure, and noble.

After the ceremony, the infant is taken to visit relatives and friends. At this time, bags of ame

(wheat gluten) are given as presents from the infant. In the past, when a mother failed to lactate a sufficient supply of milk, the baby was fed ame. Therefore, to give ame as a gift represents the infant's willingness to share his food with his friends. In return for the ame, the recipients present the infant with Inu-hariko (paper mache dogs) symbolizing hope that the child will grow as fast and be as healthy as a puppy.

Another traditional event in the child's life is the Shichigosan (Seven-Five-Three) Festival, which is said to be over 400 years old and is held yearly on November 15. On this occasion, parents with children of 7, 5, and 3 years of age go to a Japanese shrine to express their gratitude to the guardian deity for having let their children reach these critical ages and to ask for future blessings. The ages of the children correspond to the Western ages of 6, 4, and 2. The reason for the differences is that, in Japan, a child is recognized to be 1 year of age on the day of his birth.

On Shichigosan, children are dressed in their finest clothing when taken to the shrine. The color of the attire is determined by his or her age. The colors range from the very bright for the younger children and a gradual decline in colors with age. The children are also given talismans and sweet meats by the shrine authorities and receive other special gifts from relatives and friends.

Many changes have taken place with these traditional customs, particularly among the Japanese in America. In America, the events are usually combined and celebrated on the infant's first Girl's or Boy's Day, 100th day of life, or on his or her first birthday (Fig. 4). Relatives and friends are invited to the special gathering and often bring bright, colorful kimonos or futons (bed quilts stuffed with cotton), or other special gifts for the child. Upon their departure, the guests are presented with Japanese bowls or dishes from the infant.

CARETAKING

As noted earlier, Caudill and his associates investigated the relationship between maternal care and infant behavior among Caucasian American, motherland Japanese, and Sansei Japanese-American mothers and their 3- to 4-month-old infants.[13,15,16] The authors found strong cultural differences between the motherland Japanese and Caucasian American maternal caretaking styles and infant behaviors. The Sansei mothers, on the other hand, were noted to be somewhere in between—they took on a great deal of the American mother's behavior, while at the same time retained much of the Japanese mother's behavior.

Similarities between the Sansei and American mothers were observed with the amount of vocalization given to stimulate their infants. Although the Sansei mothers were observed to chat more to their infants, both groups of infants responded with a greater amount of happy vocalization and physical activity than the motherland Japanese infants.

The motherland Japanese mothers showed significantly less vocal interaction with their infants, but a greater use of non-verbal interactions, such as more lulling, carrying, and rocking in an attempt to soothe and quiet their infants to decrease their unhappy vocalizations. Their infants responded by being more physically passive and tried to attract their mothers' attention by a greater amount of unhappy vocalization.

When carrying their infants, the Sansei mothers were more like the American mothers in that they did more positioning and less rocking than the motherland Japanese mothers. However, the Sansei mothers were observed to be more like the motherland Japanese mothers in the amount of carrying done. Unlike the American mothers, carrying their infants for the Sansei and motherland Japanese mothers was not only limited to periods of feeding, but was done more often on different occasions and was accompanied by lulling.

Similarities between the Sansei and motherland Japanese mothers were also observed with the amount of play periods. Both groups of mothers did not confine play to the period involved with feeding, as did the American mothers.

The Sansei mothers, in general, were observed to be super-caretakers in terms of the greater amount of time spent feeding, diapering, and patting and touching. They were like the motherland Japanese mothers in prolonging their infants' ingestion of milk by breast or bottle (although they usually delayed the introduction of semisolid foods until the beginning of the third month), but more like the American mother who started semisolid food at about the end of the first month. Therefore, in reference to both cultural patterns of feeding, the Sansei mother did more feeding of both milk and semisolid foods. Caudill and his associates suggested that because the Sansei mothers spent more time with the intake of more food, the behavior would more likely cause their infants to need more diapering and burping, which included a large part of the patting and touching.[13]

The Yonsei infants were observed to be similar to the motherland Japanese infants in less amount of finger sucking and less engaging in play by themselves. Caudill and his associates attributed the infants' behavior to the Sansei mothers' greater basic caretaking activities and amount of time spent playing with their infants.

It is worth mentioning that the data from the studies could imply that Japanese-American mothers show a tendency to spoil their young infants according to American standards of child care. But my personal experiences with Japanese-American mothers do reveal that they are concerned about this type of spoiling, particularly when the infant cries during the suggested hours for sleep. I have observed some mothers who let their infants cry after all personal needs were met and say, "As much as it hurts me, I don't want to spoil her." Others have asked for reassurance in letting their infants cry, as they fear too much carrying when the infant cries will spoil them.

The studies by Caudill and his associates further indicated that in all cultures the mothers' concern over dressing and undressing their infants was climate-regulated rather than culturally oriented. The manner and the amount of clothing that the infant wore were dependent upon the outside temperature of the particular location.

In 1966, Caudill and Plath studied parent-child co-sleeping patterns among urban Japanese families. The father and the mother in this arrangement usually slept in separate rooms, each co-sleeping with one or more children. Extended family members, especially the grandmother, also participated in the co-sleeping arrangements.[14] In this instance, the Japanese-American families are more like the American families in that the newborn infant sleeps in his own bed or crib and continues to do so throughout his or her stay at home.

The findings from the studies by Caudill and his associates[13-16] seem to suggest that the motherland Japanese mothers interact in such a way to encourage passivity and dependency in their children, while the Sansei mothers preserved enough of their Japanese mother's or grandmother's caretaking style that their Yonsei children remained significantly more passive than their Caucasian counterparts.

Preschool Through Kindergarten

A search of the literature reveals that data on the care of the Japanese-American child of preschool through kindergarten age are scarce. The majority of the material presented in this section is rather specific to the motherland Japanese. However, certain aspects of their childrearing practices are significant, as they are observed among the Japanese in America.

APPEASEMENT AND DISCIPLINE

Takie Sugiyama Lebra, an anthropologist, reported that there is a general belief among Japanese that the preschool child should be free from frustration and tensions. Child care is largely oriented toward appeasement of the child's emotions.[46] Benedict characterized the typical life-cycle of the Japanese individual as "a

great shallow U-curve with maximum freedom and indulgence allowed to babies and the old. Restrictions are slowly increased after babyhood. . . ." Maturity and adulthood represent the peak obligation and responsibility, leaving little freedom to the individual. In America, the U-curve is reversed, with firm discipline directed toward the infant and gradually relaxed as the child grows in strength and enjoys freedom in the prime of his life.[9]

Although the family socialization of the preschool child is generally oriented toward appeasement and indulgence, training and discipline are subtly under way. Certain behaviors are encouraged and rewarded and others are discouraged and punished. Lanham noted that some aspects of the child's training are not peculiar to the Japanese culture, but are shared by other cultures as well.[45]

Lanham also identified the most frequently mentioned behaviors that were encouraged by a small sample of mothers in a small city in central Japan. The following behaviors, listed in order of frequency, were encouraged: toilet habits, polite sitting position, eating properly, washing hands before meals, using chopsticks (eating utensils), saying arigato (thank you), saying the proper words preceding and following a meal, returning things to their proper places. Playing outside without footgear, soiling clothes with urine, quarreling, letting food fall from the table, envying (wanting things others have), and throwing stones were discouraged.

The findings indicate that although socialization in Japan sensitizes the child to interdependence between himself and his socializer, he is still trained and encouraged to develop basic abilities of his own.

TOILET TRAINING

In 1946 Benedict reported that:

When the baby is three to four months old, the mother begins his nursery training. She anticipates his needs, holding him in her hands outside the door. She waits for him, usually whistling low monotonously, and the child learns to know the purpose of this auditory stimulus. Everyone agrees that a baby in Japan, as in China too, is trained very early. If there are slips, some mothers pinch the baby but generally they only change the tone of their voices and hold the hard-to-train baby outside the door at more frequent intervals. If there is withholding, the mother gives the baby an enema or a purge.[9]

However, more recently in 1976 Lebra reported that the usual steps taken in toilet training are encouraging the child to control himself physically, encouraging him to signal when his urge arises and show non-resistance when he is held over a toilet for assistance with elimination; training ends when he is able to go to the toilet by himself. She also noted that "Japanese mothers are not severe in toilet training . . . they tend to wait until the child becomes old enough to 'understand,' although they will praise the child's occasional earlier success in toilet performance."[46] The differences in methods can reflect generational changes or variations within the culture.

The following is an experience related to me by a Sansei:

> When my niece was about 3 months old, my mother, who used to care for her while my sister was at work, decided that it was time to start her potty training. She'd take my niece to the toilet on what she called a "usual basis" like after eating, after naps, etc., and just sit with her saying "sh-sh-sh" until she urinated or "un-un-un" until she moved her bowels. Since she (niece) responded so well, my mother would proudly say that she (niece) was such a good girl since she responded so well to her potty training. I used to chuckle, because it seemed like my mother was the potty trained. Nevertheless, I feel that since both seemed to get enjoyment from the experience it was all right. I'd probably try it with my own children someday.
>
> I need to mention, too, that although my mother was consistent with the training, it was not reinforced when my niece got home because my sister felt that it would come in time. She [sister] began to place more emphasis on potty training when my niece began to walk and talk.
>
> She [niece] was completely potty trained at about 2½ years old, just before she entered preschool.*

PROPER SITTING POSITION

Benedict reported that before the age of two, the child is taught the proper sitting position and is instructed to refrain from fidgeting or shifting his position.[9] The instructing of a child's sitting position along with food posture and proper eating manners is a common scene during mealtime in the Japanese-American family. Grandparents, when present, are often involved with the training.

*Personal interview, Hawaii, 1978.

EATING HABITS

Children are fed until they acquire the ability to handle a spoon on their own. When they have acquired the skill, they are encouraged to feed themselves, but parents often resort to the use of both self-feeding and adult-feeding when they have established that the child takes too long to consume his food.

As the child approaches school-age, feeding by the parents is weaned, and it is stopped when the child enters school. If the child fails to consume his food within the meal hour, discipline, which is usually verbal, is instituted.

ORDERLINESS AND TIDINESS

Perhaps more distinctly than in the American culture, orderliness and tidiness are highly stressed in the Japanese daily life. "The child is taught to be neat, not to drop food from the table, not to soil clothing, not to drop things on the floor, not to poke the paper shoji, to place shoes on the shoe shelf, to return things to their original places, to close open doors. . . . The child comes to learn that tidiness in such external forms manifests an alert and moral mind and indicates one's trustworthiness. Sloppiness is taught as a sign of moral degeneration."[46]

MANNERS AND ETIQUETTE

Cultural distinctions in childrearing are even more noticeable in the amount of stress placed on conventional manners and etiquette in disciplining the youngest member of the family, particularly in language and gestures. For example, there are proper ways in which a child needs to address his superiors and other non-formal ways in which he can address his peers. Depending on usage, the manner of address can mean rudeness or absurdity or convey respect. In polite conversation, when referring to things or persons of a certain position, the prefixes or nouns are changed to connote respect. Parents and elders are always addressed as superiors.[68]

Emphasis is consistently placed on expressing thanks for and the return of favors, and apologizing for one's wrongdoings. During mealtimes, expressions of appreciation for the food are said before (i-ta-da-ki-masu) and after (o-go-chi-so-sama) every meal. As the child grows older he learns to say "may I leave you now" (Tada-ima-itte-kairi-masu) when leaving the home and "I have returned" (Tada-ima-itte-kairi-mashita) when he returns.[46]

127

INTERPERSONAL HARMONY

When the child begins to socialize outside of the family, much emphasis is placed on interpersonal harmony and avoidance of conflict. Quarreling outside of the family is looked upon as a very serious behavior. To maintain the social control within the family, "giri" or a child's moral obligation towards others and his family is stressed. Children are trained to restore harmony after a quarrel on their own initiative, without adult intervention, particularly when the conflict involves other families.[46]

ROLE CONFORMITY

Finally, the child is trained to conform to the norms governing his prescribed role. Role behavior is defined by his sex, age, and birth order.

Sex differences in response to manners and etiquette are stressed within the Japanese culture. Such differences between the two sexes, however, have been recognized in other cultures and are one of the important conditions upon which cultures have been built.

Meredith reported that in the traditional Japanese culture, good behavior for the sexes was defined primarily in terms of obedient, conforming, and responsible conduct. The prolongation of customs, such as Girl's and Boy's Days, in acculturating Japanese groups, reinforces differential sex role behavior. For the female, particular emphasis is placed on poise, grace, and control. For the male, stress is placed on manliness, determination, and the will to overcome all obstacles in the path to success.[53]

The influence of early socialization experiences and maternal attitudes toward differential treatment of the sexes plays an important role. For example, modesty is stressed more in the rearing of girls. The female quickly learns to be modest of her nude body and to sleep straight with her legs together. Boys, on the other hand, are allowed a greater amount of freedom.[9]

The culture further reinforces sex differentiation with terms and phrases in its language. Feminine words are reserved for only females and masculine words are reserved for only males.

In terms of age, the older brothers and sisters are consistently told to set good examples for their younger siblings (Fig. 5). The older siblings are also taught to indulge the younger children. When there are quarrels, the mother will likely ask the older child to give in to the younger one. "Why not lose to win?" is a common phrase. The rationale for this phrase is that if the older child

gives up his toy to the younger child, the baby will be satisfied and turn to something else; then the older child will have won back his toy even as he relinquished it. "To lose to win" becomes an arrangement greatly respected in the Japanese life, even through adulthood.[9]

Benedict noted that in large families "the alternate children are united by closer ties. The oldest will be the favored nurse and protector of the third child and the second of the fourth. The younger children reciprocate."[9]

Role discipline increases when the child reaches school age. The child is repeatedly instructed to obey his teachers and not to bring shame to the family. He is encouraged to develop a strong sense of belonging and total commitment to the group of which he is a part, and is instilled with the motivation for status identification and role performance.

METHODS OF DISCIPLINE

Like parents of other cultures, Japanese parents manipulate the pleasure and pain directly felt by their children. The Japanese child is rewarded materially with candies, toys, or other special treats and punished by being deprived of them for his misbehavior. Physical punishment, such as pinching or light hitting, is also used. The most severe physical punishment used is "moxa," which is regarded as a medicinal technique for curing.

> This is the burning of a little cone of powder, the moxa, upon the child's skin. It leaves a lifelong scar. Cauterization by moxa is an old, widespread Eastern Asiatic medicine, and it was traditionally used to cure many aches and pains in Japan too. It can also cure tantrums and obstinancy. A little boy of six or seven may be "cured" in this way by his mother or his grandmother. It may even be used twice in a difficult case but very seldom indeed is a child given the moxa treatment for naughtiness a third time. It is not a punishment in the sense that "I'll spank you if you do that" is a punishment. But it hurts far worse than spanking, and the child learns that he cannot be naughty with impunity.[9]

A Sansei recalls the use of moxa as a child:

> When I was very young, I remember my grandfather threatening to yaito (burn) my older sister with senko (cone type incense) for using her left hand. Or he at times would set the lighted senko on the table if we failed to finish our food.*

---

*Personal interview, Hawaii, 1978.

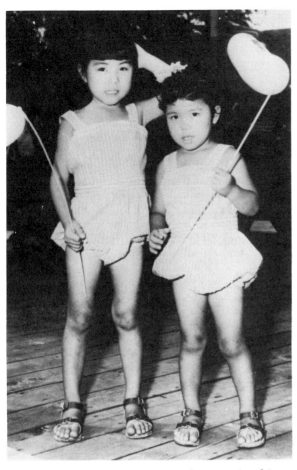

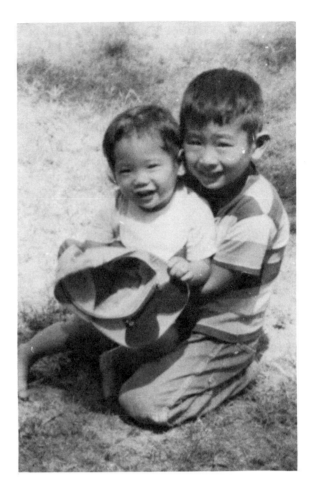

Figure 5. Sibling love, respect, and companionship.

Lebra noted that with the exception of moxa, the primary difference between the Japanese and American culture is the Japanese people's greater emphasis on reward-orientation and less severity of punishment.[46]

Verbal approval and disapproval are also used for disciplining children. Many of their social relationships and social values are manipulated and reinforced through verbal control. One method of verbal punishment is the threat of abandonment. A mother may tell her child that she will leave him, threaten to give him away and adopt someone else's child in his place, or pretend to love someone else's child more than him.[9]

The threat of kidnapping is also used. For example, if the child has a tendency to play outside too late in the evening or to wander too far away from home, he may be told that a ghost or badman will kidnap him. If his misbehavior calls for a severer punishment, the mother may threaten to negotiate with the badman.

Vogel and Vogel sighted two other methods of discipline that Japanese mothers use and that are in contrast to American practice. "One fairly severe form of punishment used in Japan is to lock the child out of the house and require him to apologize before he can come in. . . . A comparable American punishment would be to prevent the child from going out." Similarly, "whereas American mothers sometimes have to go chasing after their children, if the Japanese mother is in a hurry and can't get the child to hurry, she will run ahead, and without question the child will chase after."[67]

More subtle forms of abandonment are often used to warn the child of the unavailability of the

129

mother's help when he really needs it. For example, the mother may tell the child that his father will become very angry when he discovers the child's misconduct and say that she will not offer him any support when he pleas for help.

Another method of verbal punishment is teasing, ridicule, or embarrassment. When a male child is teased, the mother may say things such as "You're not a girl" or "You're a man." Or she may say, "Look at that baby, he doesn't cry." Or when another baby is brought to visit, she will fondle and caress the visitor in her child's presence and say, "I'm going to adopt this baby. I want a nice, good child. You don't act your age."[9]

The threat of embarrassment usually refers to someone other than the caretaker. The child is told that he will be laughed at or ridiculed by his neighbors, peers, or anyone whose opinion the child values most, or the mother may just refer to "everybody," in front of whom the child will lose face. The drawback of this method of discipline is that the child may retain an attachment for his caretaker but develop fear and mistrust of others, especially outsiders with whose ridicule he has been threatened.

The third person therefore plays a significant role in sensitizing the child to shame and embarrassment. The third person, however, is not only used as a verbal reference but as an audience present on the scene.

> The child learns the difference between the dyadic situation (with only himself and his caretaker) and triadic situation (with a third person present as audience) in terms of freedom: he feels completely free in the dyad, inhibited in the triad. This may result in sensitizing the child more to outsiders' opinions than to those of intimate insiders, to the extent that his own family may not be able to discipline him.[46]

Still another method of discipline is an appeal for empathy. The mother in this instance presents "herself as a victim of her child's misbehavior and appeals to his capacity for feeling the pain she is going through. 'If you don't stop doing that, it is I, your mother, who will suffer most. Try to put yourself in my place.' "[46] The child is thereby trained in the vicarious sharing of another person's pleasure and displeasure, so that he regards the possibility of hurting another person's feelings with fear and guilt. One of the effective means of instituting this, as in the above case of the mother, is to say a person will be displeased with the misbehavior rather than that the person will scold you.

The appeals for empathy are often used in conjunction with embarrassment for the family or members of the family. The child may be told that the mother, father, or his entire family will be laughed at by neighbors or disgraced, or that his father will lose face at his company because of his child's deviant behavior. In this situation, the child may be motivated to reform through guilt rather than shame.

Finally, praise is most often used as a means of rewarding the child for his good performance and encouraging him to repeat it. The pattern of reward is linked with the tendency for the caretaker to have the child exhibit some ability or skill as a sign of his accomplishments. The mother can also frustrate the child by praising another child, either a sibling or outsider. She may tell the child to be like that model child or use words that generate jealousy, with the hopes of changing the deviant behavior.

Therefore, the ideal Japanese child, according to DeVos, is "sunao," or docile and obedient.[22] He is possessed by a strong sensitivity to what others will think and has little concept of himself independent of the attitudes of others. The child is thus overly sensitive to being slighted, degraded, or ignored. This patterning leads to a vulnerability to any depreciatory attitude in others, and a need to constantly seek approval of others.

Through observations and personal experiences, the methods of both physical (with the exception of moxa, as it seems to have been utilized primarily among the Issei population) and verbal discipline utilized by the motherland Japanese are quite similar to those of the Japanese Americans. Variations can be seen with the nature of the situation or circumstances in which a deviant behavior has been committed.

MATERNAL ATTACHMENT

The mother appears to play an extremely crucial role in the Japanese life-cycle. From birth, the maternal-child relationship is crystallized and the relationship is imprinted on the child's memory in the course of his socialization. The works of Caudill and Doi,[12] Connor,[18] and DeVos[22] illustrate the child's close emotional bonds with the mother in the Japanese family.

Lebra analyzed Yoshiaki Yamamura's work on the child's maternal attachment among motherland Japanese. Lebra points out that the Japanese mother is unique in that her influence over her child goes beyond his infancy and continues throughout adulthood. The child's success and failures at whatever age are always reverted back to the mother.[69]

Several dominant themes were cited in Yamamura's work. First, the mother is typified as having suffered a tremendous amount of hardship. Her will to withstand such suffering comes from her endurance and dedication to her family. As a consequence of her suffering, the child feels a deep sense of guilt concerning the mother for having endured and dedicated herself in selfless acts. The child feels more guilty if he was very defiant and his mother responded with forgiveness.

Another cited theme was the child's gratitude toward the mother for having provided moral support when pursuing his or her life's goals. She was observed to have stood by her child's side in all his or her efforts to succeed and was the driving force that motivated her child to achievement.[69]

HEALTH AND ILLNESS

Through personal observations and experiences, it seems that Japanese Americans generally accept the delivery of child health care in this country. Since children are greatly valued in the Japanese-American family, parents seem to take an active part in their children's lives, particularly in their physical well-being. They seek out preventive health care services, such as well-child clinic visits, which include the recommended immunizations for children. They also practice preventive health care at home by serving well-balanced diets according to American standards, and cultural foods such as miso soup (soup made from soya bean paste) and tofu (soya bean curd cake), which are thought to be responsible for good, sound physical health.

Parents take pride in their child's good physical health. When a child is ill, parents seem to have an attitude of seeking out the proper medical assistance no matter what the cost. With less serious illnesses, some will often utilize home remedies.

Parents are greatly concerned when a child misses school as a result of illness. Subsequently, some parents may send their child to school even if he has not fully recovered from the illness.

The physical well-being of the Japanese Americans appears to be complemented by their mental well-being. Statistics compiled by Kitano show that the Japanese are among the lowest of all identifiable groups in reported incidence of mental illness. The rates of mental illness seem to be consistent, regardless of whether the data were obtained from hospital records, or from the records of "preventive" agencies, such as child guidance clinics and family service agencies, or from impressionistic evidence by professionals in the ethnic community.[39]

It is important to note that, while the data reveal a low incidence of mental illness, the mentally ill person who is hidden to protect the family image may obscure the data. Dennis Ogawa describes his mental health assessment of Nisei and Sansei families in Hawaii:

Affected by poverty, loneliness, illness, frustration, and rootlessness, some Japanese during the postwar decades had still not felt the intuitive spirit of family love. For them, the changes within the Japanese community had disturbed their patterns of well-being and security. For some the family could not keep up with the rapidly accelerating demands made upon the modern Sansei individual. Though not necessarily typical and certainly not model for the Island home, the extremes, the maladjusted, served as sobering reminders that no institution, no matter how durable, could be without its sometimes dormant but tumorous malignancies.

For the large part, the synthesis of the modified extended familial bonds and the success of social assimilation contributed to producing a Sansei personality with secure psychological, cultural, and social skills. But in some Japanese homes, as internal structures stretched in response to social changes, families failed to meet individual needs. For example, many Sansei complained that their families, while protecting the family image, had misplaced more important priorities. The couple who remained married because they feared the shame of divorce often created a family atmosphere of bitterness and insensitivity. The child whose problems were covered up because they might have caused family shame merely became more confused and socially maladjusted. A sense of pride, so often useful to the individual, could unthinkingly inhibit constructive action, thereby magnifying problems.[59]

Dr. Ogawa goes on to describe one of the more tragic consequences of the Japanese family's inability to cope with mental illness:

One of the more tragic consequences of an overweening family image was the inability of many Japanese families to deal honestly and reasonably with mental illness. Kichigai ("crazy") behavior was not viewed so much as an illness as it was an irreparable scar on the family honor. The mentally ill person had to be hidden, removed from the sight of others, so that the family was not disgraced and shamed.[59]

The circumstances described by Ogawa can also hold true for the individual himself, who recognizes that he is ill, but hides what is troubling him because of "haji" or shame. Haji connotes a sense of responsibility to the family and the Japanese community beyond the individual's personal experience of shame.

Similarly, Dr. Kitano in his study of mental illness among Japanese in Hawaii, Los Angeles, Okinawa, and Tokyo found pronounced similarities in the character of Japanese "crazy" behaviors. Kitano observed that Japanese families "resist the move towards professional labeling and categorization until the behavior literally tears the family apart. By then, it may be "too late," so that once a Japanese is hospitalized, he does acquire the characteristics of the mentally ill role, which for many becomes permanent."[38]

It was interesting to note that the personality profile of the mentally ill in each area revealed that the individual was an isolated and lonely person from a lonely and isolated family.

Ogawa indicated that the unrealistic attitudes in the Japanese family, together with their inability to overcome their pride so that they can intellectually deal with familial problems, is the source of much conflict between the Nisei parent and Sansei child. "Youngsters who were frustrated by unrealistic or self-serving familial demands felt hemmed in by threats to their independence. They were not allowed the respect to handle their own futures, to make their own decisions, to have their own friends. The family simply could not understand or deal with their problems."[59] Ogawa further reported that:

> In a modern world of information overload, the family seemed for the young to be restricting; out of touch. The Sansei had more choices, more decisions, and more information than most individuals could have hoped to sort logically—and less fundamental life roots with which to deal with personal problems. The years of religious conversions and indifference in the Nisei community, for example, had taken their toll on the Sansei. . . . The Sansei had no other institution except the family or school to help handle a personal "identity crisis"—a crisis in most cases brought on at home or in the classroom.[59]

Today, Japanese-American families seem to deal with the child's crisis in various ways. A large number respond with parental flexibility in compromising between family constraints and individual freedom. "This responsiveness of Nisei families to the needs of the Sansei, their flexibility to balance love with parental guidance and obligation, allowed the adolescent Sansei to feel that his desire for individualism was encouraged and insulated by family concern. The child could make his own decisions, make his own failures, and understand how he fit into the family unit."[59]

Ogawa describes two other means by which Japanese families respond to their child's crisis:

> Other Nisei families were not so much flexible as they were simply inert. The child did as he liked, without guidance, because the parents were usually helpless to grasp the situation. "There is nothing we can do about it" became a rationale to spoil the child with apathy and powerlessness. Still other families responded to the Sansei "identity crisis" with silence or a reexertion of overcompetition. Parental expectations for the recalcitrant youth became unusually rigid—the child was even under greater pressure to conform to the family expectations—and little room was left for failure.[59]

The data presented illustrates variations within the Japanese culture in responding to the physical and mental health and illness of the child. Certain variables contribute to the differences, such as the family's retention or rejection of traditional values or the family's acculturation pattern into the host society. It is important to note that while certain groups may tend to possess characteristic cultural patterns, these general patterns may not apply to one particular individual in the group.

Childhood and Adolescence

Much of the reported information on the preschool through kindergarten child overlaps into this age period. The childrearing lessons that extend into this age period are orderliness and tidiness, manners and etiquette, interpersonal harmony, and role conformity. Some methods of discipline are used. Maternal attachment and physical and mental health are still stressed.

SEXUALITY

Prior to World War II, a discussion of sex between the Issei parent and Nisei child was nearly impossible. Consequently, many Nisei were thoroughly misinformed on the subject. "Some thought of sex in terms of delicate, self-conscious lectures provided by the stereotypical unmarried physical education teachers, and others picked up what they could from street and gang groups. Older brothers and sisters provided the most balanced information."[39]

The male sexual attitude was reported by Kitano:

> Nisei boys, in general, tended to feel that there were two kinds of girls. The kind they would marry was usually another Nisei, of long acquaintance—either personal or through family contacts—and was "pure." She was not thought of as a sexual object. Then there was "that kind of girl," who might be non-Japanese. This way of looking at sex almost ensured that there were few "shotgun" marriages among the Nisei, despite the fact that many did not marry until their late twenties.[39]

Sex education for the young Nisei female was very restrictive. Even after marriage, she was urged not to read books on sex and believe that she was capable of sexual satisfaction.[59]

The continuation of the restrictive attitudes toward information on sex over generations was illustrated in Kitano's studies on parental child-rearing attitudes among a sample of Issei and Nisei. The studies disclosed that both generations fostered dependency and were sexually repressive of their offspring.[35,36]

Similarly, in 1966 Connor conducted a study on family bonds, maternal closeness, and the suppression of sexuality among groups of Issei, Nisei, and Sansei living in Sacramento. The responses from the three generations of Japanese Americans were matched with scores obtained from similar Caucasian American groups.[18]

The results of the study revealed that when compared with their Caucasian American counterparts, all three generations of Japanese Americans consistently scored higher on items indicating strong family ties and an equally strong emotional attachment to the mother. The Japanese Americans also scored higher on areas concerning nurturance, affiliation, succor, abasement, and order; they had lower scores on dominance, autonomy, and heterosexuality, and suppression of sexuality. Connor suggested that the lower scores on heterosexuality appear to be part of the larger pattern of maternal closeness and strong family ties, and not an isolated phenomenon.[18] This also suggests that while considerable acculturation has occurred, the lower scores among the Sansei reveal a preservation of sexual repressive attitudes from their immigrant grandparents.

The interrelation between suppression of sexuality and strong family ties and close emotional bonds with the mother is further supported in writings by Caudill and Doi[12] and DeVos.[22] Both works indicate that Japanese mothers strive to foster dependency needs in their offspring and then utilize these dependency needs to manipulate the behavior of the child. The dependency needs and maternal closeness thereby lead to a suppression of sexuality.

While the above studies indicate a greater suppression of sexuality among Japanese Americans, consideration needs to be taken of the greater emphasis of sex education in schools and variations among family attitudes.

DATING AND MARRIAGE

Current Japanese-American parental attitudes toward adolescent dating seem to fall within the same realm as those of a large number of other American parents. Their attitudes and patterns vary from family to family.

In general, during the period prior to dating, when a child begins to socialize outside of the family, Japanese-American parents prefer that their child associate with peers from his own ethnic group. They are, however, quite accepting when their child associates with peers from other ethnic groups.

Although attitudes toward interracial dating have relaxed through the years, particularly after World War II, parents still seem to place a strong emphasis on their ethnicity and in-group dating. The attitudes prevail until marriage. A recent study indicated that there is a preference for in-group marriage, even for those who married out of the group, although it was not a major issue.[34] It is noteworthy to mention that while the incidence of interracial marriages have steadily increased in recent years, there is still a high rate of in-group marital patterns.[34]

CAREER GOALS

As previously noted, throughout Japan's recorded history, high standards of excellence have been emphasized. Such standards were highly emphasized in the Issei's childhood and were one of the values that they brought with them from Japan.

Reports by Connor[19] and DeVos[22] support the view that there has been a retention of this achievement orientation among the Issei, Nisei, and Sansei. Both reports concluded that the nature of the Japanese and Japanese-American achievement is a result of a different set of reinforcements. It begins with the mother's creation of a strong dependency need within her children. Subsequently, she can manipulate the need in order to motivate her child to achieve. It is often accomplished by heightening the child's sensitivity to the opinions of significant others or by the mother's reproaching herself for raising her child inadequately, particularly when the child fails to live up to her expectations. The mother's suffering thereby induces guilt feelings in the child, which further motivate him to achieve.

IMPLICATIONS FOR HEALTH CARE PROFESSIONALS

It should be recognized that the term Japanese Americans refers to different kinds of groups and individuals, and that these groups and individuals have sometimes acculturated, assimilated, or integrated into the greater American culture in different ways. The data presented in this chapter reveal several important generalizations about the childrearing practices among Japanese Americans. Many of these practices do not appear to have detrimental effects on the healthy outcome of Japanese-American children, but are often misunderstood by Americans of Western origin. The following are important points:

1. A strong sense of gender differences in the rearing of children.

2. Emphasis on the child's need to be aware of the distinctions in status that may exist between conversational partners. Parents seem to foster this concern over authority through the child's need for deference, politeness, sensitivity toward other people, and a continuation of a formalized relationship when in the presence of superiors. Cross-cultural confusion can occur because of this differential consciousness of status, particularly as the child grows older.

3. Considerable emphasis on self-effacing behaviors (enryo). Some of the behaviors associated with this are self-abasement, modesty, and apology. The prescriptions connected with enryo direct each person, regardless of gender or station in life, to be modest, to defer to others, to play down one's accomplishments and achievements, to suppress one's feelings, and to direct attention away from oneself.

When one understands the meaning of these attitudes, a harmonious balancing can occur in which the individual's status and accomplishments can be established in subtle and indirect ways. However, if misinterpreted, the enryo behaviors can be viewed as exaggerated politeness, false modesty, unusual silence, or hesitancy to express one's feelings on any subject in the presence of people of a higher status or to articulate one's views in a group. Such behaviors can often intrude in counseling relationships. This characteristic reserve in the Japanese-American personality makes it difficult to determine where cultural patterns end and psychologically debilitating symptoms begin. When assessing or evaluating such behaviors, health care professionals should have two perceptual measures for determining "normal" behaviors: one to determine what is a deviant behavior in the Japanese-American subculture and another to determine what is aberrant in the culture at large.

4. Regulation of a child's behavior, by placing much emphasis on the opinions of significant others through shame and guilt.

5. Dependency from childhood through adulthood fostered by mother-child interactions.

6. The child's conscious need to be aware of his obligations.

7. Emphasis on the child's need to gain status and achievement.

8. Emphasis on the preservation of family name and honor.

9. The utilization of many forms of non-verbal communications. When observing the communication process among Japanese Americans, it would be a serious omission not to take into consideration the quality and explicitness of the feelings that accompany the non-verbal communications. Confusion arises between Americans of Western origin and Japanese Americans because of this apparent differential awareness of non-verbal behaviors. For instance, an American of Western origin may quite unconsciously wince, frown, or show strain with pain, which, although not intended as a negative communication, may be received as such. The Japanese American would suppress the negative facial expressions, but his very suppression may suggest that he is insincere or lacks pain.

In all circumstances, it is important to remember that neither the parents nor the child can be adequately assessed or evaluated on one behavior alone. Consideration of other variables that are significant to the situation, individual, or cultural experience must be taken.

Parents, of whatever cultural group, need opportunities to share their feelings and express how their culture dictates that children should be reared. It is equally important for health care providers to create an atmosphere that fosters trust, respect, and the sharing of information, so that mutual goals can be identified and achieved.

In general, when attempting to understand the behavior of individuals, their cultural background should always be considered. At the same time, one must be cautious in stereotyping or formulating conclusions that are based on limited knowledge about the individual or culture. While it may be true that certain groups tend to have similar characteristic cultural patterns, such general patterns may not apply to one particular individual in the group. Each person should be assessed as a unique individual.

When we speak of or look at a particular ethnic group, consideration also needs to be placed on several variables, such as age, sex, education, first generations who retain traditional cultural practices and the subsequent generations who retain or reject them, and wealth and poverty. There is, therefore, no homogeneous cultural group. In reality, people of differing cultural backgrounds who live in a geographical area may have more in common with other cultural groups in the same area than they would have with people of their own cultural group living in a different geographical location. This provides reason for some of the differences among Japanese Americans on the mainland and Hawaii.

In childrearing, the culture of the ethnic group, the geographical location, and the socioeconomic status all influence parental attitudes. Such influences are redefined by each family, thereby creating a unique environment into which children are born and reared. This home culture is greatly influential in determining the child's growth and developmental process. His home culture becomes increasingly modified as he grows older and begins to socialize outside of the home.

Certain steps can be taken to assist the health care provider in administering quality care to individuals or families:

1. The first step involves an examination of the health care delivery system itself. What are our beliefs about health care? What are our expectations of a client's behavior? What are our variations in value orientation? What value orientations do we expect from clients? What are our communication systems? Do we use words that have meaning for clients, or even other health care providers? Do we create a communication system intelligible only to ourselves? Do we impose our beliefs about health and illness on our clients, or do we attempt to discover their views first? Do our attitudes toward clients differ depending upon the client's diagnosis, his compliance with the treatment regimen, or his ability to get well? Do we include cultural variables in our assessment of the client? Do we allow for cultural variations in our plan of care?[11]

2. The second step involves an examination of the health care provider's own cultural background. Since every culture has its own set of customs and values concerning health and illness, it is important for the health care provider to be aware of his or her own cultural norms and values. A person may ask: Are my values in direct conflict with the client? If so, can I make a commitment to understand the client's culture together with his personal preferences and bias and still provide quality care?

3. The third step is the study of the client. While it is impossible for each health care provider to be familiar with the attitudes and practices of each cultural group, one should understand the concept of culture and its impact on its members, and sensitively attempt to understand the characteristics of the cultural group. What are the client's attitudes, practices, and beliefs toward health and health care? What is the client's variation in value orientation? What is his communication system? What is the client's past history with the health care delivery system? Has it affected his current progress? How has he been socialized into the client role? Has he used other health care systems in the past, or is he using one concurrently? What does the client think about his health care?[11]

The above questions are only a few of the numerous ones that need to be asked and responded to by health care providers. Such questioning and examination will help to increase their effectiveness with childrearing families. While the data presented in this chapter may be limited in context, it is hoped that the information will be useful to the health care provider who is establishing interactions with Japanese-American families.

ACKNOWLEDGMENT

I am extremely grateful to Ann Clark for providing me with this opportunity to contribute to her book.

REFERENCES

1. Arkoff, A.: *Need patterns in two gen-*

erations of Japanese Americans in Hawaii. Journal of Social Psychology 50:75-79, 1959.

2. Arkoff, A., Meredith, G., and Dong, J.: *Attitudes of Japanese-American and Caucasian-American students toward marriage roles.* Journal of Social Psychology 59:11-15, February 1963.

3. Arkoff, A., Meredith, G., and Iwahara, S.: *Dominance-deference patterning in motherland-Japanese, Japanese-American, and Caucasian-American students.* Journal of Social Psychology 58:61-66, October 1962.

4. Arkoff, A., Meredith, G., and Iwahara, S.: *Male-dominant and equalitarian attitudes in Japanese, Japanese-American, and Caucasian-American students.* Journal of Social Psychology 64:225-229, August 1964.

5. Arnold, F., et al.: *The Value of Children—A Cross-National Study. Volume I: Introduction and Comparative Analysis.* East-West Center, East-West Population Institute, Honolulu, Hawaii, 1975.

6. Arnold, F., and Fawcet, J.T.: *The Value of Children—A Cross-National Study. Volume III.* East-West Center, East-West Center Population Institute, Honolulu, Hawaii, 1975.

7. Asch, S.E.: *Social Psychology.* Prentice-Hall, Englewood Cliffs, New Jersey, 1952.

8. Benedict, R.: *Patterns of Culture.* Houghton Mifflin Co., Boston, 1934.

9. Benedict, R.: *The Chrysanthemum and the Sword. Patterns of Japanese Culture.* Houghton Mifflin Co., Boston, 1946.

10. Berrien, F.K., Arkoff, A., and Iwahara, S.: *Generation difference in values: Americans, Japanese-Americans, and Japanese.* Journal of Social Psychology 71:169-175, April 1967.

11. Brink, P.J.: *Transcultural Nursing: A Book of Readings.* Prentice-Hall, Englewood Cliffs, New Jersey, 1976.

12. Caudill, W., and Doi, T.: "Interrelations of psychiatry, culture and emotion in Japan." In Galdston, I. (ed.): *Man's Image in Medicine and Anthropology.* International University Press, New York, 1963, pp. 374-421.

13. Caudill, W., and Frost, L.: "A comparison of maternal care and infant behavior in Japanese-American, American, and Japanese families." Lebra, W.P. (ed.): *Youth, Socialization, and Mental Health.*
University Press of Hawaii, Honolulu, 1974.

14. Caudill, W., and Plath, D.: *Who sleeps by whom? Parent-child involvement in urban Japanese families.* Psychiatry 29(4):344-366, 1966.

15. Caudill, W.A., and Schooler, C.: *Child behavior and child rearing in Japan and the United States: an interim report.* Journal of Nervous and Mental Disease 157(5):323-338, November 1973.

16. Caudill, W., and Weinstein, H.: *Maternal care and infant behavior in Japan and America.* Psychiatry 32:12-43, 1969.

17. Connor, J.W.: *Acculturation and family continuities in three generations of Japanese Americans.* Journal of Marriage and the Family 36(1):159-165, February 1974.

18. Connor, J.W.: *Family bonds, maternal closeness, and the supression of sexuality in three generations of Japanese Americans.* Ethos 4(2):189-221, Summer 1976.

19. Connor, J.W.: *Joge kankei: a key concept for understanding of Japanese-American achievement.* Psychiatry 39(3):266-279, August 1976.

20. DeFrancis, J.: *Things Japanese in Hawaii.* The University Press of Hawaii, Honolulu, 1973.

21. DeGaris, F.: *We Japanese. Book 1.* Yamagata Press, Yokohama, Japan, 1950.

22. DeVos, G.A.: *Socialization for Achievement: Essays on the Cultural Psychology of the Japanese.* University of California Press, Berkeley, 1973.

23. Doi, L.T.: *Amae: a key concept for understanding Japanese personality structure.* Psychologia 5:1-7, 1962.

24. Doi, L.T.: *The Anatomy of Dependence.* Kodansha International Ltd., Tokyo, 1973.

25. Fenz, W.D., and Arkoff, A.: *Comparative need patterns of five ancestry groups in Hawaii.* Journal of Social Psychology 58:67-69, October 1962.

26. Grove, C.L.: *Nonverbal behavior, cross-cultural contact, and the urban classroom teacher.* Equal Opportunity Review 55-59, February 1976.

27. Hall, J.W.: *Japan from Prehistory to Modern Times.* Dell Publishing Co., Inc., New York, 1968.

28. Hearn, L.: *Japan: An Attempt at Interpretation.* Macmillian, London, 1904.

29. Higa, M.: "A comparative study of three

groups of Japanese mothers: attitudes toward child rearing." In Lebra, W.P. (ed.): *Youth, Socialization, and Mental Health: III.* University Press of Hawaii, Honolulu, 1974.

30. Hosokawa, B.: *Nisei: The Quiet American.* William Morrow and Company, Inc., New York, 1969.

31. Ichihashi, Y.: *Japanese in the United States.* Stanford University Press, Stanford, California, 1932.

32. Johnson, C.L.: *Interdependence, reciprocity and indebtedness: an analysis of Japanese American kinship relations.* Journal of Marriage and the Family 39(2):351-362, May 1977.

33. Johnson, F.A., Marsella, A.J., and Johnson C.L.: *Social and psychological aspects of verbal behavior in Japanese-Americans.* American Journal of Psychiatry 131(5): 580-583, May 1974.

34. Kikumura, A., and Kitano, H.H.L.: *Interracial marriage: a picture of the Japanese American.* Journal of Social Issues 29(2):67-81, 1973.

35. Kitano, H.H.L.: *Differential child-rearing attitudes between first and second generation Japanese in the United States.* Journal of Social Psychology 53:13-19, 1961.

36. Kitano, H.H.L.: *Inter- and intragenerational differences in maternal attitudes toward child rearing.* Journal of Social Psychology 63:215-220, August 1964.

37. Kitano, H.H.L.: "Japanese-Americans' mental illness." In Plog, S., and Edgerton, R. (eds.): *Changing Perspectives on Mental Illness.* Holt, Rinehart and Winston, New York, 1969, pp.256-284.

38. Kitano, H.H.L.: *Mental illness in four cultures.* Journal of Social Psychology 81:121-134, April 1970.

39. Kitano, H.H.L.: *Japanese Americans: The Evolution of a Subculture.* ed. 2. Prentice-Hall, Englewood Cliffs, New Jersey, 1976.

40. Kitano, H.H.L.: "Japanese Americans: the development of a middleman minority." In Hundley, N. (ed.): *The Asian American: the Historical Experience.* Clio Press, Inc., Santa Barbara, 1976.

41. Kometani, K.: *The Nisei and the future.* Nisei in Hawaii and the Pacific 6(1):10, 1952.

42. Kuhlen, R., and Thompson, G.G.: *Psychological Studies of Human Development.* ed.3. Appleton-Century-Crofts, New York, 1970.

43. Kuykendall, R.S., and Day, A.G.: *Hawaii: A History—From Polynesian Kingdom to American Statehood.* Prentice-Hall, Englewood Cliffs, New Jersey, 1961.

44. LaBarre, W.: *The cultural basis of emotions and gestures.* Journal of Personality 2:72, 1947.

45. Lanham, B.B.: "Aspects of child care in Japan: preliminary report." In Haring, D.G. (ed.): *Personal Character and Cultural Milieu.* Syracuse University Press, Syracuse, New York, 1956.

46. Lebra, T.S.: *Japanese Patterns of Behavior.* The University Press of Hawaii, Honolulu, 1976.

47. Lyman, S.M.: *Generation gap.* Society 10(2): 55-63, January/February 1973.

48. Maykovich, M.K.: *Japanese American Identity Dilemma.* 1-58, Totsuka, Shinjuku, Waseda University Press, Tokyo, 1972.

49. Masuda, M., Matsumoto, G., and Meredith, G.: *Ethnic identity in three generations of Japanese Americans.* Journal of Social Psychology 81:199-207, August 1970.

50. Matsumoto, G., Meredith, G., and Masuda, M.: "Ethnic identity: Honolulu and Seattle Japanese-Americans." In Sue, S., and Wagner, N.N. (eds.): *Asian-Americans Psychological Perspectives.* Science and Behavior Books, Inc., Palo Alto, 1973.

51. Meredith, G.M.: *Observations of the acculturation of Sansei Japanese Americans in Hawaii.* Psychologia 8(1):2, June 1965.

52. Meredith, G.M.: *Amae and acculturation among Japanese-American college students in Hawaii.* Journal of Social Psychology 70:171-180, December 1966.

53. Meredith, G.M.: *Sex temperament among Japanese American college students in Hawaii.* Journal of Social Psychology 77:149-156, April 1969.

54. Meredith, G.M., and Meredith, C.: *Acculturation and personality among Japanese-American college students in Hawaii.* Journal of Social Psychology 68:175-182, 1966.

55. Morsbach, H.: *Aspects of nonverbal communication in Japan.* Journal of Nervous and Mental Disease 157(4):262-277, 1973.

56. Nakane, C.: *Japanese Society.* University of California Press, Berkeley, 1970.

57. Nordyke, E.C.: *The People of Hawaii.* The

University Press of Hawaii, Honolulu, 1977.

58. Ogawa, D.: "The Jap image." In Sue, S., and Wagner, N.N. (eds.): *Asian-Americans Psychological Perspectives*. Science and Behavior Books, Inc., Palo Alto, California, 1973.

59. Ogawa, D.: *Kidomo no tame ni. For the Sake of the Children: The Japanese Experience in Hawaii*. The University Press of Hawaii, Honolulu, 1978.

60. Okamoto, N.I.: "The Japanese American." Clark, A.L. (ed.): *Culture, Childbearing, Health Professionals*. F.A. Davis Co., Philadelphia, 1978.

61. Sears, R.R., Maccoby, E.E., and Levin, H.: "The child-rearing process." Sears, R.R., et al. (eds.): *Patterns of Child Rearing*. Stanford University Press, Stanford, 1957, pp. 457-466.

62. Shand-Kovach, N.: "The earliest experience of culture: Japan and the United States." In Leninger, M. (ed.): *Transcultural Nursing Care of Infants and Children*. Proceedings from the First National Transcultural Nursing Conference. Salt Lake City, Utah, 1977.

63. Strong, E.K., Jr.: *The Second Generation Japanese Problem*. Stanford University Press, Stanford, California, 1934.

64. United States Department of Commerce, Bureau of the Census. Government Printing Office, Washington, D.C., 1930.

65. United States Department of Commerce, Bureau of the Census: *Japanese, Chinese, and Filipinos in the United States, 1970*. Census Population, Government Printing Office, Washington, D.C., 1973.

66. United States Territorial Department of Health, Bureau of Public Health Nursing: *Cultural Beliefs and Practices of the Child-bearing Period and Their Implications for Nursing Practice—Among Chinese, Filipinos, Hawaiian, and Japanese Families Living in Hawaii*. Hawaii, 1953.

67. Vogel, E.F., and Vogel, S.H.: *Family security, personal immaturity and emotional health in a Japanese sample*. Marriage and Family Living 23: 161-166, 1961.

68. Yamamoto, M.: *Cultural conflicts and accommodations of the first and second generation Japanese*. Social Process in Hawaii 4:40-48, May 1938.

69. Yamamura, Y. *Nihonjin to haha (The Japanese and Mother)*. Toyokan Shuppansha, Tokyo, 1971. Cited in Lebra, T.S., (ed.): "Early socializations," *Japanese Patterns of Behavior*. The University Press of Hawaii, Honolulu, 1976.

70. Yoshida, Y.: "Sources and causes of Japanese emigration." In Ogawa, D. (ed.): *Kodomo no tame ni. For the Sake of the Children: The Japanese Experience in Hawaii*. The University Press of Hawaii, Honolulu, 1978.

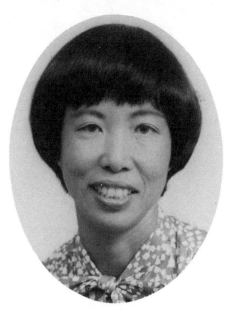

Chapter 6

At a recent national women's convention I listened to a Black Women's caucus urging minority women to unite. When the speaker very emotionally beseeched "our downtrodden Asian sisters to join us," I turned and looked around the room to see whom she was addressing. As I realized she was looking at me and the other members of the Hawaii delegation, my unspoken response was, "Who, me? I'm not a 'downtrodden' Asian."

During my intermediate and high school years I was an Air Force "brat." Living among predominantly White Americans I can vividly recall the shock I occasionally felt when I passed a reflective surface and saw my Chinese face looking back at me. I thought, felt, acted like a "Haole," a Hawaiian term that refers to the Caucasian. To be reminded that I was Chinese was unsettling—I didn't think I knew what a Chinese was, and I didn't want to be one. While living in the mainland United States I was aware that I didn't really belong with the "Haoles," and I also didn't identify with the mainland Chinese Americans. I was different from them, too, and I didn't understand why. Twenty years later my son went from Hawaii to the mainland United States for college and his comments made me remember those long forgotten feelings of being "neither here nor there." "Hawaii kids are different," he wrote. As I delved into the history of the early Chinese immigrants I learned about the cruel discrimination they encountered in the continental United States while my ancestors in Hawaii were welcomed with open arms and presented with many opportunities for advancement. Growing up in such diverse environments, of course we were different!

My husband is also of Chinese ancestry; he was born and raised in Hawaii and educated in the Islands and on the mainland. During the early years of our marriage, a major adjustment for me was doing things according to Chinese customs and practices, such as distributing roast pork to friends who gave us baby gifts, staying home for 1 month after delivery, and attending frequent family gatherings. As I matured, I was better able to accept doing things Chinese and I gradually acknowledged that much of my life was influenced by my parents' Chinese values and beliefs, even though our home life was extremely Westernized. My married life was very much influenced by the values and customs of my husband and his Chinese-American parents and large extended family.

When presented the opportunity to research and write this chapter I thought it would be a good chance to learn some history about the Chinese coming to America. That I did. In the course of writing this chapter, I set it aside many times to do family things and came to realize that those things were definitely

The Chinese American

Evelyn L. Char, R.N., M.S.

Chinese family practices. Two days were spent shopping for and cooking various food for Chinese New Year. I ran errands for my parents, took care of my ailing grandmother for a few hours, cleaned house for my widowed father-in-law, and attended family gatherings. In learning about the concept of familism I have increased my understanding of my parents, my husband, my parents-in-law, and their respective families and have been able to see more clearly how the value of the family has persisted through our generations in many adapted patterns. My husband and I have some of the same desires for our five children that the interviewees in the chapter identified, and we foster their educational values and close family ties.

I made some interesting discoveries about myself and the things our families have done for years. I was amazed that I had stored in my memory so many practices and observations from my childhood and later years. It was amusing to learn the beliefs behind the things we "had" to do; had I known earlier I might not have been so contrary. Bits and pieces of information fell into place along with remembering and I realized I knew a great deal about being Chinese, but never admitted it. I discovered that I had assimilated what I valued and did not need to feel obligated to practice everything. In assimilating what I choose from each cultural system, I do not select one culture over the other; neither is judged good nor bad. Over the years my strong belief and value in individualism has clashed so many times with the familism concept. I am pleasantly surprised to realize that along the way I have found a peaceful working agreement with myself. I am an American person with a Chinese heritage.

Researching the literature stimulated recall of what I had stored in my memory bank. The publications demonstrated practices that were identical to those with which I was knowledgeable or personally familiar. Some examples in the text are drawn from personal experiences and those of my Chinese-American friends.

Professionally speaking, I have a Bachelor of Science degree in Nursing from the University of Hawaii, a Master of Science in Maternal-Child Health Nursing from Boston University, and a Master's degree in Psychiatric/Mental Health Nursing from the University of Hawaii. My professional experience has included pediatric office nursing and staff positions in pediatrics, obstetrics, and psychiatry; I have also instructed baccalaureate nursing students.

At the moment I am independently practicing as a clinical specialist in psychiatric/mental health nursing, working with individuals, couples, and families. I am conducting the ENCORE program in Hawaii, which is the national YWCA postmastectomy group rehabilitation program.

A cultural system is adaptive, dynamic, shared, and transmitted from generation to generation, consciously and unconsciously.[1] Becoming knowledgeable of the cultural system of the patient or client and sensitive to the variations of that culture can aid the health professional to understand his patient and utilize that understanding in developing patterns of intervention. Having knowledge of the main dimensions and how they are demonstrated in behaviors related to a specific area, such as childrearing, will assist the provider of health care in all aspects of his contacts with the patient. "The dominant value orientation of a society determines the process of socialization by which children are inducted into the existing value system."[2] Childrearing practices influence child development and behavior.

This overview is intended for health professionals who encounter Chinese Americans and their families. In order to more fully appreciate the Chinese American of today it is important to know a brief history of the Chinese, especially their values and beliefs, way of life in China, and their beginnings in America. Detail about the culture and history is offered because the old esteemed cultural values continue to permeate the Chinese-American way of living. The beliefs and practices may have changed greatly with the passing of years and acculturation, but the basic values of a strong family group, education, and achievement persist.

HISTORY OF THE CHINESE IN AMERICA

As early as 1788 the first Chinese immigrants arrived in the United States. They came as sojourners, solely for economic gains, with plans to return to China after their fortunes were made.[3] Life was very difficult and many families were starving in Southern China. The men left their families and homes to seek ways to make money that they could send back for support or save for a return to China in affluence. They were hired on sailing ships as crew and made many voyages across the ocean. Sometimes a man would find work and remain in a visiting port.

In the late 1800s, thousands were imported as contract laborers for construction jobs, to work on the railroads, and in the mining camps of California and the Rocky Mountain area.[4] Listed among their attributes as railworkers were that they "learned quickly, were cleanly in habits, did not fight, were quiet, peaceable, patient, industrious, economical, as efficient as white laborers,

and did more work than the white people. They lived on less and quarreled noisily among themselves."[5] At the mining sites they initially panned for gold, but the White men soon denied them claims and places to work, so they began doing "women's work," cooking and laundering, which was needed by the predominantly male population and was the least competitive.[6]

After building the Central Pacific Railroad, the Chinese filled in and created the fertile farm region in the California delta, but they were not allowed to own the land they farmed.[7] They looked, acted, and sounded different from the White people. Their foreign dress, unfamiliar language and customs, and threat of competition for work and money resulted in total discrimination. Laws were passed that denied them employment, housing, and land. They were discouraged from settling anywhere and people who assisted them were jailed or fined.[8,9] They were taxed when others were not, barred from work in other industries, and from becoming citizens.[10] Crimes, including physical abuse, were committed against them, not by them, but the Chinese could not testify in court. Being heathens, their oaths were considered worthless.[11]

By 1860 the coolie trade had increased the Chinese population in the United States to 34,933. They were concentrated primarily in California, with an overwhelming ratio of 2000 males per 100 females.[12] The women were wives who had gained entry from China or the few women who had been born in America. The men made return trips to China to visit their families, but for the most part could not bring their children and wives to America. The separations were long and it was not uncommon for a child to be a teen-ager before he met his father.[13] American women lost their citizenship if they married a Chinaman.[14] For many years the Chinese in America were a bachelor population; the few existing families were coveted and treasured. Children were especially cherished because they were so scarce.

By 1880 there were 105,465 Chinese in America, the largest number to that date. Of these, 1000 had been born in the United States.[15] The steady increase in population and discrimination resulted in the Chinese Exclusion Acts of 1882, in which only nonlaboring classes of Chinese were allowed limited entry to this country. The granting of citizenship was still prohibited. From the enacting of that legislation the Chinese population in America decreased to a low in 1920 of 61,639.[16] After the Civil War the Western politicians who wanted laws against the Chinese joined with the Southern lawmakers who wanted ways to control the newly freed slave, and together they enacted racist laws that restricted education and allowed murders and lynchings. This plight of still not being allowed to testify in court, yet being the repeated receivers of abuse, gave rise to the phrase, "not a Chinaman's chance."[17]

Just as the words Englishmen and Frenchmen denote the country of origin, men from China proudly termed themselves Chinamen.[18] But the Whites could not see the common humanity beneath the pajama pants, gowns, high collars, and hair worn in long queues and stereotyped them as exotic, mysterious, inscrutable Orientals.[19] For centuries, Chinamen had grown the queue, or pigtail, as a sign of subjugation to the Manchus and their successors. At the turn of the century, the Sun Yat Sen revolutionaries in China and America cut off their queues in defiance of oppression.[20]

Forming of Chinatowns

The rough and uncultured frontier of the West contrasted sharply with the refinement and order so highly valued by the Chinese. They lived by the White man's rules, restrictions, and prejudices in clusters of families or groups of men in family-like situations.[21] They found solace in grouping together and sharing a familiar way of life, voluntarily segregating themselves from a hostile and cruel larger society.[22] Chinatowns were formed to provide mutual aid to recently arrived immigrants and safety and protection for each other, just as villages in China had done.[23]

Living in close physical proximity is a common practice for an immigrant population. This serves as a boundary-maintaining mechanism, a powerful anti-acculturative force.[24] Within the Chinatown boundaries, a highly structured society developed with the establishment of ethnically oriented institutions, which kept alive the ancient Chinese cultural heritage.[25]

As seems to be very commonly the case when immigrants reside in an area in large enough numbers, the Chinese established a number of Associations and institutions patterned after those of their native land. These Associations, composed of persons with the same name, from the same district of China, or speaking the same dialect, were formal and chartered in most cases and formed the basis of an elaborate social structure which was the Chinatowns of the United States. These Associations plus others such as the Chinese-language press, entertainments, schools, and churches, Chinese-style shops and goods and services, kept alive in many sections of this country, "islands" of a China-derived subculture.[26]

The social structure within the Chinatowns exerted a great deal of power and influence upon the residents. Each family unit was represented by a clan or organization that provided protection, settled disputes, and solved problems. Only when unable to reach agreement, did they refer themselves to the American courts of law. In order to succeed, any major undertaking within Chinatown sought the aid and approval of these essential units of power. Over the years, these clans and associations were less supported by the American-born Chinese, and since World War II they have lost their power and position, existing today in name only and as social clubs.[27]

The Chinese placed a high value on education and white collar jobs, but outside the Chinese community most jobs, other than menial, were closed to them. They supplemented the larger economy without competing directly within it, by choosing occupations such as laundries and eating establishments, and looked to their own Chinatown community to satisfy their social needs.[28] Because they did not trust the White people or their government, the Chinese tried to hide and be as inconspicuous as possible. Yet the more they tried to be hidden, "the more mysterious they appeared in the eyes of the Americans."[29]

San Francisco's Chinatown was established as early as 1860 and has continued to be the largest and best known. As the Chinese dispersed eastward from California to the Midwest and Eastern states, they demonstrated a tendency to settle in large metropolitan areas, which is how New York's Chinatown developed. Today it is over 100 years old.[30] Smaller Chinatowns exist in Chicago, Boston, and Canada. Kuykendall traces the evolution of Chinatown from a small service center in its earliest days, to a powerful and influential ghetto.[31] In the late 1940s and 1950s Chinatown changed. The veterans of World War II returned and insisted on living in the general community, wherever they chose.[32] Only the old stayed in Chinatown. In order to survive, Chinatown became a supplier of specialized goods to a larger population.

In 1943 Franklin Roosevelt repealed the Chinese Exclusion Act of 1882 and from 1945 to 1950 over 6000 Chinese women and 600 infants entered this country (Brides Act) as new families. Since then, the number of Chinese immigrants has increased each year, with more women entering than men.[33] During the centenary from 1860 to 1960 the total was never more than 237,000 Chinese in the whole United States. The 1970 census listed 435,062 Chinese in America, with a projection of 750,000 by 1980—still a small minority.[34]

The Chinese in Hawaii

While some Chinese were being imported to build the railroads in the West, others were brought to the Hawaiian islands as contract laborers for the sugar plantations.[35] The usual contract was for 5 years at 3 dollars per month, and it included passage money for the trip over, food, clothing, and lodging. These laborers were also hired as merchants, sugar masters, and shopkeepers. In contrast with the continental United States, these newcomers were welcomed and recognized as needed by the island people. They were urged to come to Hawaii and free to leave at the end of their contracts. Some purchased land and soon the Chinese were plantation owners as well as employees. Some reached out for the independent livelihood of small farming.

When they were isolated in plantation camps, the Chinese followed their own life-styles and traditional practices. The formal Chinatown in Honolulu was more a supplier of Chinese goods than a ghetto for displaced families. Honolulu's Chinatown has never been entirely occupied by Chinese because the Chinese in Hawaii live, work, and play as do all the other citizens of that state. They have never needed to live in clusters or be set apart. The lack of racial restrictions on land ownership and residential occupancy throughout the state accounts for the wide residential dispersion.[36]

The social and economic climate of Hawaii encouraged equality, and island-born Chinese are recognized as good examples of acculturation and assimilation. Owing to the rapid expansion of Hawaii's economy, there has been an increased demand for skilled and professional services, and the Chinese have been well received in these occupations. Today the Chinese comprise 6 percent of Hawaii's total population and they have one of the highest median incomes among that state's ethnic groups.[37]

Recent Immigrants

In more recent years the Chinese immigrants to America have been those escaping the political struggle between the Nationalist government in Taiwan and the Communist government, which came into power in Peking in 1949.[38] Some are laborers like the early immigrants to this country, but many of today's arrivals are well educated or specially trained and are given a preference to enter the country. Some may be better educated and have special skills, but they do not know the English language. They may feel helpless or fearful in the larger American community, so they are drawn to the familiarity of Chinatown, which now has old, dilapidated buildings. The latest quota (1965) of 20,000 Chinese immigrants annually has pushed the existing boundaries of Chinatown to new expansion. The newspapers have reported unsanitary living conditions in Chinatown and increased occurrences of hostile incidents among the new immigrants themselves.

Geographical Distribution

Today two out of every three Chinese living in America reside in the coastal states of California, New York, and Hawaii. They are concentrated in large urban centers of San Francisco, Los Angeles, Chicago, Boston, New York City, and Honolulu. The Chinese live in every state of the union, but are least visible in the central states.[39] The highest percentage of Chinese Americans, 20 percent, are service workers and 18 percent are in professional occupations, which is higher than the percentage for White Americans. Managerial, clerical, and operative positions follow closely as major areas of employment.[40]

CHINESE CONCEPT OF FAMILISM

The Chinese have long been considered the most familial people in the world. The family was the basis of Chinese culture and way of living; therefore, an in-depth understanding of their familial concept is necessary for an appreciation by the health professional. For over 2500 years a remarkable social and cultural continuity has characterized Chinese social institutions.[41] The traditional family existed without significant structural change among these institutions, maintaining a characteristic form—patriarchal, patrilineal, patrilocal, extended, located within the broader social organization of the clan and district associations, and integrated within a system of ethicoreligious beliefs centering

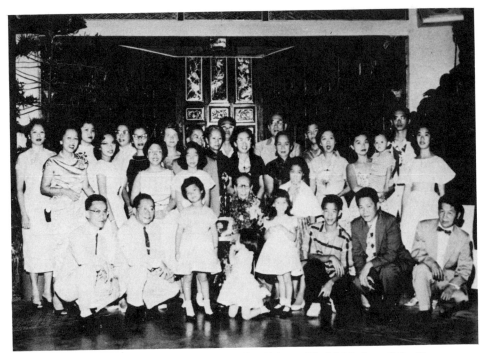

Figure 1. Four generations gather to honor the Chinese Model Mother of the Year.

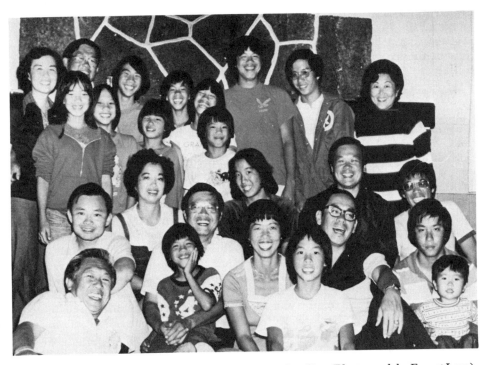

Figure 2. Modern and progressive Chinese-American families. (Photograph by Ernest Lam)

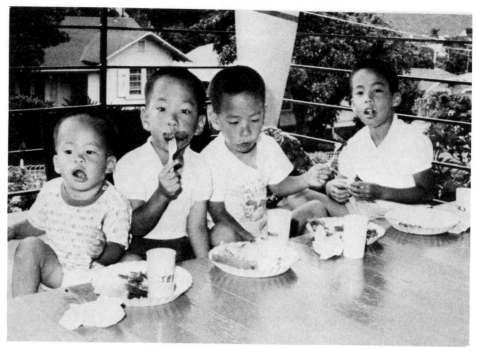

Figure 3. A man with many sons was considered truly blessed.

around ancestor worship. The whole Chinese social structure was based on the family, and the value orientation of the Chinese was bound into the concept of familism (Figs. 1 and 2). This concept can be better understood by closer examination of the forementioned characteristics of the Chinese family.

Characteristics of Traditional Chinese Family

The father was the autocratic head of the family and household. As head of the household and usually the oldest male, he was responsible for the management of all domestic affairs as well as the behavior of the family members.[42] As the economic principal, all things regarding financial matters were carried out under his direction.[43] His sons called him "yeh," the symbol of dignity and sternness.[44]

A man with many sons was considered truly blessed because males ensured the continuity of the family name and line (Fig. 3).[45] To die without a male offspring was the worst misfortune of all. Authority, property, and craft skills were passed from generation to generation along the male line, in descending order from eldest to youngest son. The first-born son held a special

importance as the extension, inheritor, and later principal caretaker of the family.[46]

There was greater emphasis on the parent-child relationship than the husband-wife relationship. The wife was considered an outsider to the family group until the birth of the first son. When a girl married, she automatically lost her position in her childhood home and became a member of her husband's family.[47] The synonym for marriage in Chinese is "taking a daughter-in-law."[48] Ties of blood, common ancestry, and shared childhood experiences were more valued than the relationship resulting from the marriage contract and sexual union.[49] A wife who did not bear sons was worthless and had no position or standing.

The traditional Chinese family system placed equal filial obligation upon all sons, enforcing this by patrilocal residence for all males, including the requirement that wives remain in the home of their parents-in-law even when the husband is absent.[50] Many of the early immigrants to America were married immediately prior to their departure to ensure an attachment and commitment to the family and the return of the sojourner. The new bride went to live in her husband's family home for the remainder of her life, even though her husband returned only infrequently to visit. Marriage was a vital concern of the family and the parents were responsible for arranging a proper marriage for their children. Children obeyed the selection and detailed arrangements made by the parents of the respective families, with the fathers exercising the most influence in the decision making. Sons were usually married by the age of 20, daughters by 18 years. Marriages were arranged for the laboring men in the United States with native women in China. The early immigrant families in America arranged marriages for their children until the end of World War II. By that time most of the children were acculturated and insisted upon the Western way of selecting their own marriage partner.

In China the singular importance of male progeny and the encouragement of reproduction gave rise to polygamy and concubinage.[51] If the legal wife delivered too few sons it was permissible for the husband to acquire additional wives or a concubine for procreation. Any children resulting from these liaisons were officially considered children of the first wife and subject to her.[52] It was not uncommon for female infants to be killed or given away at birth, as females were considered of low value and economically burdensome. Divorce was virtually non-existent, but allowed if a wife was barren. An elderly woman who had many grandsons was respected and honored.

THE EXTENDED FAMILY

The domiciliary unit in China consisted of the head of the household, his wife or wives, his children, and other kin, such as married sons and their wives and children.[53] Such an ideal family of as many as five generations under one roof was possible for those who could afford it, that is, the upper class. The peasants and farmers had considerably smaller households, which consisted of the husband, wife, and children, but the value of the extended family was held as the model and desired by all. The whole Chinese social structure was built upon the principle of the extended family organization. The first Chinese families in America did not have as many kin in the household; often they were a nuclear family. However, the principles of familism were still maintained and practiced.

The formal structure of the family dedicated the lives of the members to the continuity and welfare of the family group. A sense of collective responsibility was fostered by teaching children at an early age the necessity of cooperation, courtesy, patience, self-control, and self-sacrifice in family relations. Individualism was discouraged and denied. Everyone was taught to work for the honor and glorification of the family name.[54] Because each member felt responsible for the security and good name of the family, caution was exerted before taking action that would reflect on the family name. Approval of the individual by the family and the good reputation of the family were very important.[55] Members strove to "gain face" for the family, while any personal "loss of face" reflected on the entire family group and was to be avoided at all cost. These factors combined to exert considerable pressure within the family and extended to the clan.

All tangible property was equally divided among the sons, except that certain special privileges were sometimes shown the eldest son. Individuals did not own property or keep money for themselves; it was shared with the whole family. In Chinese etiquette someone might properly have been greeted with, "What is your occupation?" An equally acceptable reply would have been, "My uncle (or other relative) is a such-and-such," meaning "he makes good money, has enough to eat and therefore I am also well provided for." Wealth was shared in very concrete ways. It was required that the males remain together to share the property, which also encouraged patrilocal residence. While the husband was alive, the wife had no absolute ownership of anything. When he died, the widow received a share of the property settlement and went to live with one of her sons.

CLANS

A clan was the recognized grouping of families with the same surname and ancestors.[56] Clans included direct descendants or those related through marriage. They functioned as a larger extension of the family and actively influenced behavior, roles, expectations, and duties of family members. The clan defined rights, privileges, obligations, and ranks of individuals to each other. A clan maintained and held property for its members and financed economic institutions, including schools. Participation in family and clan affairs was not only desirable and preferred but was often the only real social existence one had. Persons with the same surname were generally considered to belong distantly to the same clan, even when a relationship could not be traced. Marriage between persons with the same surname was forbidden, even in cases where the family history and ancestors were known to be different.

The clan concept was highly developed in Southeast China, the area from which came most of the immigrants to the United States. In the new country the clan system maintained assumed ties of blood. Today when strangers meet and discover they have the same surname, a special closeness is felt between them, and one will usually comment, "We come from the same family." In Chinatown they united families with the same surnames into family associations. If there was a paucity of families in the family associations, then district associations were formed by the conglomeration of several family associations. Clan or association members united against other clan members with the most powerful group in each Chinatown generally ruling that domain. The clan system maintained isolation of the immigrant Chinese from the larger society.[57] After World War II they lost their power and existed only as social groups. Since 1960 there has been increased clan-like warring among the new youthful immigrants of San Francisco and New York.

ANCESTOR WORSHIP

The religious life of the Chinese was an integral part of the family's life. Their religion was expressed in the context of ancestor worship and practiced in the home and ancestral temples where they worshiped.[58] Great worth was ascribed to the ancestors and it was important that they be given due respect and honor. The Chinese believed that the "lineage from the remotest ancestor to the most recently born progeny formed an unbroken line which theoretically interacted regularly."[59] The concept of familism includes respect and obedience to one's living and dead ancestors, plus reverence and propitiatory activities for the deceased. The family was perpetuated through the father-son link—from the living sons to the patriarch, and then he to his deceased father. The relationship between the worlds was believed to be close and reciprocal. The link between the remotest ancestors and posterity was dramatized and symbolized in filial obligations and ancestral worship. It was believed that the spirits of dead ancestors hovered about, looking after the welfare of their descendants, and it was vital that they were as-

sured of their proper respect. The respect of the father to his ancestors is duplicated by the filial piety of his own offspring.

In *Sandalwood Mountains*, Jah spoke to her dead mother through a spiritual medium to seek advice for perplexing problems.[60] The dead were consulted because it was believed that once they had entered the higher world their knowledge was unlimited and their judgment always correct.

Each family kept a genealogy—information which gave the origin of the family, its collateral lines, marriages, births, deaths, official honors, burial sites, and generally a record of the male issues of the family.[61] Every 30 to 50 years that generation brought the book up to date. The genealogy was used to distinguish between families and to regulate marriages. Present-day families keep records of happenings to both males and females, as well as family trees. The genealogy resulted from an imperial decree that all people must have a family surname. As mentioned earlier, marriage between persons of the same family name was forbidden. A few years ago when a son from a family in Brooklyn, New York, wed the daughter of a family in Honolulu with the same surname, the more traditional family strongly objected. Family records were carved on stone tablets and kept in ancestral temples or family altars to perpetuate the eternal life of the family name. Each birth of a male, no matter how far away, was recorded with no break in lineage records. With the invention of the camera, the Chinese not only wrote their names on plaques but also hung portraits.[62] Chinese societies hung pictures of respected members and homes displayed portraits of ancestors. When the Communist government took control in China, they systematically destroyed the ancient tablets to discourage ancestor worship, but the people still maintain pride in their genealogy.

FUNERAL PRACTICES

Funerals had many rituals and practices that the immigrants continued to observe in the new country. Death was a natural occurrence, accepted as part of the life-cycle.[63] At the funeral, relatives burned paper images of clothing, dishes, a house, servants, horses, cows and other animals, spectacles, tobacco, pipes, money, and other articles that might be used in the spirit world.[64] The author has seen a television set among these items! The elaborateness of the articles indicated the wealth of the deceased. Each family tried to provide their best for the departed member. Special musicians were hired to play gongs and cymbals while firecrackers were burned to drive away demons and evil spirits. Flaming candles placed near the bier lighted the way to the afterworld. Those buried in America desired to have their bones excavated after a few years and carried to China for a permanent burial. Upon returning home from a funeral, a mourner walked over a small fire before entering his house. This was to ensure that no evil spirits or demons gained access to his home. He also purified himself by washing his hands in water, upon which floated leaves of the pomelo tree. The death date of the deceased was then commemorated annually thereafter because it signified his birth into the spiritual world.

The clans were involved with ancestor worship by financially contributing to the upkeep of graveyards and temples.[65] Ching Ming was the yearly gathering of the clan at the gravesites to honor their dead by burning paper offerings and decorating the graves. Cooked food was placed before the name tablets or gravestones in the same spirit as Christians placed floral offerings on their ancestor's graves. When the graveside activities were completed, the clan gathered for a banquet, at which clan affairs were discussed.[66] Contemporary Chinese-American families commemorate Ching Ming in late spring and gather for a social meal after the visit to the cemetery.

The Christian belief in only one God with emphasis on the individual's relationship with God was very alien to the Chinese concept of familism. In the early days of the Chinatown, the Christian mission churches did not have many members from among the Chinese, yet they protected the residents of Chinatown from outside attacks and spoke out against the injustices that occurred. The Christian missions provided medical care and helped greatly to acculturate the immigrants by teaching them English.[67] As more Chinese in America became Christians, the traditional funeral practices diminished in elaborateness and ritual.

CHINESE FAMILY IN AMERICA

The Chinese brought their ideal of a large extended family to the United States, but were seldom able to realistically achieve the same kinship-clan existence of China. The American-Chinese family has taken many altered forms, owing to several factors. Immigration restrictions, which diminished the number of Chinese women available for marriage and forced the lengthy separation of husband and wife, resulted in very few families prior to 1930. The increased number of American-born Chinese from 1930 to 1950 indicated that these few families produced many children. Children were very important and vital to the Chinese family (childrearing is considered in another section of this chapter). Early families in America remained traditionally similar to those in China, though diminished in size.

Early Chinese-American families preferred living in Chinese neighborhoods and associated primarily with other Chinese people.[68] The associations and clubs they joined were composed exclusively of Chinese. Many families conducted small businesses as family enterprises and those who worked for others tended to work for relatives. Close financial relations existed between relatives. A person needing money would approach a grand-uncle or fourth cousin for a loan before applying to a bank.

The people of China once exalted the scholar, and education has always been the means to higher economic, political, and social status.[69] The scholar was considered to be of the highest class and most respected. The Chinese have always had a respect for learning, and the immigrants realized that it was the answer by which their children could gain security and the admiration and respect of others. They expected their children to learn and do well in school, even in a strange land.[70]

The immigrant children were educated in English-speaking public schools within Chinatown. They became bilingual and acculturated at a more rapid pace than their parents, especially the mother who might never have occasion to learn English. The father might have learned a smattering of English from his work contacts, but the mother usually remained home and had limited association with other Chinese women in the ghetto.[71]

The children also attended Chinese language school after the daily English school was over.[72] Families insisted on the dual education to ensure that their Chinese heritage, language, and values were learned and perpetuated. The adept Chinese-American student read English on a horizontal plane from left to right during part of his day and then shifted to Chinese, which read vertically from top to bottom, moving in the opposite direction of right to left. The flowing English

149

script was also very differently formed than the Chinese strokes for characters. Each character was square-shaped, equivalent to a one-syllable word. Written Chinese began as a picture language.

A study done by Liang identified the ideal Chinese-American family in 1951 as one in which the father had a higher status than other family members and usually made the family decisions.[73] The mother remained in the home not seeking outside employment and had few social relations. Boys were superior to girls because of their potential as income providers and continuing the family name, while daughters-in-law were subservient to their parents-in-law. Working children contributed their earnings to the family income; sometimes they were allowed a portion for personal expenses. Liang concluded at that time that the Chinese families in Chicago were moving along a continuum of acculturation and assimilation and were becoming more Americanized. The above ideal characteristics were found to be consistently present in only a few families, which were considered more traditional. The second-generation family was significantly more Westernized than that of the first-generation, resembling the White American middle-class family. Chinese families engaged in American occupations were more acculturated than those who worked in restaurants or laundries. The practice of ancestor worship was declining and Chinese holidays were less observed. There were more numerous families, half of which were residing away from Chinatown. The average number of family members was four. The median age for marriage was 26 for males and 21 for females. A very small percentage of the Chinese moved to rural areas but engaged in non-farming occupations. The two most famous Chinese businesses were the hand laundry and the exotic restaurant.

Betty Sung describes modern Chinese-American families as being very different from those in China and early America.[74,75] Today's kinship family includes father, mother, children, and sometimes grandparents who reside with the eldest son. The mother may work outside the home, creating a new problem of unsupervised children at home after school. The problems of the working mother are not new to this country, but they are novel to the Chinese family if they are unaccustomed to the mother being employed by an outsider. The younger people have moved to the suburbs and socially interact with other ethnic neighbors, leaving the elderly and newly arrived immigrants in Chinatown.

The present day Chinese-American family seems to closely resemble Rothschild's description of a modified extended family, which involves residential separation of the nuclear family from other kin, while simultaneously maintaining a close relationship between the couple and their parents.[76] This is accomplished through frequent visiting and communication, mutual financial assistance, babysitting and housework services, and a variety of other exchanges and obligations. By maintaining a closer relationship with the parents, a couple can enjoy the advantages of psychological and financial security provided by extended family relationships. Residential separation affords more privacy and the choice of how, when, and what degree of interaction will occur between parents and offspring.

Like many other American families, the Chinese have become more mobile, leaving their childhood environment to accept work and reside in other areas of the country. They join the increasing ranks of nuclear families existing alone, without any kin nearby. As subsequent generations of American-born Chinese live outside of Chinatown, socializing and interacting with other Americans of mixed ethnic backgrounds, they will be influenced by and adopt many American ways. They may observe some of the Chinese customs, but it will be increasingly difficult to preserve the family in its traditional, defined form. Family conflict has increased with the children refusing to accept the values and customs of a China they do not know and rebelling against strict parental control. Increasing interracial marriages have also changed the physical identity of the Chinese. One out of four Chinese marries outside of his race nowadays.[77]

Woman's Role

Woman's role in old Chinese families was very rigid and utilitarian.[78] Girls were not highly valued.[79] Families of means had many domestic servants and poor parents sold their daughters to the wealthy anywhere between the age of 3 to 10 years; the price ranged from $10 to $100. When the girl was married, the cost of her upbringing was recouped from wedding presents arranged through the marriage broker. As an unmarried daughter, she helped with all domestic duties, especially child care and cooking, in preparation for her role as wife and mother. If raised in her

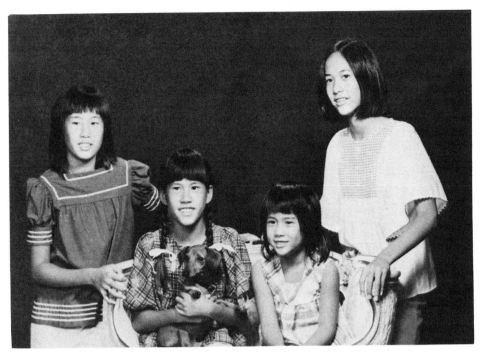

Figure 4. Chinese-American daughters are appreciated.

family home she relinquished those ties when she married and became a member of her husband's family. If her husband was wealthy and took another wife, the first wife was expected to accept the new wife as another member of the household. Second and third wives also knew their designated roles in the system. The only alternatives for an unhappy wife were returning home to her parents, bringing utter disgrace to herself and them, or suicide.

As an immigrant wife in Chinatown she worked with her husband if he had a business and also managed the household and children.[80] Limited social contacts and confinement to a small geographical vicinity retarded her acculturation. She learned the new ways from her children. Although it is generally believed that Chinese women were submissive and weak, studies of Chinese-American families have shown that the mother was a very powerful person within the family unit.[81] The husband was usually too busy attending to the economics for the family and the mother was responsible for the actual child care and managing the household. Working together with her children provided many opportunities to mold personalities and influence thinking. She took care of all the house-

hold details. Although the father retained ultimate authority for major decisions, the mother had great influence in many of the decisions.

The depth of the husband-wife relationship was not readily apparent to a stranger. In Chinese culture it was improper for a husband to express intimate feelings, including those for his wife.[82] She was not mentioned in his conversation and even when working in the family business was not introduced to others.[83] The Chinese had the expectation that those who wed as virtual strangers will develop personal bonds in the course of married life.[84] Although the Chinese emphasize maintaining composure and pose and much of their expression is formal, the love of parents for their children and for each other is definitely not inhibited to the point of extinction (Fig. 4).

Modern Chinese-American women have been educated and are highly acculturated. Arranged marriages have ceased to exist in America; young people are marrying for love. Wives are no longer subservient to their husbands, although he may still have the edge on authority. A recent study found that foreign-born Chinese mothers have more restrictive attitudes toward child-rearing and higher acceptance toward their childrearing and maternal roles than the American-born mothers, whose attitudes tended to be more democratic and permissive.[85] With increased acculturation the foreign-born mothers have become less restrictive and also less accepting of their childrearing and maternal roles. American-born Chinese women consider themselves equals with their husbands in family matters, including decision-making, child-rearing, and economic opportunities.

CHILDREARING PRACTICES

> The child is born as a white linen cloth and the design which eventually appears upon it is due to the kind of training that he has had.[86]

Childrearing is a very important function of the family. The Chinese believe that during the years the child lives with his parents and other family members he should be learning the values of his family and proper ways of behaving, as preparation for his future participation in society.[87] Early immigrant families especially cherished children because of the paucity of families and children. Having children meant increasing their numbers and more important, perpetuation of the family name. The Chinese first nurture and protect the infant, then train the older child to bring honor to himself and the family.[88] Nurturance of the very young borders on indulgence, and combined with an extremely protective environment builds a reservoir of trust and security. Sollenberger attributes the school-age child's conforming and accepting with minimum hostility the rigid demands made upon him as he grows older to this secure foundation in his early years.

The values of the traditional family are still conveyed to the children of the modern family.[89] In 1971 Nancy Young observed childrearing practices and interviewed families in Hawaii for her doctoral thesis. In this author's opinion the Chinese in Hawaii are further along the continuum of acculturation and assimilation than those Chinese families in mainland United States Chinatowns and probably are very similar to those mainland Chinese-American families that have become very Americanized in their mode of living. Young's findings are apropos to Chinese-American families in general because the values have remained the same, while the practices vary in degree or style depending upon the family's acculturation. The enduring values that Chinese families maintain are emphasis on the family, educational attainment, high occupational status, diligence, and economic attainment.[90] The strategies that the parents utilize to teach these values and attain their goals are the childrearing practices of providing a nurturant environment, administration of early and firm discipline, definitive statements of sanctioned and non-sanctioned behavior, maximum exposure to models of exhibited sanctioned behavior, restriction from models that exhibit non-sanctioned behavior, and the expectancy of a relatively late age at which the child will informally interact with his peers.

The first year for the infant is warm and secure. He is lavished with attention by everyone—mother, father, siblings, grandparents, and other relatives (Fig. 5). The extended family members may not reside in the same house, but if they live nearby, a close relationship provides the infant with frequent contact with them. If he cries, someone immediately checks to see what the reason might be. Physical causes such as a wet diaper, or excessive or inadequate clothing, are promptly remedied. Carrying a baby to relieve crying varies with the mother's orientation. If she is of the belief that crying is good for the child and carrying will spoil him, then she will usually allow him to cry in his crib after having checked for physical discomforts. If the mother does not consider carrying detrimental to the child's development, she will pick him up. This area seems to be one of great conflict between mothers and grandparents and it does not seem confined to Chinese families. However, in traditional Chinese families infants were not allowed to cry. They were immediately carried in the arms by a family member, carried in a sling on the back, put to breast, or rocked in the cradle.[91]

Breastfeeding is usually directed by the infant's demand rather than the mother's schedule. The child may be eating solid food and drinking from a cup before weaning occurs. The incidence of breastfeeding seems to diminish as the mother becomes more Americanized. Bottlefeeding mothers anticipate the infant's awakening and feeding and will have a bottle in readiness so the baby does not have to wait.

The very young infant frequently sleeps in his parents' bed or the same room at night.[92] If the infant cries or is sick, he shares their sleeping arrangements. Often the baby is allowed to fall asleep in his parents' bed and later is carried to his own bed. Parents say it is more important at this age to provide a sense of security and allay

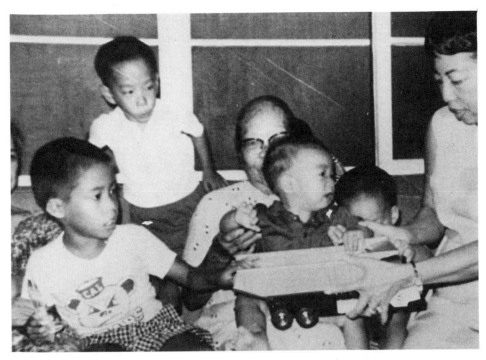

Figure 5. Great-grandmother and grandmother involved with childrearing.

the child's fears than for him to be brave and show independence.[93]

During the early years a permissive attitude prevails and the infant and very young child are not put on a rigid schedule in regard to any biological function. They eat and sleep according to their own needs, not according to the clock. The Chinese mother trains herself to recognize the child's needs and to take care of them,[94] as she has been previously trained to anticipate the needs of her husband and parents-in-law. She teaches the young child to use the bathroom by placing him on the toilet as he demonstrates readiness, but there is usually no punishment for lapses in toilet training before 4 years of age.[95] An informal comparison made over the years by this author has shown that Chinese mothers change their children's diapers more frequently than their White American counterparts. This may be related to the anticipation of the infant's needs.

There is little or no enforcement of eating habits at the toddler age.[96] As he wanders about, the parent or older relative may follow the toddler around with rice bowl in hand, feeding him occasional mouthfuls.

Children are taught behavior and values mainly through observation, participation, and imitation. The parents' sense of complete responsibility plus the belief that the child's behavior reflects his training encourages Chinese parents to keep their children under careful surveillance.[97] This includes taking them everywhere with the parents or limiting the parents' social activities to those to which they can bring children. Children are included in family and social gatherings, where they have a wealth of opportunity to observe the behavior of adults and to interact with them (Fig. 6). The extended family provides models for acceptable behavior. If the parents cannot be accompanied by children, the preference is for one parent to remain home with them.[98] When absolutely necessary for both parents to leave the children at home, only grandparents or relatives are relied upon and trusted as parental substitutes. This accounts for the presence of many children, even very young ones, at social gatherings and out shopping. The permissive attitude about bedtime and the desire to keep children close by also explains children being seen out late at night with their parents.

The Chinese delight in the antics of babies and young children. Parents may give in or indulge children in consideration of their needs or demands; however, a firm discipline is maintained.

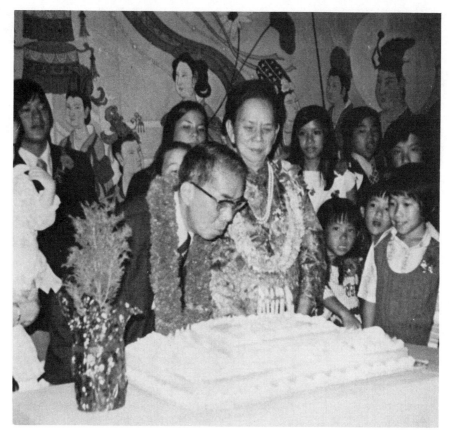
Figure 6. Children are included in celebrations and social gatherings.

As the child becomes mobile he is taught to avoid certain objects. This is accomplished by a sharp verbal "no," frequently accompanied by a slap on the hand or buttocks and physical removal of the child from the undesirable object. At an early age he learns to avoid such things as hot or breakable objects and especially areas that the parent deems unsafe, such as steps or high places.

Respect for their parents is a primary virtue taught to Chinese children.[99] This is manifested by the child's obedience to his parents and an attitude of honor and deference towards them, even when the child is grown and has his own children. This respect extends to older persons in the family; each uncle or aunt is addressed in a specific manner, such as "my father's youngest sister," or "mother's older brother." Modern families are not quite as precise, but adult males and females are called "uncle" or "aunt" to indicate respect, whether or not they are kin.[100]

Parents feel totally responsible for their child's behavior, which is considered a reflection on them. If a child misbehaves, he has not received proper training at home. Sollenberger relates an incident in which the teacher sent home a note reporting an infraction of the rules by a Chinese pupil.[101] The father personally went to school the next day to apologize to the teacher for *his* failure in the proper upbringing of his child. Such action on behalf of the father would probably be rare today; more likely the child would be chastised at home and the parent would remind him of the shame he has brought to the family name. "One person's disgrace results in shame to the entire family"[102] and similar admonitions are repeated early to the young Chinese.

Education has always been stressed as a means of achievement and continues to be an important value. Immigrant children were told to "study hard, then life will be easier for you than it is for us." Implicit in statements made nowadays is a similar chain of events: if you study hard you can go to college, which will help you get a better job, resulting in more income and a higher standard of living. American schools have reinforced this by stressing academic achievement, effort, and good conduct. They also indicate models of famous people who have earned their fame by this behavior.

The absence of overt parental praise and reward has been identified as a childrearing practice designed to teach a child humility.[103] Young's study confirmed this and also found that reward for desired behavior was not totally lacking.[104] Mothers were unable to describe positive incentives for good behavior, but they acknowledged that substantial recognition from peers, teachers, and relatives served as encouragement. Non-verbal indicators of pleasure, such as a slight affirmative nod or the glimpse of a smile on the parent's face, are obvious to the child from an early age. The absence of a scolding may also serve as positive reinforcement to the Chinese child. Immigrant parents preferred to give material rewards, such as money or a food treat, rather than praise. Modern parents give material rewards and in addition are more generous in verbal praise.

Verbal communication has increased between Chinese children and their parents. Immigrant families had stilted, formal contacts, which were commands or scoldings. The child remained within hearing range of an adult and was ignored as long as he did not exhibit rough behavior or unnecessary loudness.[105] Children did not speak unless they were spoken to. Chinese families today have more small talk and children voice their opinions in discussions.

Parents convey the importance of certain values verbally and through their actions. First-generation parents were strict authoritarians and their commands were never questioned.[106] "If my parents disapproved, it was wrong," was a guideline for second-generation children. Hard-working parents demonstrate through their own actions their belief that diligence is a desirable trait and leads to success. Industrious parents reiterate to their children, "We work hard so you can have this and even better. You must also work hard to maintain what you have and strive to improve."

Spanking and scolding are common methods of punishment. Immigrant families were accustomed to beatings with a bamboo rod from either parent but modern families spank or threaten spankings. Shaming or lecturing are other usual forms of punishment. The young child may be temporarily removed from the social life of the family or deprived of certain privileges or objects. Rarely is the child ridiculed.[107] Undesired behaviors are disobedience, aggressiveness, fighting, messiness, and poor school work. Desired behaviors are obedience, sharing, non-competitiveness among siblings, and achievement, especially in school work.[108,109]

Chinese children are incorporated early and relatively fully into the daily life of the family. They are taught that everyone works for the welfare of the family, so they, too, must be useful at an early age.[110] They are assigned specific chores not only to demonstrate that their help is needed at home, but as proper training for their future life (Fig. 7). The children are given a great deal of responsibility at a comparatively young age.[111] Older children are responsible for teaching and supervising younger children and assisting with food preparation. Older siblings are encouraged to set the example for younger ones by giving up pleasure or comfort in favor of someone else, to give in during a quarrel, and to politely refuse in favor of someone else.[112] Although given responsibility for tasks at home, the Chinese child is not encouraged to have independent activity outside the home or with other non-family children until late childhood.

The young child is dependent on his parents for food, shelter, clothing, and other aspects of his physical existence, as well as his emotional security. As he grows older and ventures outside the family and home, his parents are insistent upon knowing details about his friends. Peers are carefully screened and the child is not allowed playmates who exhibit undesirable traits or behavior. Other Chinese children of similar economic and social status are highly encouraged as associates.

Chinese children enjoy playing, but it is not overtly encouraged by their parents. Little girls in China did not play with dolls because they were regarded as having magical powers. In the Chinese language, the word "doll" comes from the same root word as "idol" or "fetish." "Dolls were used as ritual objects to be held during confinement or placed as a temple offering when one hoped for the birth of a child."[113] Exuberant physical activity is not highly valued among traditional parents, who prefer games and puzzles that challenge the mind and the individual's

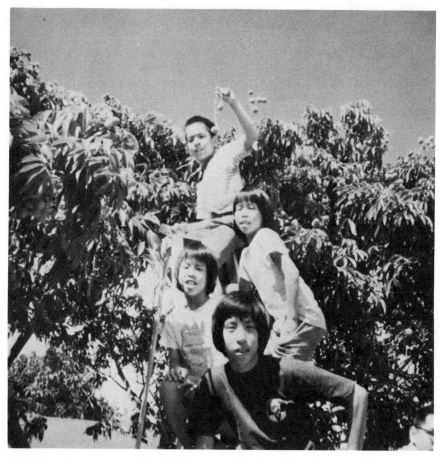

Figure 7. Chinese-American children are given chores at an early age.

abilities.[114] Chess, go, cards, and mah-jong are popular games among many adults. Wealthy women in China played these games for hours and were interrupted only to nurse the infant. Children of American-born Chinese have been exposed to a great deal of physical activity and their play is like that of other American children. Suburban teams of baseball, football, and soccer include Chinese-American members.

After World War II the American-born offspring reacted strongly against the traditional values and practices and displayed enthusiasm for the concept of individualism. As the younger generations assimilate more American culture, the gap widens between the old and young.

Kuykendall[115] found that acculturation-oriented Chinese Americans were proud of being Chinese and considered themselves "modern and progressive." They were not trying to become Anglo-Americans but described themselves as being "like everyone else."

A recent interview of several young Chinese-American adults revealed that they embrace and perpetuate the strengths of their heritage, shunning the parts they term rigid, and combining their selected cultural system with their Western learning.[116] Expectations of their parents that they had fulfilled included attending prestigious colleges, becoming teachers, physicians, or lawyers, marrying their "own kind" and into the "right" family, and advancing their position on the social ladder. A corporate vice-president said that in his family of origin the idea of his attending college was a foregone conclusion. In his family of procreation he tries to expose his children to "things Chinese," attempting to give them some sense of identification with their ancestry. Fluent in the Chinese language, he no longer speaks it to his children because they do not understand it. They laughed at his previous attempts to speak it to them and subsequently avoided his further attempts.

Contemporary Chinese-American youths are more vocal than those of previous generations. They are less hesitant to champion a cause, speak out, protest, or demonstrate against what they deem inequities or injustices. A youthful political activist related being ostracized more by his own family than by outside society. "They didn't throw me out, they just iced me and then surrounded me, that really did the job."

Those interviewed described some of the acculturative changes that they observed. The young adults are no longer pressured to date only Chinese. Social interaction among people of different racial backgrounds is acceptable; the Chinese no longer need to band together for protection. These young adults want to perpetuate certain aspects of their heritage. They want their children to learn the cultural ways and the tradition that binds them. They also want their children to experience the closeness, sense of belonging, and acceptance that is part of the extended family. An example given was the immediate inclusion of a new wife into the family grouping. She was a White American married to a Chinese American, and upon first meeting his aunts, they invited her to a family cooking lesson because she was now "part of the family."

CULTURAL BELIEFS AND PRACTICES

America's culture has been enriched by the folklore, customs, and ideas that the various immigrant groups have brought to this country. The Chinese in America kept their social customs and practices, which they remembered from the "good old days" in the villages of China. Their insular existence in Chinatown encouraged this preservation. In some instances the Chinese in Hawaii observe more traditional practices than the Chinese in the mainland United States, even though the Hawaiian Chinese have assimilated more American culture. Perhaps it is their way of demonstrating their Chinese heritage while they otherwise appear very American. Second-generation Chinese may continue certain practices without knowing or understanding the original reason or belief. They learned the practice from their parents, and not to continue doing it might bring bad luck or offend the spirits. Recent arrivals from China have not recognized the old practices that some of the overseas Chinese, those who live across the ocean from China, continue to keep.

Western calendar months are reckoned by the earth's revolving around the sun.[117] The Chinese lunar calendar months are determined by the revolutions of the moon around the earth. The Chinese use the lunar calendar on a recurring cycle of 12 years.[118] Each year is designated as belonging to a certain animal and characteristics of that animal are attributed to persons born in that year.[119] For example, persons born in the Year of the Rat have great charm and attraction, and are diligent perfectionists. Dog people are loyal and honest; they can be depended upon to keep secrets. Emotionally cool, they do not mix well in social gatherings.

Holidays

Chinese families in America celebrate both the traditional American holidays and also certain Chinese holidays (Fig. 8). The most common are Chinese New Year, Full Moon Festival, Ching Ming, All Soul's Day, and Dragon Boat Festival. Some families commemorate anniversaries of an ancestor's birth or death days, while others observe only a few of the preceding holidays. The focal point of the year's celebrations is Chinese New Year. Thanks is given for the past year and supplication made for the coming year. It is a time to start anew, to wipe the slate clean. Chores left undone are finished and all debts are paid before one can begin the new year.[120] Whatever happens on New Year's Day determines the events for the coming year. Sweeping the floor that day is forbidden, to protect against the family luck being swept away. Spanking, crying, and washing of hair are not allowed on the first day of the year.

Red is the predominant color for New Year's as well as weddings and birthdays. Red is the sign of joy and happiness, symbolizing virtue, truth, and sincerity. White is the color of mourning. Early Chinese in America were very puzzled to see American brides in white!

Firecrackers are an important part of many celebrations. "Gods and men delight in the noise while devils fear it and stay away."[121] Traditional Chinese believe the noise serves to honor the immortals and scare away evil spirits. Chinese-American children have great fun being risky and making loud noises without being reprimanded. Today's children value firecrackers for their daring fun.

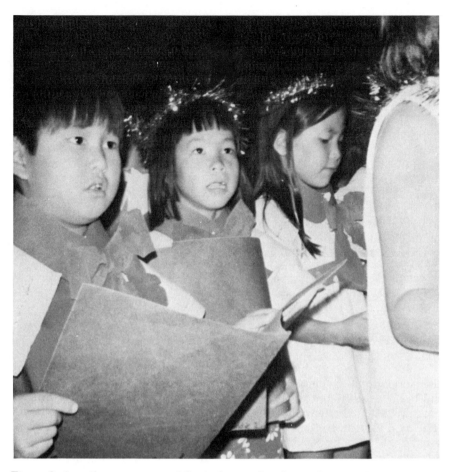

Figure 8. American customs and festivals are also observed.

Not only at New Year's but whenever one greets friends, the traditional posture is with both hands joined together and raised before the breast. This stance is to imply the hands are not employed in a hostile manner but held forward in a token of friendliness.[122]

Food

As with any culture, food is an integral part of celebrations as well as daily living. As one group becomes acculturated to another's way of living, the changes are manifested first in clothing, then language, and lastly food.[123] The Chinese consider food to be not merely for existence but as an art that can always be enjoyed.[124] Gifts of food denote that the giver has more than the bare necessities of life and wishes to pass on good things to others. Chinese do not think of whole roasts of meat, entire chickens, or ducks. Rather, preparation is based on inventiveness and in-

genuity. High in vegetables, low in fats and sweets, cooked in a manner that preserves vitamins, it is one of the healthiest of diets. It is served in bite size pieces to enable easy access with chopsticks. Porcelain spoons are used for semi-liquids or soups, as they do not conduct heat or alter the taste of delicate foods. A college student newly arrived from China described being nauseated when served a thick American steak for dinner. The sight of such a huge slab of meat on the platter offended her palate and her throat constricted at such a barbarian practice.

The Chinese in Hawaii, being residentially dispersed, freely mingled with the many ethnic people of the islands. They assimilated foods of other cultures, such as the Japanese, Filipino, Hawaiian, and Korean, as well as the predominant American. It is not uncommon for a Chinese-American family in Hawaii to sit down to a meal that consists of rice, a meat dish prepared in a Chinese manner, a Japanese vegetable, Korean pickles, and ice cream for dessert.

Proper etiquette ordains receiving and giving food with both hands. Poor table manners resulted in a quick rap across the knuckles from the father's chopsticks. Dinnertime conversation was considered very rude among immigrant families. Kingston remembers in her family that silence while eating was inforced with the declaration, "Every word that falls from the mouth is a coin lost."[125]

Rice symbolizes life and fertility; hence the origin of throwing rice grains at newly married couples.[126] Rice and vegetables are served at each meal among families from Southern China. Families from Northern China, where it was too cold to grow rice, are more accustomed to noodles, pancakes, or wheat products for their staple. A birthday party is not complete until the noodles are served because they symbolize longevity.

Tea is poured and served for all occasions.[127] Tea pouring can be an elaborate ceremony, as it is for weddings, welcoming a new wife, visitors, or friends, and celebrating birthdays. Or it can be the accompaniment to a simple meal. There are many medicinal teas. On special occasions the receiver of tea gives the pourer money wrapped in red paper.

Health Care

In China people associated the high death rate from smallpox with doctors and they were reluctant to seek medical care or be vaccinated.[128] Some early immigrants feared and refused vaccination also, but subsequent Chinese in America have accepted Western professional medical care. The hypothesis that Asians are reluctant to use medical facilities was not substantiated in Kurokawa's study.[129] His findings were that traditionally oriented people living in the midst of non-traditional society handled familiar situations themselves. If the condition was unique to them they were willing to seek medical advice. The predisposition to medical care was positively correlated to the degree of acculturation.

The balance of yin and yang is foremost in maintaining optimum health, according to the Chinese.[130] Harmony and moderation are stressed in relation to the philosophy that elemental forces pervade all aspects of an individual's life.[131] Illness is attributed to an imbalance of either the yin or yang forces, and a cure is the result of restoring the balance. Folk medicine was based on yang factors of warmth, light, and heat to the body, and yin elements of cold, dark, and cooling to the body. For thousands of years the Chinese cured their sick with skills and medicinal herbs. From experience they learned that certain barks of trees, roots, or plants will reduce fever, build up blood, or clear away infections. Certain foods are also said to retard healing, increase inflammation, and form keloids and scars. Pharmacology has substantiated the usefulness of many of these herbs.

Acupuncture, the use of needles inserted into key points of the body to restore health, has been practiced by the Chinese for centuries.[132] Recent exchanges with the current government of China have resulted in Western doctors and newspapermen reporting on its use in Chinese hospitals. Research in Europe and the United States is being done to determine its principles, methodology, and effectiveness. Licensed acupuncturists are available and practicing in Hawaii. Further information about them has not been investigated at this time.

Childbirth Beliefs and Practices

Birth, marriage, and death are considered the three vital stages of the life-cycle. Awaiting the baby's arrival is an exciting time, full of anticipation and anxiety. In the old days many beliefs and customs were brought from China and practiced by the immigrant mothers. An unpublished study by the Public Health Nurses in Hawaii described many interesting childbirth beliefs and practices.[133] They recognized that being in good health, receiving medical help, and observing the fertile period were aids to conceiving. Other means they tried for becoming pregnant were adopting a child, making offerings to the gods, taking male images to bed, and sleeping in certain postures after intercourse. Contraceptives were not used, since large families were desired, yet some women told of knowing the contraceptive effect of certain herb teas and extracts that would induce abortion.

If the woman carried the fetus high and close, her abdomen was rounder in shape, and she appeared happy, the baby was predicted to be a male. An unhappy countenance, protruding abdomen, or the facial "mask" of pregnancy were indications of a female child. During pregnancy the woman ate a high protein diet, which emphasized eggs, meat, and bean curd. Too many fruits and vegetables were considered weakening to the mother. It was also believed that shellfish caused indigestion and poisoned the baby's blood, resulting in boils. Hot herb or ginger tea relieved the nausea and vomiting of pregnancy. During the second and third trimesters, herb tea was taken daily to strengthen the mother's body. Chewing beetlenut was thought to be good for her teeth.

Delivery at home with the assistance of a midwife was customary in China and among the first generation in the new country. If the woman was ill she consulted a medical doctor who examined her indirectly through the aid of an ivory figurine of a reclining woman.[134] The patient pointed to the area on the doll that corresponded to her area of discomfort and described the pain or symptoms. The doctor then made a diagnosis and treated her accordingly. For delivery, the mother squatted on the protected floor. The umbilical cord was kept for good luck and to brew medicinal tea if the child became ill. The placenta was buried deep in the ground so harm would not befall the infant. A baby born with a caul was believed slated for fame.

The mother was held responsible for an infant born prematurely or with defects. A physical anomaly was punishment for the mother's wrongdoing during pregnancy, such as nailing, pounding, lifting heavy furniture, or looking at ugly animals. A harelip was thought to be the result of cleaning ditches. Any defect represented injury to the child's spirit and physical self. Avoiding the subject of deformities was held as a preventive measure by some. The Mongolian spot, an acceptable mark, meant the baby had been born dead to another family and spanked back to life by the gods; then his spirit was reincarnated and he was reborn into this family. Twins were welcomed but multiple births of three or more were regarded as animalism.

The idea that the mother was solely responsible for birth defects placed an unusual burden of guilt feelings upon her and deprived her of the helpful effect of shared responsibility. The beliefs in evil spirits gave additional fear to the natural anxiety of pregnancy and childbirth that is experienced by all mothers. Fortunately, neither of these beliefs exists today.

The baby was put to breast immediately after delivery and placed on a self-demand feeding schedule. An oil bath was given to cleanse the infant. A Chinese baby is considered 1 year old at birth. This relates to the Chinese way of reckon-

ing and the 12-year cycle. At the New Year following his birth, the child is then calculated to be 2 years old. The health care provider might want to determine the family's method of counting when given a young child's age.

It was thought that during the first month the infant's spirit wandered, and many precautions were taken lest he became possessed by evil spirits. A party was given at the end of the first month to celebrate the union of the child's spirit with his body. The mother also took special care of herself during the first month. She ate pig's feet cooked in vinegar, which was thought to have a cleansing effect, and drank chicken-wine soup, which was strengthening and promoted lactation. Vegetables and fruits were avoided because they were considered weakening. Second-generation mothers tell of sneaking fresh fruits and vegetables to eat to combat constipation during pregnancy and after delivery—unseen by the older women. A woman was considered in an unclean state when having menstrual or lochial flow. During those periods she remained at home and did not socialize with others. Intercourse was restricted for a hundred days after delivery.

A practice on the one hundredth day after birth was to place the infant on a sticky pancake on a chair, to make him a quiet child and one who "stayed put," and feed him bits of solid food. The same food was offered to the gods in thanksgiving and supplication for blessings on the child.

Eggs have a great deal of symbolism for the Chinese.[135] They represent good luck, happiness, and fertility. Their oval shape is pleasing and implies well being; the lack of corners denotes tranquility. The yolk and white are likened to the positive and negative forces of yin and yang. Eggs are dyed red, the color of joy and happiness, and given to friends who have given gifts to the newborn.[136] Buns with black sugar stuffing and slices of roast pork garnished with pickled ginger are included with the red eggs. The friends reciprocate with a small monetary gift wrapped in red paper.

Naming the baby was a very important undertaking. Learned men, temple monks, or respected persons were consulted as givers of names.[137] Chinese have two character names; frequently the first character is identical for all sons in one family. Children born in America were given American first names and also Chinese two-character names. "The Chinese name must reflect his individuality, convey a good meaning, be suitable for his social status, and not duplicate names of relatives."[138]

IMPLICATIONS FOR HEALTH PROFESSIONALS

"Making sense out of human behavior is an important skill for a health specialist."[139] The behavior of the Chinese-American patient may be different from that of the health specialist or the larger society, but with a knowledge of the cultural system the care provider can better anticipate and understand the behavior of the patient. When meeting the patient of Chinese ethnic origin, the health professional needs to consider where that person is along the continuum of acculturation and assimilation. Is he newly arrived in the United States? What generation is he? If American-born, how close are the family ties? The American-born Chinese is more likely to be highly Westernized and, indeed, may more closely identify with the White American of his social and economic level than with his Chinese racial background. Consumers may not carry the cultural system that their external appearance suggests. Talking with the patient and members of his family and observing their interactions and behavior are ways in which the health provider can learn about and understand his client. Having a background of knowledge about the cultural system aids the professional in his assessment of the client's needs and in planning and implementing interventions.

The indirect, non-assertive method of interaction that is more traditional with the Chinese may be misleading to the health professional. The high regard and respect for an educated and learned person includes the doctor, nurse, or specialist with whom the Chinese person meets. Any advice, instructions, or opinions from the professional may be accepted without question, even though the patient may not understand or agree. The latter will not ask for clarification or inquire further because he fears to do so may be exhibiting rude, disrespectful behavior. The professional may interpret non-conformance as negativism or resistance when in reality it is a lack of understanding.

Clear understanding by the patient of prescribed health care is necessary for interventions to be carried out and effective. Strange and different activities may produce puzzlement and fear, with resulting uncooperativeness by the patient. A first-generation grandfather recollects his family being given an analgesic that fizzed when combined with water. They refused to drink it because they thought they were being poisoned.

Another manifestation of non-assertive interaction may occur if there is conflict between directions or interventions suggested by the professional and the beliefs or practices of the client and his cultural system. The Chinese patient may not verbalize his disagreement; instead he will quietly wait for the health specialist to depart and then observe the practice that he prefers. He may not inform the specialist of his actions because he does not want to admit to disobeying the authority of the specialist. Again, tactful inquiry is important for health care to be beneficial.

A common occurrence among people living in two cultural systems is that practices from both cultures will be observed. A child with diarrhea was given the medication prescribed by the pediatrician. He was also fed Chinese rice gruel, made by his grandmother specifically to counteract the diarrhea, and a warm cloth was wrapped around his abdomen by his Chinese-American mother. When the different practices call for opposing actions, then conflict arises.

A great deal has been said about the Chinese concept of familism. The traditional clan concept of China no longer is practiced but the ideology of family still persists and is found in various forms among the Chinese Americans. It may exist only as an ideal with a nuclear family long separated from other relatives, or it may be present as the modified extended family described by Rothschild. Here, too, the health worker needs to appraise the family configuration, because treating the Chinese-American individual includes treating him as a member of a family, regardless of its size.

Family members may be in conflict with each other regarding interventions or instructions given by the health professional. For example, the parents of a child with a dermatologic condition that does not seem to be responding to treatment may be pressured by the first-generation family members to discontinue the therapy and try a folk remedy. The parents are caught between doing what the expert outsider has prescribed and the authority and good intentions of the older family members.

Reflection of the individual's behavior upon

the family reputation continues to be of high significance. In the area of mental health, there may be reluctance to seek professional services. Mental illness connotes "something wrong" with the family member, which in the concept of familism includes the family, and shame is felt. Acquiring professional services means acknowledging a "shameful" situation, and when this is done, the family tries to protect its secret by not informing others.

Kurokawa found that acculturated Asian children have more accidents than those who are non-acculturated, because of increased exposure to possible hazards.[140] They are out of the home more and less protected by their parents. Young Chinese children may be less daring and less adventuresome than their classmates. By the time they are of school age they have been advised for many years to beware of dangerous or potentially harmful situations. They learn to be cautious of new situations and look to the teacher for permission and safety before attempting the unaccustomed. The close family ties and rigid authority accounted for a lower delinquency rate among Chinese-American children in years past. As acculturation progressed and the family influence decreased, the rate of delinquency increased.

Kurokawa also stated that Asian children use the mechanism of separation as a defense against anxiety.[141] They suppress feelings, especially those of physical aggression, as a means of adaptation to many conflict situations. Avoiding conflict and confrontation decreases anxiety, with a resulting sadomasochistic orientation towards the body. The tendency for Chinese to use their bodies as scapegoats for their adjustment failures is exhibited in somatization and physical illness.

"Homes are for families and for friends who are almost family."[142] The Chinese are reluctant to invite strangers into their home. If a home visit is part of his interventions, awareness of his intrusion into the privacy of the patient and his family will help the specialist to present himself as one seeking to help a family member rather than a foreign authority who is invading their domain.

The health care provider may experience frustration when encouraging Chinese patients to attend group activities, especially those of a social nature, such as health education. The extended family often provides the major social contacts for the patient and he may not consider additional contacts beyond his kin to be valuable or applicable to himself.

The aged were respected and cared for by their family in the traditional system. Having a large family ensured the elderly of comfort and care. The old Chinese person in America, without relatives to support or provide for him, is eligible for medical care and economic and other public assistance. He rationalizes that it is a necessity and although he qualifies to be a recipient, accepting public charity is a great loss of face and resented by him.[143] The aged patient in clinics or on "staff care" may be experiencing these conflicting emotions and values. His behavior may manifest these conflicts and be difficult to understand.

The current Chinese population in America is very diverse. Old timers cling to traditional ways and values. Newcomers searching for a life in this country are often highly skilled and well educated. Some newcomers are of the laboring class and need training as well as education. The native born think of themselves as Americans, but their physical features distinguish them as Chinese. Their dual identity must be integrated and reconciled, so they may acknowledge their Chinese heritage as well as their American birthright. "The variations among individuals of similar cultural heritage enlarge the complexity of providing quality health care."[144] This chapter has been written to promote understanding of and appreciation for the Chinese American, with the sincere hope that the knowledge gained will assist the health care professional, or other reader, in his interactions and relationships with those who are Chinese and American.

REFERENCES

1. Aamodt, A.: "Culture." In Clark, A.L. (ed.): *Culture, Childbearing, Health Professionals.* F.A. Davis Company, Philadelphia, 1978, p.16.
2. Kurokawa, M.: *Acculturation and Childhood Accidents Among Chinese- and Japanese-Americans.* Unpublished doctoral dissertation, University of California, Berkeley, 1967, p.89.
3. Liang, Y.: *The Chinese Family in Chicago.* Unpublished doctoral dissertation, University of Chicago, 1951, p. 17.
4. Kuykendall, K.: *Acculturative Change in Family Structure Among Chinese-Americans.* Unpublished doctoral dissertation, University of Colorado, 1972, p. 64.

5. Dowdell, D., and Dowdell, J.: *The Chinese Helped Build America*. J. Messner, New York, 1972, pp. 46-47.
6. Lee, R.: *The Chinese in the United States of America*. Hong Kong University Press, 1960, pp. 33-34.
7. Kingston, M.: *San Francisco's Chinatown*. Sponsored by the American Association for State and Local History, Society of American Historians. American Heritage 1(30):47, 1978.
8. Ibid.
9. Sung, B.: *The Chinese in America*. Macmillan, New York, 1972, pp. 22-23.
10. Kuykendall, p.75.
11. Hoyt, E.: *Asians in the West*. T. Nelson, Nashville, 1974, p. 13.
12. Liang, p. 17.
13. Lee, p. 240.
14. Kingston, *San Francisco's Chinatown*, p. 39.
15. Kuykendall, p. 72.
16. Ibid., p. 74.
17. Dowdell and Dowdell, p. 59.
18. Kingston, *San Francisco's Chinatown*, p. 37.
19. Ibid., p. 38.
20. Ibid., p. 47.
21. Kuykendall, p. 85.
22. Lee, p. 56.
23. Kuykendall, p. 76.
24. Ibid., p. 4.
25. Sung, *Chinese in America*, p. 53.
26. Kuykendall, p. 91.
27. Ibid., p. 80.
28. Ibid., pp. 75, 90.
29. Sung, B.: *An Album of Chinese Americans*. Franklin Watts, New York, 1977, p. 27.
30. Kuykendall, p. 74.
31. Ibid., pp. 85-87.
32. Hoyt, p. 94.
33. Sung, *Album*, p. 29.
34. Sung, *Chinese in America*, p. 44.
35. Char, T.Y.: *The Bamboo Path: Life and Writings of a Chinese in Hawaii*. Hawaii Chinese History Center, Honolulu, 1977, pp. 209-219.
36. Young, N.: *Development of Achievement Oriented Behavior Among the Chinese of Hawaii*. Unpublished doctoral dissertation, University of Hawaii, 1971.
37. Char, *Bamboo Path*, p. 208.
38. Sung, *Album*, pp. 28-34.
39. Sung, *Chinese in America*, pp. 44-46.
40. Ibid., p. 92.
41. Queen, S.A., Habenstein, R.W., and Adams, J.B.: *The Family in Various Cultures*. J.B. Lippincott, New York, 1961, p. 97.
42. Kuykendall, p. 52.
43. Char, T.Y.: *The Sandalwood Mountains*. The University Press of Hawaii, 1975, p. 122.
44. Liang, p. 54.
45. Sung, *Chinese in America*, p. 64.
46. Mann, E., and Waldron, J.: "Intercultural Marriage and Child Rearing." In Wen-Shing, T., McDermott, J., and Maretzki, T. (eds.): *Adjustment in Intercultural Marriages*. The University Press of Hawaii, Honolulu, 1977, p. 66.
47. Char, *Sandalwood Mountains*, p. 121.
48. Kingston, M.: *The Woman Warrior*. Random House, Inc., New York, 1977, p. 8.
49. Kurokawa, p. 78.
50. Ibid., pp. 102-103.
51. Queen, Habenstein, and Adams, p. 99.
52. Char, *Sandalwood Mountains*, pp. 120-121.
53. Queen, Habenstein, and Adams, p. 100.
54. Ibid., p. 123.
55. Kuykendall, pp. 51-53.
56. Ibid., p. 52.
57. Kurokawa, p. 103.
58. Queen, Habenstein, and Adams, p. 123.
59. Kuykendall, pp. 50-51.
60. Char, *Sandalwood Mountains*, p. 125.
61. Char, T.Y.: *The Char Family Genealogy Book*. Private publication, Honolulu, Hawaii, 1972, p. i.
62. Kingston, *San Francisco's Chinatown*, p. 47.
63. Dowdell and Dowdell, p. 78.
64. Char, *Sandalwood Mountains*, pp. 124-134.
65. Kuykendall, p. 59.
66. Sung, *Chinese in America*, pp. 80-82.
67. Sung, *Album*, p. 55.
68. Liang, p. 86.
69. Char, *Bamboo Path*, p. 215.
70. Sollenberger, R.: *Chinese-American child-rearing practices and juvenile delinquency*. Journal of Social Psychology 74:19, 1968.
71. Kuykendall, p. 133.
72. Sung, *Album*, p. 48.
73. Liang, p. 86.
74. Sung, *Chinese in America*, pp. 63-70.

75. Sung, *Album*, pp. 55-60.
76. Rothschild, C.: *Trends in the family; a cross cultural perspective.* Children Today 7(2):38-43, 1978.
77. Sung, *Chinese in America*, pp. 70, 96.
78. Char, *Sandalwood Mountains*, p. 247.
79. Kingston, *Woman Warrior*, pp. 54-55.
80. Dowdell and Dowdell, p.67.
81. Kuykendall, p. 89.
82. Liang, p. 53.
83. Dowdell and Dowdell, p. 67.
84. Queen, Habenstein, and Adams, p. 124.
85. Law, T.: *Differential Child-rearing Attitudes and Practices of Chinese-American Mothers.* Unpublished doctoral dissertation, Claremont Graduate School, California. Dissertation Abstracts International 34:4406-A, 1974.
86. Sollenberger, p. 21.
87. Liang, p. 76.
88. Sollenberger, p. 20.
89. Young, p. 16.
90. Ibid.
91. Ibid., p. 123.
92. Mann and Waldron, p. 64.
93. Young, p. 134.
94. Mann and Waldron, p. 64.
95. Sollenberger, p. 16.
96. Ibid.
97. Ibid., p. 21.
98. Young, p. 160.
99. Sung, *Chinese in America*, p. 65.
100. Kingston, *San Francisco's Chinatown*, p. 37.
101. Sollenberger, p. 21.
102. Sung, *Chinese in America*, p. 69.
103. Dowdell and Dowdell, p. 68.
104. Young, p. 14.
105. Ibid., p. 181.
106. Sung, *Chinese in America*, p. 69.
107. Sollenberger, p. 17.
108. Young, pp. 150, 152.
109. Sollenberger, p. 17.
110. Char, *Sandalwood Mountains*, p. 122.
111. Kuykendall, p. 209.
112. Sollenberger, p. 16.
113. Fawdry, M.: *Chinese Childhood.* Barron's, New York, 1977, p. 168.
114. Ibid., pp. 60-74.
115. Kuykendall, p. 7.
116. Lum, A.: *How young Chinese view their heritage.* Honolulu Star Bulletin, July 13, 1970, Section B-6.
117. Sung, *Album*, p. 45.
118. Fawdry, p. 170.
119. Jones, A.: *Door to Chinese Festivals, Feasts, Fortunes.* Mei Ya Publications, Taipei, Taiwan, 1971, pp. 144-170.
120. Sung, *Chinese in America*, p. 77.
121. Jones, p. 17.
122. Ibid., p. 21.
123. Liang, p. 32.
124. Jones, p. 58.
125. Kingston, *Woman Warrior*, p. 13.
126. Jones, p. 93.
127. Char, *Sandalwood Mountains*, p. 125.
128. Liang, p. 80.
129. Kurokawa, p. 320.
130. Dowdell and Dowdell, p. 75.
131. Rose, P.: "The Chinese-American." In Clark, A.L. (ed.): *Culture, Childbearing, Health Professionals.* F.A. Davis Company, Philadelphia, 1978, p.57.
132. Sung, *Chinese in America*, p. 60.
133. Territorial Department of Health, Bureau of Public Health Nursing: *Cultural Beliefs and Practices of the Childbearing Period and Their Implications for Nursing Practice Among Chinese, Filipino, Hawaiian, and Japanese Families Living in Hawaii, 1953.* Unpublished report, 1954.
134. Sung, *Chinese in America*, p. 60.
135. Jones, p. 125.
136. Char, *Sandalwood Mountains*, p. 133.
137. Kingston, *Woman Warrior*, p. 223.
138. *Cultural Beliefs and Practices*, p. 5.
139. Aamodt, p. 16.
140. Kurokawa, p. 325.
141. Ibid., pp. 118-121.
142. Kingston, *San Francisco's Chinatown*, p. 47.
143. Kuykendall, p. 89.
144. Aamodt, p. 4.

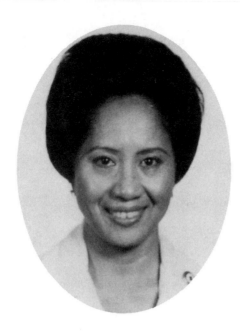

Chapter 7

The youngest of four children, I was born in Barrio Caybiga, about 15 miles from the city of Manila, the old capital of the Philippines. I grew up in the beautiful and serene atmosphere of a Spanish style home surrounded with verdant grasslands, varied tropical fruit-bearing trees, rolling hills, huge rocks covered with green foliage and ferns, bamboo trees, a banana orchard, a brook, and sprawling, wide open rice fields. From these surroundings I learned to love nature; I felt like I had my own "forest shrine" where I could daydream and find solace and peace.

Owing to circumstances within the family, I was oriented to a matriarchal family with a large kin group. My grandfather died when I was four; my mother, being the only child, and because of their culture, had to stay with grandmother. My father, a mining engineer and geodetic surveyor, was always assigned to the gold mines in Surigao, the mountain regions of Luzon and Mindanao; later he became the Assistant Director of the Bureau of Mines in Cebu, and was therefore constantly away from the family.

Both my grandparents were of Spanish-Malayan heritage. Active in civic and community affairs, a senator, a governor, a vice-governor, an agriculturist, and a philanthropist emerged from my father's side of the

family; physicians, dentists, accountants, a pharmacist, and educators from my mother's side. The socialization processes during my early childhood, with a cohesive, bilateral kin system, taught me the concepts of sharing, caring, respect, loyalty, gratitude, and adaptability at an early age. I learned the family traditions through observation and participation, and "to do my best and God will do the rest."

My maternal grandmother, a strong-willed person with good managerial abilities, taught me the meaning of hard work, and the concepts of leadership. Her home was always a center of gathering for relatives, neighbors, and friends. Harvest season brings in vendors, tenants, harvesters, and field workers. During typhoons, thunder storms, earthquakes, and air-raids (war-time bombings), Grandmother's home was a refuge and shelter for the needy. At the height of the war, her yard and meadows became camp-sites for weary and hungry soldiers whom she fed by the hundreds. At 7 years old, these experiences provided me with precious lessons in life.

I was speaking and writing in English before I went to the Barrio school, was accelerated to the higher grades, and was in the fourth grade at age 7 with Mother as my tutor. When not involved with adult education, Mama spent

The Filipino in America
Consuelo J. Aquino, R.N., M.P.H.

most of her time nursing sick relatives in their homes. The unique medical bag she carried around fascinated me as a child. Mama died before my eighth birthday, and a few months before World War II. The family activities implanted the seeds of caring, nursing, and serving humanity within me in early childhood.

My formal education was interrupted during the war. Using the family library, I became acquainted with Greek, Roman, and world history, English literature, Oriental philosophy, Filipino corridos in verse forms, and poetry. Grandmother taught me to be home for Angelus at 6 P.M. She also taught me how to read the Life of Christ in Tagalog and how to cope with fear by praying in my own words, even at the point of a bayonet and with bullets soaring by my ears.

When peace resumed, Grandmother died before I completed high school. At the age of 12 I have observed, knelt, and prayed at the bedside of three loved ones, and learned the meaning of death and dying. My intense desire to see the Pope and Parthenon in Athens, and to become a medical missionary were reinforced after Grandma passed away. With the help of our parish priest, I entered the convent, where I performed social work with disadvantaged children, family counseling, and education. I also learned the art of the contemplative life, fine arts, music, and embroidery. Ill health pre-

vented me from completing the religious profession. I went to Colegio de San Jose, then to the School of Nursing in Southern Islands Hospital in Cebu, where I became a registered nurse. I then went to the United States for postgraduate study in obstetrics in New Jersey and worked as a registered professional nurse.

After working as an operating room nurse in medical/surgical, pediatrics, labor and delivery, nursery, postpartum, clinical instruction, and industrial nursing, I married a penpal whom I never met until 4 days before the wedding. Letters, long-distance calls, a dear friend, and perhaps a miracle brought us together. This marriage in 20 years has brought us five lovable children and has taken us around the world twice. With a thirst for knowledge, I studied, worked part-time, and performed volunteer works. I also taught mother and baby care, disaster nursing, first aid, and home nursing, and trained nurses aides for the American Red Cross in Japan and Europe.

My husband's tour of duty brought us to different parts of the world and gave me the opportunity to work in different areas of nursing; it also gave me the chance to work with different cultural and ethnic groups, which enriched and broadened my understanding of "human needs," a very important aspect of nursing.

I obtained credits towards BSN from the Uni-

versity of Maryland and the University of the Philippines. With my husband as a classmate, we obtained our degrees in Social Sciences, and a Master's degree in Public Health (a wonderful, challenging experience because of cultural differences). My professional experience includes work in intensive care units, emergency nursing, orthopedics departments, and outpatient clinics, along with research in maternal and child health, and family planning. I have been a visiting professor at George Mason University in Virginia, an Occupational Health Nurse in the DHEW, Washington, D.C., and a Clinical Nurse in Urology and Oncology at Walter Reed AMC, Washington, D.C. These experiences have provided me with valuable tools in communication and the delivery of health care.

In a span of 23 years, I have been fortunate to be able to serve the cultural minorities of my country—the Negritos of the Philippines through volunteer public health work; the Americans in America and overseas; the Japanese in Japan; the Puerto Ricans in New Jersey; the Mexicans in Texas; the American Indians in Arizona; and the French, Italians, Germans, and Turkish children in France and Turkey. I also provided critical care for Vietnamese children, infants, adults, and elderly people during the Vietnam crisis and "Operation Baby Lift" (all volunteer services). At present I am working as an Adult Medical Nurse Practitioner and Diabetic Nurse Educator at Kaiser Foundation Hospital.

THE HOMELAND

Lying on the western rim of the Pacific, a close neighbor of the countries of Southeast Asia, is a string of 7100 islands with a land area of about 115,707 square miles known as the Philippines. During the Pleistocene era land bridges connected the southern parts of the Archipelago to mainland Asia, Borneo, Celebes, Java, and Sumatra. Today, the land bridges are submerged, though some of the peaks are still visible in Palawan. In this part of the world where winter never comes, there are some of the greatest unused natural resources in land, minerals, fish, forests, and power. The country is richly endowed with timber, copra, sugar, abaca, and tobacco. It is one of the three great areas of tropical potential in the world (the two others are Africa and Latin America).

The 7100 islands were grouped into three major islands—Luzon, Visayas, and Mindanao—which have 52 provinces and 28 chartered cities. Of the 7100 islands, only 2773 had been named so far. Luzon and Mindanao are the largest islands. The substantial, rich rice lands are in the Central Plain of Luzon and Cagayan Valley; Mindanao has the rolling plains of Cotobato and Agusan Basin. The fragmented character of the Archipelago, with great contrasts of types of landscapes, forests, volcanic formations, elevations, coastlines, mountain slopes, and different rainfall patterns, creates the particular beauty of the Philippines. Picturesque palms lean over coral reefs and rocks along the white sand beaches.

When a typhoon spills its enormous load of rain it encourages the growth of varied tropical fruits, flora, and fauna. The Archipelago has a longer coastline than that of the United States.

Physical barriers, remoteness of many islands, inadequate roads, poor inter-islands communication, and inadequate commercial distribution are some of the factors that hinder economic and social progress. Inhabitants of remote islands and mountainous areas remain isolated and remotely linked to the modern thinking of the people around Manila, the old capital city of the islands.

During the 3 centuries of Spanish domination, from 1521 to 1898, the Filipinos were the object of the most intensive Christian Missionary effort in the Orient. As a consequence the Philippines became the only Christian nation in the Far East.

The Stars and Stripes of the United States were raised over the Archipelago in 1898 following the war between Spain and America. Americanization was carried out through public education. Democratic ideals and ideas implanted a concept of freedom. In 1935, the Philippines became a Commonwealth of the United States. American policies were implemented and socioeconomic, political, and educational reforms were carried out. The Filipinos assimilated nearly all these cultural and political changes without losing their sense of dignity and identity. Attitudes, values, customs, and traditions that were established among the natives long before Magellan discovered the Philippines were retained and blended with Western concepts. Free enterprise, social mobility, and industrialization did not change the role of the family as the primary concern of the Filipinos.

The new era of Americanization was interrupted by another war, this time, by the Japanese invasion in 1941. In the war-torn country, a puppet Republic was set up. After 5 years of chaos, atrocities, dehumanization, death, starvation, and deprivation, the Japanese invaders were driven out of the Philippines by the Americans. Constitutional government was promptly resumed. The Americans kept their promise; on July 4, 1946, independence, the national aspiration of the Filipinos, was officially inaugurated. Tagalog was proclaimed as the national language by President Quezon. English continues to be the medium of instruction and the universal language of the islands, while Spanish remains the language spoken by a minority of 2 million Filipinos.

The young republic experienced economic, social, and political problems and growing pains, but remained democratic until the proclamation of martial law. The Filipinos participated in world affairs and became active members of international organizations such as the United Nations, World Health Organization, and Southeast Asian Organizations.

The problems of the Philippines as a new country are similar to the problems of any new developing nation in the world: rebuilding, clearing up the ruins of the war; rehabilitation; relocation; social and psychological problems as an aftermath of destruction, fear, and horror; disease; unstable government; development of reliable exports; lack of manpower and technology to develop natural resources (e.g., gold mines, copper, coal, ore); national development; and an exploding population. Despite all the struggles, the Filipinos have not lost their vitality in nation-building and have not lost their capacity to enjoy the experience of daily life. The remoteness of the other islands and physical barriers pose a special problem in speeding economic progress and social reforms. Land travel continues to be a problem in many areas, but a modern super-highway in Luzon connecting several provinces has improved travel time and opened economic opportunities for a greater number of people in the barrios.

THE PEOPLE

There is evidence of human settlement in the Philippines as early as 20,000 B.C. The Negritos were probably the first group of people to arrive. They crossed the land bridges that connected the Philippine Archipelago to the Asian mainland. The brown-skinned Malays were the later immigrants who came by sea. They settled in the lowlands and the coastal areas of the islands. They are the ancestors of the present day brown-skinned Filipinos that make up the predominant population of the Philippines. Other inhabitants came from Indonesia, Malaysia, China, Celebes, Borneo, and India in various waves of migration. Ancestors came from Southeast Asia by way of island chains to the south and across the China Sea. Arabs and Indian traders added their blood to create a Muslim population in Mindanao. During the Spanish regime there was a blending of diverse racial strains, and linguistic differentiations continued until the 20th century.

The population of the Philippines is composed of a considerable number of cultural and linguistic groups. Forty million Filipinos represent 90 languages and dialects with 135 sub-dialects, the result of varied historical circumstances and racial intermixture.

About 85 percent of the people live in rural areas. Agriculture is the main source of livelihood; fishing, arts and crafts, raising live stock, and small cottage industries are other sources of income. Because of the nature of land use and availability of resources, houses are scattered in small clusters of two or three and are often close to the farmer's field. In some areas, houses are built close to each other. Heads of households speaking the same dialect group together in one place; they tend to follow an ethnolinguistic pattern, which is unique.

The minority people of the Philippines inhabit the mountains of northern Luzon, parts of the Visayan Islands, and Mindanao, where they practice upland agriculture. Their lack of knowledge about health and nutrition make their existence increasingly marginal. A National Integration Commission has been created to provide health and education to these people.

THE BARRIO

The Philippine countryside is marked by small communities known as the "barrios," where daily life has remained virtually the same with very little change, if any, over the last 100 years. With the agrarian character of the islands and with agriculture as the main source of Philippine economy, 83 to 85 percent of the people live in the rural communities or barrios.

Life in the barrio is simple. People are occupied with farming activities, such as vegetable gardening, poultry raising, hog raising, and raising carabaos or water buffalos for their work animals. For extra income they also engage in small cottage industries, such as weaving, pottery, wood-carving, fishing, and part-time occupations. Settlement patterns set centuries ago are still the same today, influenced by the availability of resources, the use of the land, location of rivers, and family affinity.

A bond of common interest exists in the barrios. The people participate in church activities with colorful ceremonies and pageantry. Christmas and Holy Week are very special occasions celebrated with elaborate feasts, music with marching brass bands, processions, and dancing. Christenings, weddings, and deaths are also occasions for celebrations. Customs and traditions associated with burial rites and ceremonies as a final tribute to the departed are still practiced.

The barrio Captain chosen by the people is usually a successful businessman or a prominent member of the community. Together with a group of Councilmen, he manages the barrio affairs. The people function according to the group norms. Values developed through group interaction influence the manner in which the barrio people live: how they migrate; agree or disagree about civic duties and responsibilities; agree on certain beliefs and actions; vote; observe marriage customs; and raise their children. Leadership and authority are based on tradition, local beliefs, and existing practices in the barrio; the legal basis for leadership and authority is based on the laws of the Republic of the Philippines.

Municipalities are the administrative unit over the barrios. They were known in the Spanish era as the "poblacions," where there is a church,

a municipal building, a public market, a grade school, elementary and secondary schools, shops, and a town hall.

Children of the barrios attend the primary schools in the barrios; in some areas, they complete their elementary and high school education in the towns, while others complete their high school education in the cities.

Teachers are very influential in the barrios, where they are highly respected by the people. They help implement programs in health and sanitation, beautification of the surroundings, and horticulture, and provide first-aid care for minor cuts and bruises for the barrio children.

The towns are supported largely by the agricultural communities around them, and are grouped into provinces. Barrios, towns, cities, and provinces are the basic units of the Philippine Republic.

Barrio fiestas are the highlight of barrio life. Filipino customs and traditions are a mixture of religion and fun; traditional practices blend devotions to the Saints with fanfare and merrymaking. Each barrio has a Patron Saint, and afternoon novenas for 9 days in thanksgiving for a bountiful harvest and good weather (some areas of the Philippines get more crop-destroying typhoons than other areas) are offered to God through them. On the ninth day of the novena, people dressed in their best attire after being awakened by the joyful ringing of church bells and brass marching bands parade along the street to remind the people that Mass celebration is about to start. The whole day's activities include open-air entertainment, beauty contests, sports contests, fireworks, and candle-lit processions in honor of the Patron Saint. Ladies with colorful attire and their escorts, representing the Hermana Mayor, are another center of attraction in the procession.

On the eve of the fiesta, there is usually the coronation of the queen and her court, followed by a coronation ball.

Friends, relatives, and guests from neighboring towns and cities and other provinces take special trips to attend the festivities. These fiestas are also occasions for relatives to visit each other, interact in a more festive mood, and exchange goods (relatives love to bring "pasalubongs" and they are given "pauwi" when they go home). Relatives from the provinces generally bring food items and produce, such as chickens; fruits from their orchards, like bananas, mangoes, pineapples; eggs; a pig or a young turkey;

vegetables; and large sacks of rice. These goods are used for the fiesta, and visiting kin help in the cooking and cleaning up. When they are about to return to their homes, they are given presents or "pauwi" in the form of money, home preserved fruits called "cusilva" in Tagalog, leche-plan (custard), cookies, or special bread, sugar, and other commodities.

Hospitality is at its height during fiestas, baptismal parties, weddings, and funerals. Lavish preparation of food is undertaken with great expense. Home and yard beautification and street decoration are community affairs. People work together to make the feast a colorful and memorable occasion.

A procession in honor of the Patron Saint is the climax of the fiesta. There are towns in the Philippines that are famous for their fiestas. People from all parts of the country visit Santa Clara in Obando, Bulacan, and San Roque in Polo, Bulacan, where childless couples perform fertility dances. The Patron Saints there are reputed to be very influential in asking God to give children to childless couples.

THE FILIPINO FAMILY

Cooley describes the family as "the cradle of human nature."[1] As an institution, it is the basis for group life, which deals with human interaction. Its members form an organization with the concepts of authority, role, status, and social stratification. As a primary group, it plays a significant role in the personality development of the individual; it is influential in determining the social organization of the entire society it belongs to.

The family has been characterized as the most universal institution; it ensures the continuity of the society through its reproductive functions. The basic family is composed of husband and wife, bound in a union recognized by society, and their children. In the Filipino culture, other collateral relatives reside with the nuclear family. The members form an organization commonly known as the extended family. They interact with each other in their reciprocal roles and maintain a common culture.

As a group, the Filipino family is regulated by means of the rule of descent, rule of inheritance, and rule of residence; as a social unit it is regulated by customs, traditions, beliefs, and law. Reciprocity is the basis of social cohesion; in the Filipino family, reciprocity among its members is maintained through mutual concern and economic cooperation, and mutual love and respect.

One of the powerful elements of the family social organization is the kinship system. Dr. Landa Jocano describes kinship as "the structured relationships in which individuals are bound to one another by complex interlocking ties."[2] It is through kinship principles that family rights and obligations are defined, expressed, and regulated. They are the basis for rules of conduct, management of family affairs, interpersonal relationships, intermarriage with different groups, intergroup movements of the people, and management of community affairs. Kinsmen are consulted and serve as intermediaries in resolving difficult questions, making decisions in important matters, or achieving an important goal. When desires and aspirations are thwarted, conflict among the kin group arises. Although kinship solidarity unifies families, it also generates conflicts. Aspirations, attitudes, preferences, and even prejudices are influenced by the kinship system. Mutual respect, consideration, loyalty, sense of belonging, acceptance of the members without question, certain individual rights and privileges, and protection and support in time of need are among the important benefits the kinship group enjoys. In turn, members of the group are obligated to help older kinsmen when they need assistance. The smooth interaction within the family system is in part the consequence of bilateral kinship; this means that the children of a particular set of parents are equally related to the kinsmen of the father and the mother. The individual may indicate closer ties with kinsmen from one parental side and may establish residence close to a particular kin group.

Kinship is also generational, which means that the members of the group are recognized according to the order of descent. The individual's generation consists of his brothers and sisters and cousins; the first generation above him consists of his parents, uncles, and aunts; the generation above his parents is his grandparents; the first generation below the individual consists of his children, nephews, and nieces; the second generation below him is his grandchildren. Rules of inheritance, emotional ties, hierarchy of values, respect for elders, social etiquette, and administration of social control are established, clarified, and interpreted through the generational kinship system. Seniority demands respect and affectionate consideration.

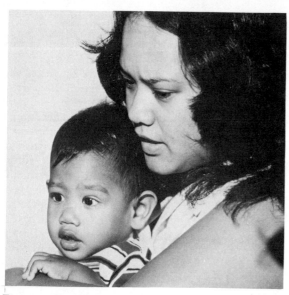

Figure 1. The Filipino mother keeps the family closely knit. Her relationship with her children is highly valued by the entire family. (Photograph by Brad Powell)

The task of providing for the support of the family rests on the man. In some situations parents of the groom help out the newly-weds in their new venture in life. Sometimes the newly-weds stay with the girl's parents until they are able to be self-sufficient. The husband's income is the source of the family's support. He is expected to aspire to higher economic security, provide for his children's college education, help provide support for his aging parents, and improve his social status. The family looks up to the father for leadership and authority. He voices decisions on important matters; serious problems of discipline are referred to him, and he may impose certain punishments on his children if they bring dishonor to the family.

The wife, besides the role of mother, performs other functions beyond household tasks. She assists her husband in enhancing the economic security of the family. With remarkable skill and initiative she looks for opportunities to achieve this, sometimes becoming a small-scale businesswoman.

Family Authority

The father is the acknowledged head and has the patriarchal control of the family. He is obeyed and respected. The mother is the spokesman, household manager, the one who keeps the fam-

ily closely knit, and the husband's partner, and her role as family treasurer is a high and respected position (Fig. 1). The husband consults the wife and asks her approval before he undertakes any important activities or enters into contracts. She has the same educational privileges and suffrage rights as her husband. She is free to dispose of the property she brought into the marriage, and to transact business independently. Her high status in the family is unparalleled in the Far East. Through her influence, the family traditions and values remain intact. She is the most influential member of the family.

Authority in the family is also influenced by age. Grandparents have a very important role in family authority. Even now, children and grandchildren consult and seek their advice on important matters and significant events in their lives.

After the parents' deaths, the oldest child takes over the family. He or she takes care of family matters regarding property, care of the younger siblings, management of family income and expenditure, and distribution of goods and inheritance.

Social Relationships

Each child begins life at the bottom. The younger ones show respect and obedience to older ones; nevertheless, the young look up to the older siblings and older members of the family for affectionate regard and protection. If harsh words are used, they are immediately corrected and discouraged. Every domestic act in the household is performed with courtesy and kindness. A special rank with status is given to the oldest child and the next, and so on down the line. The youngest usually gets away with many things, but he is also reminded to be mindful of his elders. Sometimes the youngest is shown special treatment, which, although it is accepted, creates inner feelings of animosity and sibling rivalry. The first born has the say about inheritance. If the oldest child properly adheres to the "equal distribution" concept, then the younger siblings will not have any problems; if the eldest is authoritarian, then there will be conflict with the younger ones regarding inheritance.

Owing to the nature of the extended kin system, the Filipino child is cared for by a number of individuals with whom he develops trust, affection, a feeling of security, and intimate relations. A special relationship exists between the parent and the child; between the child and the grandparents; and between the child and the maid or domestic help. The maids may be replaced occasionally; however, the child learns to adapt to each maid after a period of time. The maid's values often influence and sometimes interfere with the child's upbringing. The children that are brought-up in a household where there are no maids or domestic help learn to adapt with their grandparents, aunts, cousins, and other members of the extended family.

A working mother entrusts the care of her children to her mother, aunties, or other relatives who are willing to babysit them. In a household where there are other relatives living with the working mother, child care is not a problem. Day care centers and nursery schools are also utilized by families who do not have live-in babysitters. Other mothers work only part-time or make arrangements with their husbands to look after the children when the husbands come home from work. Most husbands prefer their wives to be home while the children are still small, and the more affluent families do not allow their wives to work at all. Of course there are exceptions to this, depending on the husband-wife relationship and the wife's educational attainment.

Significant findings obtained through the Thematic Apperception Test done by Bulatao and associates[3] showed important values that affect the Filipino family:

Value A—Emotional closeness and security in a family.

A1. The interest of the individual must be sacrificed for the good of the family.
   a. Parents must strive even at great cost to themselves to give their children an education.
   b. Older children must make sacrifices for younger children.
   c. Even marriage must be put off at times to help the family.
A2. Parents should be very strict in watching over, protecting and disciplining their children who otherwise might meet with disaster.
   a. Watch the child closely, for physical harm may befall the child.
   b. If left by themselves moral harm might befall the children, especially the girls.
   c. There is a fear that when the children leave the house, they may meet an accident.

   d. Accordingly, parents believe that while their daughter is still young she can still be taught by spanking or frightening her.
   e. Somehow or the other, this concern for bodily safety is linked to the drive for family security.
A3. Women are valued for their qualities as Mothers and Housekeepers; they are primarily the ones expected to keep the family close together.
   a. Women are undemanding, they love once and only one.
   b. A marriage should be kept intact no matter what the husbands do; the woman should forgive an unfaithful husband.
   c. Away from their family, women are insecure; they worry about their loss of chastity.
A4. Tender relationships, "carino" or lambingan, are highly valued.
   a. Husband and wife are close to one another. Wife pleads for her son.
   b. Even in unconscious moments a man thinks of his loved one.
   c. A man parts with pain from his wife. He leaves her with his parents.
   d. A girl when jilted has recourse to mother.
   e. Marriage to a simple Filipino is preferred to a foreign marriage.

Childrearing

Childrearing is one of the most important functions of the family. Influenced by social traditions and Christian principles, the Filipino family recognizes that the primary purpose of marriage is procreation. Children are desired as the natural outcome of the union of husband and wife. The Filipino parents do not have any scientific methods in rearing children; much is left to chance, common sense, and the influences of customs, traditions, education, beliefs, myths, legends, folklore, and prevailing practices. Sometimes childrearing is done haphazardly, but whatever method is used abounds in love, politeness, and respect.

RESPECT

The socialization process starts through kin-group orientation. Childrearing is permissive and gentle. Close family ties of the extended family system develop desirable characteristics in early childhood, such as gentleness, hospitality, kindness, respect for elders, politeness, obedience, loyalty, friendliness, teamwork, and suppression of hostility. The child learns to accommodate the many figures of identification. He learns to recognize and respect authority in early childhood. Reference terms are used to address elderly brothers and sisters, elderly relatives, family friends, neighbors, and strangers. Two of the reference terms are "Ate," for the oldest sister or female cousins; "Kuya," for the oldest brother and male cousins. Some regions in the southern and northern Philippines use the term "Manang" instead of Ate and "Manong" instead of Kuya. Other reference terms used to show respect are Ditche, Sanse, Ka, for the other sisters according to chronological order of age; that is, in a family with five girls, the oldest will be called Ate by the younger ones, the second girl will be addressed Ditche, the third Sanse, and the fourth one will be called Ka or Dette. The youngest daughter is subject to the elder sisters, but respect is with affection and there is mutual love and consideration. The older sisters are obligated to care for the younger ones. In a family with boys the order of address is Kuya for the oldest, Dico for the second boy, Sanko for the third, and Ka for the fourth one. All these titles confer status, certain privileges, responsibilities, and expectations on the children. The elders are expected to be good examples to the younger ones; they help in the care of the younger siblings, and in many instances, the older children are expected to help the younger ones finish college education.

THE NEWBORN

After birth, the newborn is physically cuddled, fondled, sung to, talked to, and rocked to sleep. The baby is picked up immediately and nursed whenever he cries and for as long as he wishes. The first 4 weeks after birth, the mother's time is wholly devoted to the infant. Friends and relatives come to help with the household chores to free the mother from doing the work; she is not allowed to lift heavy things. Her postnatal care requires complete rest to assure the complete healing of the womb and to assure adequate production of breast milk.

While waiting for the mother's milk to flow, the baby is given boiled water. At intervals, the baby is allowed to suck the mother's breast to stimulate milk flow. As soon as the milk starts to flow, a small amount is collected and poured on a corner post inside the house; hence the first secretion of milk is not given to the baby because of certain beliefs.

The mother nurses her baby lying down on one side, a common practice among Filipino mothers. Both mother and child fall asleep during the process, but there is always much contentment for both. Mixed feeding is resorted to if the mother decides to go to work; she breastfeeds the baby before she goes off and during the night. Formula is used during the day. When the baby is 4 months old, rice gruel, broth, soups, mashed sweet potato, and mashed banana are given. The mothers from the urban areas use the commercially prepared baby foods. The baby usually sucks his mother's breast until he is 1½ to 2 years old, or until his mother becomes pregnant again.

As soon as the baby is able to sit on his mother's lap, he is held by his mother and joins the family during mealtime. He is given a taste of the food prepared for the meal and learns to eat what is desirable by tasting. As he grows older he occupies a space at the table with the rest of his brothers and sisters. If he dislikes certain foods, he is trained to decline the food gracefully and politely without making a fuss. Some parents prepare special dishes for the child, others prepare the favorite dishes, but generally, the child adapts the family's eating habits early in life.

Filipinos attach a sacred symbolism to food. They regard food as a sacred gift from God, and since food is a gracious gift from God, eating is partaking of God's blessings. This concept rules out quarrelling at the table, loud or boisterous conversation, unruly behavior, and scolding. Mealtime is to be regarded as a happy occasion in which a pleasant atmosphere is encouraged and wasting food is considered wasting God's gifts. Children learn these concepts through observation and participation.

WAYS OF WEANING A BABY

The manner in which the Filipina mother weans her baby varies from the first baby to the next. The surveys done by Jovita de Guzman and colleagues revealed that the methods used by Filipina mothers are either learned from their parents, from experiences, or from the experience of others (relatives and friends).[4] The most common methods used are the application of bitter extracts from ampalaya leaves, garlic, onion, ginger, or pepper to the mother's breasts to discourage the baby from sucking. Some use physical separation: the baby is entrusted to the

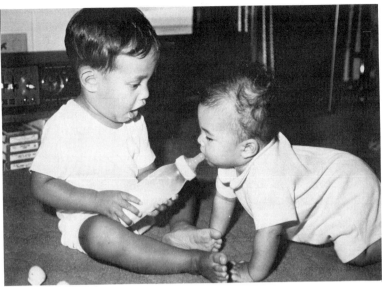

Figure 2. The older child learns early to assist the younger. (Photograph by Brad Powell)

care of his grandmother, or other willing relatives. The baby usually cries for a period of time after weaning. He is given supplementary feeding or substitute feeding. Another popular method is by reduction of frequency of breast-feeding and training the child to drink from a cup early (1 year old).

Most parents bring their children to social functions, parties, baptismal ceremonies, weddings, festivals, and church. It is common to see mothers nursing their child wherever and whenever the child needs feeding, which is an accepted practice among Filipinos.

DISCIPLINE

Parents discipline their children in various ways. The process varies from one social class to another, from region to region, and depending on the parents' educational attainment and prevailing sociocultural practices.

Close family ties of the extended family system develop gentleness, politeness, modesty, loyalty, friendliness, and supression of hostility in early childhood (Fig. 2). Close associations with family members also may foster imitation, dependency, irresponsibility, "hiya," "bahala na" (leave it to fate or chance), extravagance, inferiority, and procrastination.

Harmony and smooth interpersonal relationships are highly valued. Most of the Filipinos'

actions are motivated by the desire to conform and to avoid shame or disgrace. The children's behavior is controlled by fear of censure. Whenever there is a real cause for concern or correction, adults or elders take the child aside and correct him; the child accepts the correction without argument. If the child argues, other measures are resorted to, such as spanking or a lengthy talk. Resentment can vanish as quickly as it appears; however, resentment that is not mitigated immediately by some act of conciliation or a gesture can be a cause of an explosive display of behavior. Enthusiastic efforts are taken immediately to make amends.

Filipino parents are generally authoritarian. As a rule, children of all ages are not allowed to answer back to their elders when they are scolded. Depending on the circumstances, the children are not scolded openly in public for their mistakes; they are taught in early childhood to learn to accept corrections with humility. Parents seldom ask the opinion of their children; this conditions the children to doing only what they are told to do. In situations in which spanking is necessary (most parents believe that "sparing the rod will spoil the child"), the parents use their bare hands; slippers or the belt are used occasionally for older children, or a ruler-sized stick. Spanking is approved as long as it is not brutal. If a child is spanked severely, a neighbor may feel free to admonish the parent to prevent serious consequences.

Some parents equate love for their children with complying or giving in to the children's whims and wishes; some believe that if the parents love their children, they must practice firm but gentle discipline. Many believe and practice consistent, practical, and firm discipline, which gives room for self-direction, creativity, and efficiency. A number of personal practices are religiously defined, for example, kissing the hands of the elders as a sign of love and respect, and the rule of no quarrelling, shouting, or boisterous language during mealtime, for such actions show irreverence to God.

Methods of punishment used by parents, according to the studies of Guzman,[5] reflect the personality of the parents, especially the mother. Harsh physical punishment is rarely used. Aggressive behavior that is punished severely produces more aggressive children; it is not an effective technique.

One and two year olds are usually scolded and shouted at. Other methods of discipline used are verbal appeal and silent treatment. At these age levels, mothers are generally over-protective. Children usually react by crying, but sometimes they keep quiet.

Three to six year olds are either submissive, silent, pleasant and agreeable, or indifferent. Verbal appeal, shouting, silent treatment, scolding, and spanking are the disciplinary methods used by parents and elder members of the extended family for this age group.

For 7 to 10 year olds, Filipino parents use corporal punishment when disruptive behavior, disobedience, or a disrespectful show of rebellion is in evidence. Reasonable restrictions are imposed; silent treatment, scolding, verbal appeal, ignoring, and disowning are also used. When wild behavior emerges, fathers generally intervene. Mothers are the center of inspiration and the manager of the household; serious matters that require firm intervention and heavy parental artillery are referred to father.

The Filipino father emphasizes the development of survival instincts in his sons. Important aspects of anger, dependency, and sexual drives are handled in a subtle way. Early in life, when a male child falls (from regular or usual play activities), he is admonished to "get up by himself, because he will be all right and should take it like a man." He is taught to defend himself if another child beats him or fights him harshly, for it is cowardly to run away from an enemy. In the same token, the child is taught not to offend or create a scene. Outward harmony is highly regarded more than "being right." Westerners regard this as voluntarily giving-up one's rights, but the Oriental way must be learned first before denigrating its value.

Most Filipino parents forbid their children to fight back, but if the family honor is at stake, the children's prerogative is to defend that family honor. The child's opportunity to express anger is circumscribed; he may throw fits or tantrums occasionally, but he is thoroughly forbidden to talk back to his parents or strike back. There is very little room for a rebellious attitude. Children learn early in life to obey humbly. Suppression of hostility is balanced by a set of other childrearing practices, such as gentleness, permissiveness, close parent-child relationships, and other aspects of kindness.

Most parents welcome the early independence of their children. They take pride in the child's early accomplishments such as brushing his teeth, combing his hair, washing his face and hands, feeding himself, dressing himself, and picking up his toys after playtime. In many instances, Filipino parents that employ domestic help or maids have children that stay dependent too long. Preschool children normally can perform the tasks mentioned above for themselves, but because the maids are expected to help them, the child ends up relying on the maid to perform those simple tasks. Most often the child's initiative and effort is curtailed. The child is deprived of the freedom he needs for his continuing development. However, the child finds time for other play and activities that interest him.

In the barrios the baby is considered a very precious thing. As the baby grows, he is watched closely with loving concern. Expectations are kept below the child's potential. He is removed from danger rather than instructing the child to avoid the danger. All problems are met indirectly by distracting and pacifying the child. This leisurely maturation process influences the mother's action in feeding, toilet training, and modesty training. Baby talk is carried on and positive reinforcements are used in the child's nurturance. Children tend to be dependent, but this is an accepted norm within the culture.

PRAISE

Filipino children are not usually praised openly or publicly. Social customs frown on parents who praise their children in public, but it is acceptable for someone outside the family circle to praise the child publicly. Parents praise their children at home; this is a most welcome gesture whenever there is an occasion to do so. Outside the home children are easily embarrassed and require positive reinforcement. They are shy and do not want to be laughed at. They are conditioned to be praised in private; when the children are praised publicly, they want their peers' approval.

Praising in private is more or less reinforced in schools. After their feeling of shyness diminishes, children learn to accept praise in front of their classmates. But whenever an achiever is ridiculed or laughed at, his enthusiasm and effort are affected; as soon as the achiever's feeling of embarrassment levels off, he will continue to perform to the best of his ability to earn more praise and to prove that he deserves it.

Rewards come in various forms of praise, words of encouragement, acknowledgment from parents and significant others, special treats of favorite desserts, toys, special trips or outings, clothes, or a bigger allowance. Most families give affectionate gestures as a form of reward. Children from large households learn the "bayanihan spirit," a spirit of cooperation and helping one another with mutual respect and affectionate regard; for them, the welfare and happiness of each member of the family is already a reward. Depending on the social and economic circumstances, children from urban areas may receive material rewards, such as a new pair of shoes, an expensive toy, or foreign made or imported articles. (Imported goods are highly desired by the Filipinos even if the same articles are locally produced or manufactured. Status is attached to anyone who possesses imported goods.)

When parents take trips, they come home with "pasalubong," meaning special presents that are given out to the children when they arrive home from the trip. The pasalubong may be in the form of food or special delicacies that the children love, such as pastries, cakes, cookies, apples, or grapes (usually imported fruits). The trip may be long or short—it could be just a trip to the city or the market. The pasalubong conveys a message of love and care, "I miss you," a reward for the child for staying behind; the pasalubong elicits joy from both the giver and the receiver.

PRINCIPLES OF HABIT FORMATION

Filipinos help their children develop good habits and proper conduct. Parents are the child's first teachers; the child learns how to write the alphabet in his native language or dialect and learns how to speak and read the vernacular be-

fore he goes to school. Parents use tales, fables, quotations, proverbs, legends, folklore, and stories from the Bible to teach the young a lesson or a moral. They hope to instill ideas and ideals with a philosophy that will endure. Popular stories and quotations are learned by heart; they illustrate charm, loyalty, respect, truthfulness, bravery, cooperation, obedience, and reverence for God. Parents are expected to prepare the child for social efficiency and realization of his potential. They teach their children desirable characteristics and prepare them for meeting the challenges of life with determination and efficiency.

An old custom in the Philippines that is still evident today is the Angelus. As a reverence for God, people from all walks of life and all ages pause for a moment as soon as they hear the church bells at six o'clock in the afternoon. Wherever they are, they stop to say the Angelus or to make the sign of the cross. As a rule, children should be at home with the family to say the Angelus together. After the short prayer they kiss the hand of their elders—parents and grandparents—as a sign of respect and affection.

"MANO PO"

Kissing the hand of the elderly is a symbolic Filipino custom. It is a practice handed down from generation to generation, a sign of respect and reverence. It expresses a form of salutation, kind regard, an expression of gratitude, affectionate greeting, and fond goodbye. Children and younger members of the family greet their elders during Christmas, New Year's Day, Easter, birthdays, after the Angelus, special occasions, and at any other time by taking the right hand of their grandparents, parents, and significant others and gently placing the hand on their forehead or their lips, saying "mano po." The elderly will in turn impart blessing to the young ones by saying "God be with you" or "God bless you." It is a cordial and affectionate exchange of greetings. The custom is highly valued by the Filipinos.

Since the Filipino child is conditioned and trained early in life to be respectful, humble, and obedient, he easily conforms to the norms and expectations within the culture. Childrearing practices that conform to the mores of the society are sanctioned by the members of that society as correct and imperative. When the accepted norms are violated, it generates doubt, guilt, and a loss of the sense of belonging.

Adolescence

Certain practices associated with the onset of

menstruation are still observed in the rural areas. On the first day of the menstrual flow, the girl is told to stand on the third step of the stairs, say three "Hail Marys," and then jump to the ground. It is part of the folk-belief that by doing so, the menstrual flow will only last for 3 days. Sour food such as tangerines, lemons, or any food containing vinegar is forbidden, and taking a bath during the menstrual flow is taboo—she can bathe on the last day of her period.

Boys are generally circumcised when they reach the adolescent stage. The procedures vary according to the prevailing practices within the community or barrio. Some are done at the health centers, others are done at the hospital, the rest are performed by someone who is an authority with a great deal of experience, known as the "manunuli."

Sex education, the handling of overt behavior, and important aspects of emotional development associated with sex vary greatly. Sex is a very delicate matter and is not discussed openly. Inference is often used. Girls and boys between 11 and 14 years of age do not feel free to discuss subjects pertaining to sex; fathers and mothers, likewise, do not feel comfortable in discussing the matter. Sons and daughters usually prefer to get sexual information from a more detached source, such as the school counselor, magazines, movies, health education teachers, and peers. Girls receive instructions regarding hygiene and what to do when menstruation comes. In the same manner, the boys undergo special care after the circumcision to prevent infection. An open and uninhibited child may ask his father or mother intimate questions about sex, but this rarely happens. Questions about sex are discussed in a hush-hush manner. Some parents consider questions about sex as taboo—to them sex is a deeply personal, honorable matter, a relationship between a man and a woman that is private.

Mothers are highly concerned about their daughter's sexual behavior as soon as they reach the age of puberty. The young girls in the barrios are generally chaperoned at parties, fiestas, carnivals, dances, theaters, picnics, and other activities that occur outside the home. Colorful celebrations such as fiestas, Christmas, and Easter are part and parcel of the Filipinos' way of life. These affairs are a blend of devotion with religious ardor and festive spirit, merry-making, eating specially prepared foods, dancing, song-fests, and sports. Children enjoy these events, partic-ularly the teen-agers and the young adults. They take part in the activities and preparations with a special feeling of jubilation and a special sense of tradition. These events provide opportunities for young ladies and gentlemen to interact with minimal restraint from the watchful chaperones.

Courtship

When a boy from the barrio gets attracted to a girl, he visits her house two or three times. He usually pays his respects to the parents and talks to them before he is introduced to the girl. If he knows the girl before the house visit he is not allowed to talk to the girl directly. As soon as he gathers enough courage to express his love to the girl, the boy generally asks the help of an intermediary or a "go-between." The "sala," or living room, or the balcony is the part of the house where the boy and girl are allowed to see each other. The parents do not approve of the young man sitting close to their daughter. The interaction is modified in certain situations, such as parties, fiestas, and other social gatherings. Exchanging glances generally suffices in expressing emotions. Exaggerated display of affection, such as holding hands in public, is frowned upon.

To win the girl's affection, and the approval of the parents, the boy must show the sincerity of his intentions by performing tasks for the family, for example, helping in the fields during planting season or harvest time, clearing the orchard, gathering firewood, fetching water, and other tasks around the farm. When the girl's parents show acceptance or become more friendly with him, he then gets other privileges, such as an outing with the family, or he gets invited to family social gatherings. The girl may then go with the boy to fiestas and social functions, if properly chaperoned.

Family influence is important in outings and social affairs. Girls are chaperoned whenever an affair is outside the limits set by the parents. "Time in" is carefully considered. School outings chaperoned by teachers and other grown-ups are acceptable. Many groups still regard the close scrutiny of a chaperone as very important in preventing infractions on the mores governing premarital behavior. Romantic impulses are subject to personal restraint and censure. Free association of the young is not accepted. Philippine society still considers free association of the young as a threat to the concept of chastity before marriage. The bride's chastity is considered the greatest virtue she can uphold before she gets married. Even today, any association with the opposite sex beyond the most formal type of association makes the bride a victim of criticism and negative sanctions. However, this attitude is modified in situations in which the girl has some informal association with the barrio's young men during special activities and at work.

Another way of courting the girl is through the romantic custom of expressing the boy's love with the *harana,* or serenade. He invites the young men of the barrio, and with a guitar, he serenades his lady-fair with songs that express his love and devotion. The songs are still popular today, such as "Dungawin Mo Hirang," which means "look at the window beloved one;" "Natutulog ka Man, Irog Kong Matimtiman"— "even if you are asleep, wake up and give me a glance." The harana are usually done on moonlit nights.

Marriage

Marriage in the Philippines is a complex of customs centered on the relationships of the associating pair of young adults. It unites two people plus a network of extended kin who influence family life. Behavioral expectations, reciprocal obligations, and the socially accepted restrictions are defined and communicated to the participants. A series of traditional preparations before the wedding are undertaken by both families. The boy's family, besides paying the dowry, pays the expenses for the wedding feast. Relatives and friends of the groom perform the tasks of cooking; decoration; arranging for the orchestra or band; building a banquet hall on the premises of the bride's residence; building arcs with intricate designs out of bamboo; making decorated baskets for the "alayan" (offering); purchasing a cow or pig and butchering it for the occasion; and preparing for the wedding procession. The bride's family takes charge of the wedding ensemble, the choice of sponsors, bridesmaids, and flower girls; the groom chooses his best man and ring bearer. Both families participate in the decoration of the church. The announcement of the wedding, the arrangement between families, and the customs observed vary from region to region and from one social class to another.

Arranged marriages were prevalent in the past. They are still practiced today in some regions but are less prevalent in urban areas. Contracts are made between two families usually with a "go-between." The bride's price is determined during a series of two meetings: the first meeting is the "pautos"—when the boy's parents ask for the girl's hand in marriage; the second meeting is called "pamamalaye" or "padulog"—which means the girl's parents will make the decisions and agree on the proposals of the boy's family. The dowry may be in the form of money, land, a brand new house, or land titles. The boy's family usually gets a very influential or prominent member of the community as go-between. If the girl opposes the contract the go-between loses his integrity. If a contract is broken it is usually for practical reasons; however, depending on circumstances, the go-between sometimes uses drastic measures to consummate a marriage, even before the gift-giving and the wedding feast take place. The highlight of the preparations and negotiations is the marriage ceremony and the wedding feast. Valuable gifts are presented to the girl by the boy's family and the girl's family are the guests of honor.

The Filipino family recognizes the sacred functions of marriage. Childbearing is a natural desire. There is a religious implication in the manner children are regarded: they are the outcome of a sacred union, God's blessings. Even with the advent of modern problems caused by over-crowding, malnutrition, hunger, and overpopulation, children are desired. In the rural areas, large households are still evident.

Large households in the Philippines are set up as a cooperative unit. The young are cared for by the elders and the adults look after the very old. The non-productive and those that cannot earn sufficiently on their own are helped by the household. Mutual love, respect, and concern exists. Although there are advantages and disadvantages in this type of set up, there is no trauma evident.

The dramatic impact of modernization has affected the Filipino family. The pressures of modern trends are reflected on the aspirations of the younger generation. The dynamic forces of change awakened the masses to acquire better things in life; their desire to achieve improved working conditions, higher wages, better health benefits, and better distribution of resources created social unrest. However, the Filipino family remains steadfast in its kinship tradition, and kinship solidarity still remains intact.

Values Attached to Having Children

Social scientists, Filipinos, and Western scholars who studied, measured, and classified Philippine value systems, have made important contribu-

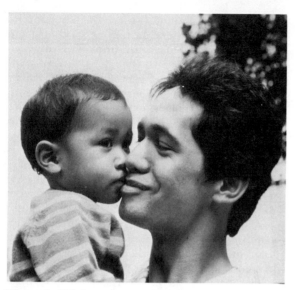

Figure 3. Filipino parents value their children highly and perceive them as signs of God's blessings. (Photograph by Brad Powell)

tions by identifying values that Filipinos attach to having children.

Several definitions of the term "value" by scholars, sociologists, anthropologists, economists, and psychologists were applicable in the description of the values studied in the Philippine setting. Kluckholn characterizes value as a "conception explicit or implicit, distinctive of the individual or characteristic of the group; means and ends of actions."[6] Vernon and colleagues classified values as theoretical, aesthetic, economic, social, political, and religious.[7]

Value refers to what the individual regards as important. It is affected by family relations, socioeconomic status of the family, education, religious beliefs and customs, and prevailing sociocultural practices within the community. Like attitude, values determine how the individual will respond to his environment; they help determine what is right and wrong.

Important values regarding children demonstrated in Bulatao's survey are happiness that children bring, incentives to succeed, inspiration to strive for a goal that children bring, help in household work, companionship, comfort and care in old age, relief from strain, play and fun with the children, distraction from problems, continuity of family name, strengthening of the bond between spouses, fulfillment, extension of self and own values, continuation of family tra-

ditions, satisfying religious obligations, and social benefits.[8]

Guthrie's work in 1968 revealed that Filipinos value their children as a sign of God's blessings; a source of pleasure to parents, siblings, and other relatives; a necessity to complete the atmosphere of a home; the basis for a mystical feeling of continuity between generations; and a source of security in old age (Fig. 3). Thus, one's child is one's wealth.

To provide more companions for other siblings is the most common reason why Filipino parents want additional children. The need to have a family of the right size with the proper combination of boys and girls, associated with concern over having a harmonious environment for bringing up the children, is another reason for wanting more children. Other motives for having another child are that mothers enjoy having a small baby; parents want to have a girl or a boy; there is a desire to have another girl or another boy; parents want to carry on the family name.

EDUCATION IN THE PHILIPPINES

Informal education starts at home. The parents are the first teachers and are assisted by other members of the kingroup. The moment the child is born he learns to socialize along the accepted patterns of behavior within his family circle. As he grows older, he learns the accepted norms of the community in which he and his family live.

Formal education through the public or private school system is a highly specialized process, which prepares the child to become a productive member of society and later on to become self-sufficient. The expectations of the family are similar to society's expectations from an educated individual: that he may contribute and participate in the betterment of his family and the society to which he belongs.

The educational system in the Philippines has been influenced by the colonial imperialists, chiefly by the Spanish and American systems of education. The Spanish influence had been largely in the area of religion and morals. The American influence was directed towards the duties of citizenship, the management of community affairs, and the introduction of English as the basis of instruction and the means of communication in the management of national affairs and important functions.

Education is undertaken by government and privately owned schools and supervised by the state. There are three levels: the elementary level, which is 6 years; secondary, 4 years; and the collegiate level. The new trend now includes prep schools in various categories, for example, 4 year olds may be enrolled in the prep school; 5 year olds go to kindergarten; some private schools have seventh grades. Vocational education is also offered as mandated by the 1935 Constitution.

Formal education is greatly valued by the Filipinos, especially those belonging to the low-income groups and the middle-class families. They consider education as the key to upward mobility on the social ladder. In the Far East, the Philippines has the highest literacy rate, but the unemployment rate is also high, according to the 1972 survey (taken by Romeo Pajarillo of the *Manila Times*).[10]

The language problem in the Philippines is largely a political and cultural one. Until 1936, English was the only language taught in the schools. With the coming of the Commonwealth government, the national language based on Tagalog was taught in all grades in elementary school, high school, and college. In 1952, legislation included 12 units of Spanish as a requirement for graduation in college. As a result, college graduates know at least three languages besides their own.

The Philippine educational system still uses English as the medium of instruction. Imported Western and American books on all levels of education; American trained teachers and professors; American oriented materials, curriculum, and audio-visual aids have all caused a confusion in the identity and orientation of the Filipino.

SUPERSTITIOUS BELIEFS IN HEALTH AND DISEASE

Unique aspects of superstitious beliefs about health and the treatment of diseases persist in the Filipino's way of life in spite of the prevailing high literacy rate. Progress in health education, detection and treatment of diseases, preventive measures, health maintenance, and nutrition programs have not eradicated superstition.

Children are frequently the victims of superstitious practices, because of the rapid onset of common diseases among them, unusual symptoms, unknown causes, the children's inability to express what is ailing them, rapid course, and sudden death. Most of the childhood diseases are believed to be due to supernatural causes.

One belief that contributes to a high incidence of gastroenteritis is the belief that diarrhea is associated with teething. The diarrhea is not treated, as the parents wait for the tooth to erupt, hoping that the ailment will disappear as soon as the tooth appears.

Minor cuts, skin abrasions, and wounds are cleansed by a concoction prepared by boiling young leaves from the guava tree.

Prickly heat, a skin condition peculiar to the summer season, afflicts children and adults; it affects the neck of babies, the back and sides of the trunk, the abdomen, and crevices. It is characterized by red pimple-like eruptions about the size of millet seeds and is treated with "gaugau," a common laundry starch similar to corn starch. Prickly heat is known as miliaria rubra or heat rash.

There are other unusual beliefs regarding the newborn. The baby can not have a full bath until the cord is dry; babies are not to be laid on their tummy when they are sleeping. Herbs are placed on the stomach to prevent gas pains. Mother and child must stay within the confines of the home until the baby is baptized, so that the baby is protected from evil spirits. Mothers put tight binders around the abdominal area so that the baby, especially if it is a girl, will have a waistline. Supplementary feedings given to 4- to 8-month-old babies are prohibited; it is believed that they will cause parasitism, since the baby cannot digest the food (only rice gruel is allowed).

Concepts of Illness

According to folk belief, illness occurs when the balance of elements outside or inside the body is disturbed. Changes in season, improper diet, sorcery, witchcraft, general conduct in life, and accidents disturb the equilibrium. It is also believed that supernatural powers cause disease. This explains why some Filipinos perform rituals and say special prayers, and why they wear protective devices such as charms, amulets, medals, and crucifixes as a protection against disease agents from the physical environment.

The official teachings of the Christian religion have been modified to suit the Filipino's way of thinking, believing, and doing things. The crucifix, the prayers, the holy water, and many of the church rituals are used by the traditional healers—faith healers.

Folk Beliefs Associated with Pregnancy

During the period of "lihi," which means maternal craving for special food during the first few weeks after the cessation of menstruation (it may also be a special liking or dislike for a certain individual or object), the conceiving mother's longing or strong desire for the particular food has to be satisfied. Husbands and other members of the family oblige the wishes or craving of the wife. These are some of the folk beliefs: if the mother eats twin bananas she will have twins; eating crabs will cause deformity on the hands of the child; if an expectant mother shows a special liking for the statue of the Virgin Mary, the child will be very beautiful; if she happens to like a neighbor's child, that child will get sick until the second trimester of the pregnancy.

There are other superstitious beliefs related to illness and health:

1. Taking baths on Fridays will cause illness.
2. A person with big ears will have a long life.
3. A girl must not take a bath during the menstrual period, for this will cause insanity.
4. Combing the hair at night is bad; it will cause eye problems.
5. Sleeping with wet hair will cause blindness.
6. Babies should have a cross, a medal, or a charm to ward off evil spirits and to protect them from harm.

FILIPINO IMMIGRATION TO THE UNITED STATES

The Filipinos came to America in three waves of migration. The first group came in 1903. They were called the Pensionados. William Howard Taft, the first civil governor of the Philippines, affirmed the Pensionados Act of 1903. This educational plan for talented young Filipinos was used to send them to the United States to learn American democracy and later use their training in reforming the Filipinos. The first group was chosen from 20,000 applicants. They were enrolled in major universities such as Purdue, Harvard, Cornell, Columbia, Stanford, Yale, and USC in a variety of professional programs: education, civil and mechanical engineering, medicine, and agriculture. The first group all returned in 1910. They assisted in implementing reforms and took their places in Philippine society. They played important roles in improving agriculture, business, government, and education. Most of them became prominent provincial and national leaders. The achievements of the first group of

Pensionados attracted other Filipinos to go to the United States. Between 1910 and 1938 almost 14,000 Filipinos came to America on their own to further their studies. There were some that returned home successfully. Many remained in the United States, but owing to the high cost of living, discrimination, and discouragement, many of these Filipinos did not complete their education. They were forced to drift into cheap labor and remained in the United States. Those that succeeded returned to the Philippines. They joined the earlier Pensionados in implementing change and improving conditions in the homeland.

The second group of Filipino immigrants belonged to the working class. They were ambitious laborers recruited to work on American farms and plantations. Most of them were single males under the age of 30. When they reached America they often became victims of riots, hatred, and discrimination. They faced hostility and exclusion from economic and social benefits. Many of these immigrants ended up living in the "oriental ghettos" and sought the companionship of undesirable White prostitutes. They were forced to live at low levels of economic and social existence. The impact of prejudice and discrimination did not match the ideals and teachings the Americans had implanted in the Philippines: those of freedom, liberty, justice, equality, fraternity, and opportunity for all. The Filipinos came to feel that the Americans do not practice what they preach.

Between 1940 and 1960, 78,000 more Filipinos entered the United States. The increasing number of immigrants came with varying political and economic reasons. "Seeking a share of the American dream," they came with high hopes and determination, willing to challenge whatever opportunity awaited them. Many of the Filipinos aspired to go to America after learning that "America is a land of promise"; educational reasons merely increased their aspirations. Additionally, those Filipinos who wrote about the good life and the "high wages" in the United States and the successful return of some workers motivated more Filipinos to leave their homeland.

In 1965, some female immigrants were beginning to be attracted to the "land of promise." The majority of them were nurses, physicians, pharmacists, dentists, and other health professionals. Some of them came under the "Exchange Program" and later on changed their status to immigrants. An estimated 25,000 Filipinos that were on the West Coast by 1930 were Navy enlistees. Their requests to be assigned in the Pacific Coast areas were granted. Their presence added to the pool of "cheap labor" in California and they were regarded as another threat to the White working class of America.

As the number of Filipino immigrants increased, their image became less and less favorable. They continued to be subjected to many types of discriminatory processes, including hatred and denial of citizenship and naturalization, even at a time when the Filipinos were still American Nationals. In 1935, President Roosevelt signed a Repatriation Act to transport Filipinos back to the Philippines. This was a measure sought by anti-Filipino agitators and exclusionists. The provision included denial of re-entry to the United States. The Filipinos believed that the color of their skin prevented them from assimilating into White society, not just their threat as a labor force replacing White laborers.

The desire to adapt to White standards of success, the desire to regain their self-respect, prompted the Filipinos to unite and to seek honorable means of resolving their grievances, to stop the dehumanizing processes and unjust labor practices against them. They formed Filipino clubs and organizations to protest the unfair legislative measures and policies of exclusion by the American government. Wary and disillusioned, many of the Filipinos did not know which way to turn; it would not be of any consolation to go back home since they knew that the Americans still controlled the Philippine economy. Their high sense of pride also prevented most of the immigrants from going back as "failures." With the endless fight for a right to life and pursuits of happiness, the Filipinos challenged the hardships and remained in a society hostile to them. They were forced to live at the lowest levels of economic existence and found themselves "double social outcasts," for the other Orientals discriminated against them also.

Filipino immigrants that were admitted to the United States after 1957 encountered many of the same difficulties as the early immigrants. Most of them belonged to the working class and were subjected to racial, economic, social, and job discrimination. The impact of prejudice forced many of the educated immigrants to accept menial jobs that were below their abilities and professional training. It is common today to

find a professional working as bus boy, pantry worker, dishwasher, servant, or hotel maid. They were restricted from performing according to their capabilities, opportunities for job advancement were always lacking, and wages were always lower. As a result, many of the educated Filipinos underachieved; frustrated and disillusioned, they still remained in the United States without realizing their potentials and professional fulfillment.

The immigrants who came after 1965 are employed in semiprofessional occupations, many are employed in unskilled jobs, and a few are able to secure professional licenses. With the changing regulations of labor unions in the United States in the 1960s, some Asian minorities were slowly admitted into unions. This change does provide an opportunity for the Filipinos to obtain economic and social benefits. However, the Filipinos' struggles for better wages and equality of working hours, working conditions, and pay continues. They are still restricted in what they are able to do.

Filipinos speaking the same language or coming from the same region in the Philippines tend to follow the same ethnolinguistic pattern of grouping as in the Philippines. They establish closer ties with the people from the same ethnic group, whom they identify with. They form an ethnic subsociety, which is a large group of people with a "shared feeling of peoplehood."

Impact of Immigration on the Family

The problems encountered by the immigrants when they started their "new life" in America created psychological, social, and economic disruption of family life. Segregation, exclusion, prejudice, an alien culture, unfamiliar norms, and the diversified culture that they brought with them caused problems. Campaigns of hatred aimed at the early Filipino immigrants are believed to have reduced their enthusiasm and achievement. They were forced to a low level of livelihood. Some of them have become irresponsible, aimless, and not free to engage in the process of acculturation. The feelings of inferiority, inlaid by the Spaniards, later reinforced by the American conquerors, and now perpetuated in America, caused many to internalize a very low self-concept. Economic deprivation affected family functioning, nutrition, and health. Crowded dwellings and ghettos emerged for the Filipinos when they were denied access to decent housing. In order to survive, several persons often shared a rented house or one room. Some of the boarding houses that accepted Filipino tenants and areas where Filipinos dwell were often disparagingly referred to as "Little Manila."

The family structure in America more or less follows that in the Philippines with some modification and some variation. Those immigrants who get married in the United States usually sponsor their parents to come, and later the rest of the siblings are sponsored by the mother or father. They form a simple extended family system. Parsons defined "system" as an organization of units or elements united in some form of regular interaction and interdependence. Aspects of kin-group solidarity still exist.

The nuclear family is the system into which most of the Filipino families in the United States could be categorized. The system stresses marital ties in which man's primary duties are to his wife and children. The form of authority is generally patriarchal; with the case of a highly industrialized American society, authority is usually egalitarian. The family customs in the homeland, influenced by social traditions and the Christian religion, are practiced in America.

The Filipino immigrants brought their diverse cultural backgrounds from the Philippine barrios to the United States. Their rich cultural heritage, regional differences, customs and traditions, beliefs, folklore, and diverse languages are evident in the Filipino settlements and communities in America today, but because of racial, political, social, and legal discriminatory practices, Filipinos have not been really assimilated into the American mainstream.

Melendez[11] and Rabaya[12] revealed interesting accounts of present day Filipino feelings. The young Filipinos may attach shame to their Filipino heritage; they may express a desire to break away from any "old timer" Filipino identity; and they yearn to be totally assimilated as Americans. Very few American-born Filipinos appreciate their rich cultural heritage; existing educational processes deprive the Filipino-Americans of learning about the Philippines and its people.

FAMILY FUNCTIONS IN AMERICA

Living in a modern industrial society, the Filipino family attempts to adapt and carry out its functions. To some extent the Filipino nuclear family has become specialized, as have other social institutions. A variety of functions are performed by a smaller number of people, compared with the functions performed by a larger number in the extended family system. In childrearing, father and mother are exclusively responsible for primary socialization and socialization for family participation. Aunts, uncles, cousins, grandparents, and maids, who took active roles in the life of the child in the Philippines, can no longer do the same in the American setting, except for very few exceptions in which the family of orientation and the family of procreation are living in the same household.

Parents discharge basic functions of personality formation, tension management, status conferral, religious training, character development, and formation of desirable traits. In the kin group, the child may draw many kinds of support from the many figures of identification; in turn, the child is expected to assist or offer help to the members of the kin group as soon as he is capable. The child's achievement and success will be regarded as the family's success, and his failure will be considered a disgrace to the family. This is modified to some extent in America. Although the Filipinos maintain close ties with the families back home, their major economic, political, religious, educational, and household maintenance duties have become more important.

The family in America, trying to live up to the standards of family life according to the norms of the surrounding community, has continued a series of interchanges with the kin group in their homeland. These interchanges link both families; they exchange goods, financial support, moral support, love, and thoughtfulness. Sometimes the flow of goods is one way, for example, when a member of the kin gets married, more gifts are expected from the family in America, and when the newlyweds have a baby, the expectation for more presents increases. Oftentimes, the interchange consists of behavior and behavior response. In some cases, the interchanges may be negative, such as withholding of goods, a hostile attitude expressed in letters, and even in silence. Although the interchanges vary, the relationships between the nuclear families in America and the kin group in the Philippines remain closely knit.

Characteristics of the first-generation adult immigrants follow:

1. Respect for elders, authority, school rules and regulations, and teachers are outstanding characteristics of Filipinos wherever they may be.
2. Modesty in dress, speech, and manners.

3. Politeness in interaction within the family, the group they identify with, and others.
4. Hospitality, regardless of social status, is a special trait; when visitors drop in, they are accorded a cordial welcome; be it stranger or non-kin, the Filipino home is almost always ready to receive a guest.
5. Loyalty to family, friends, and group is manifested in the way Filipinos defend their family honor. Family disasters or problems are resolved by enthusiastic efforts to make amends. They show genuine concern and sympathy for any member of their group whenever they are in need. They offer immediate assistance according to their abilities when friends are having difficulties; for example, in situations in which someone loses a job, relatives and friends give economic assistance in the form of money, food, or shelter until the disadvantaged person is able to find another job. Another instance is when someone gets sick—friends help by cooking, performing errands, or doing some of the household chores.
6. Gentleness is evident in the Filipinos' mild manners and easy-going attitude; they are very gentle when they are caring for their elders or young children; they show gentleness when they are assisting a person in pain.
7. Love for music, dancing, and pageantry.

Social Control

Social control is a primary factor in the family organization. As a member of the organization, the child gains much and learns much from his involvement and interaction within the family; and as a member of society, which is a much larger organization, the child is subject to all forms of social control. He pays the price of acceptance of restraints (laws and regulations), obedience, conformity, and limitations on the freedom to do as he pleases. The child learns to face the consequences when he deviates from the accepted norms set by the family and society.

The Filipinos use hiya, bahala na, saka na, and utang na loob as forms of sanction. Other kinds of sanctions the child gets accustomed to are:
1. *Negative*—reprobation by a community towards a person whose conduct is disapproved.

2. *Satirical*—met by ridicule by other members of the group.
3. *Religious*—involves the belief that uncleanliness and sinfulness can be appeased by penance and charity.
4. *Legal*—primary and secondary. Primary is imposed by constituted authorities, such as ecclesiastical, political, and military authorities. Secondary is involved in procedures carried out by a community when an individual disobeys the regulations and rules set up by the community.

Factors That Affect Family Life in America

Rapid changes have focused attention on the problems of the families in America, particularly the problems of poverty, unemployment, adequate housing, health, divorce, and juvenile delinquency. Early in the twentieth century, family forms were changing and more problems were emerging. Just as disturbing as poverty, the problem of divorce and separation increased, and there was a decline in birth rate. More women were spending longer hours outside the home, and the existence of the family as a group was seriously challenged.

Values, economic pressures, health problems, health maintenance, communications, and educational needs affected the mother's traditional role in the home. The need for supplementing the husband's income to meet the family's finances became apparent, and working mothers and working wives brought about serious problems. There were the problems of housekeeping, child-care, fatigue, emotional outbursts, maladjustment of children, and limited communication, which sometimes led to family disintegration. The Filipino families were not spared from these problems; however, their value system, religious ardor, and traditional beliefs help them cope and meet the demands of contemporary society.

Childrearing of Filipino Children in America

The permissive, gentle atmosphere of the Filipino home allows for the leisurely maturation of the child. Early achievers are admired, suppression of hostility is emphasized, fighting is discouraged, and the child is compelled to suppress his aggressiveness and anger, but he is encouraged to express himself in a respectful manner. Smooth interpersonal relationships are highly valued by the Filipino parents in America also. Mild forms of spanking, verbal appeal, admonition without the use of vulgar words, threatening, silent treatment, ignoring, and distraction are among the methods parents resort to when disciplining the child. As the children grow older, some types of deprivation are effectively used, such as limiting the child's favorite activities (e.g., shorter time for watching cartoons if the child neglects to finish his school work), or sending the child to his room when he shows an exaggerated display of tantrum.

When the child's behavior gets out of control, the punishment is generally done by the father. In the absence of the father (who is away or at work), the mother uses the slippers, the belt, or a ruler for spanking the child. Back talk is not allowed. As long as the tension is high in situations in which parents are aroused to anger, the child is trained to remain silent until the parents' anger subsides; then he may explain his side and the problem is immediately mitigated. Children learn and accept correction with humility; parents and child make up with enthusiasm and affection after a conflict.

Parents encourage their children to tell them everything, especially the teen-agers; mothers feel that they should not have secrets. In like manner, parents encourage their children to be dependent—another aspect of their way of life that is accepted in Philippine society. The dependency pattern is balanced by the reciprocal pattern that comes into play because of the nature of the value of kind regard, gratitude (utang naloob), love, and respect that the child learns early in life. When an older brother helps a younger sister or brother to finish college, the sibling receiving the support obligates himself to help his brother in time of need, including emotional support and loyalty.

Household chores are delegated to the children according to their age. Picking up their toys after play time; performing their own self-care, such as washing their hands and face before meals; watching younger siblings play; and running errands and other simple tasks that provide help and relief to their parents are assigned to the children. They are trained to perform their tasks cheerfully. There is no room for resentment. These divisions of labor give children a sense of accomplishment, responsibility, and well-being. Parents dispense positive reinforcement and verbal praise generously. Family solidarity requires the individual to sacrifice his interests for the sake of better interests that will benefit the family as a whole. Belongingness and acceptance of individual members promote self-esteem.

When the child reaches the adult stage and becomes self-sufficient, he is expected to provide economic support for his parents and to look after the welfare of the other siblings after the parent's death. This task is usually undertaken by the oldest child.

MORAL TRAINING

How do we assess moral responsibility in the area of human sexuality? Because of the limitation of the Filipino family's ability to express their concepts about sexuality, we can only infer or make statements about their responses regarding the subject. Most of them feel that sexuality has a religious dimension, a dimension that opens up to the holy and wonderful mystery of God. This religious dimension influences their attitude toward sex—why certain stances must be taken on how far parents should control and limit their children's activities and behavior, the way they dress, the way they carry themselves, the way they relate with their friends, and the places they go to. As soon as the child reaches the age of puberty, indirect forms of control are implemented through persuasion, verbal appeal, and setting up rules and restrictions. Because of early conditioning in regard to respect and obedience, conflicts are minimized and there is a high level of compliance.

CULTURAL HERITAGE

In terms of learning the cultural heritage of the parents, the Filipino child has to be exposed to other forms of educational processes, which are very limited in America. There are no museums, parks, or children's books that are representative of the Filipino way of life except for a few displays of artifacts in the Smithsonian Institute in Washington, D.C. Participation in the activities of some professional organizations with Filipino members, joining Filipino clubs that are already in existence, and forming groups that will promote educational and cultural benefits for the American-born Filipinos will help disseminate knowledge and understanding of their parents' homeland.

SUMMARY OF CHILDREARING PRACTICES

The general characteristics of Filipino childrearing practices can be summarized as follows:

1. Parents are generally permissive.
2. Baby talk is sometimes carried on.
3. Respect is taught early in life.
4. There is hardly any spanking.
5. Positive reinforcements are used.
6. Children sometimes are dependent too long.
7. The pattern of discipline is influenced by the concept of "walang malay."
8. There are no set expectations from the child.
9. High ideals are inculcated in the child.
10. Harmony is stressed over being "right."
11. Social acceptance is highly valued.
12. Just a look from the parents sometimes suffices to bring a message or action.
13. Threatening is used.
14. Childrearing is shame oriented (hiya).
15. Parents sometimes compare children with siblings or important others.
16. Obedience is emphasized.
17. Fables and tales are used to teach a lesson or moral to the child.
18. Sharing and helping one another ("bayanihan") are taught early in life.

Negative sanctions of adults, which serve as a form of social control, are characterized by the following:[13]

1. *Amor propio*—functionally, this is not merely a response to any attempt at casting doubt or questioning an individual's action, integrity, or honor; it is a validation of one's self-image.
2. *Hiya*—this has been translated by Western observers as "shame," "shyness," or "losing face." Other dimensions of hiya are:
   a. *Nangingime*—which means an individual is unable to express what he feels for varied reasons (e.g., a poor boy is ashamed to express his love to a rich girl).
   b. *Atubili*—hesitation to perform an action or say what one wants. It involves caution; one studies the situation first. A person beats around the bush and does not say what he really wants to say directly.
3. *Utang na loob*—(Charles Kaut, 1961) a feeling of gratitude, this consists of a series of positive and negative behaviors. It defines the limits of socially meaningful relations among individuals. When a person asks the help of his landlord to pay a doctor's bill for a seriously ill child, he obligates himself to reciprocate by offering services to his landlord even after he repays the money he borrowed.
4. *Saka na*—which means later on, is an expression of procrastination; it may mean one has no time or no inclination to do something now. It also connotes one's dislike for something or possibly disgust for something. When an aunt wants to take a niece to a movie that the niece does not care to see, she'll usually respond "saka na po."
5. *Hinanakit*—means displeasure when a person does not fulfill long-term obligations, displeasure when certain expectations are not met. In other cultures, when a person pays back what he borrowed, it ends there; in the Philippine culture, the obligation goes beyond payment. When a person fails to acknowledge his debt of gratitude (utang na loob), that person will be ostracized or treated negatively because of hinanakit.
6. *Mañana habit*—putting off until tomorrow what one can do today.
7. *Bahala na*—one who is frustrated will undertake certain actions not knowing what the outcome of those actions will be; he will then face the consequences later on. This concept applies in situations such as when a person with an incurable disease, frustrated from all the expensive treatment he has undergone, desperately tries the technique of folk healers and says "bahala na."
8. *Niñgas cogon*—short-lived enthusiasm or lack of perseverence, one gets discouraged easily. This characteristic is demonstrated when an individual starts a project that requires special technique, materials, and man-hours, initiates effort but not enough to complete the project, then stops halfway through the project. *Niñgas* means heat of the fire, burning, ardor, enthusiasm. *Cogon* is a type of grass that grows in the Philippines. It is used for thatched roofing of shelters in the fields where farmers rest from the heat of the sun, and also has other uses. It burns easily and the fire dies down quickly.

EFFECTIVE DELIVERY OF HEALTH CARE

In dealing with the Filipino child, the nurse (and other health workers) will also deal with the par-

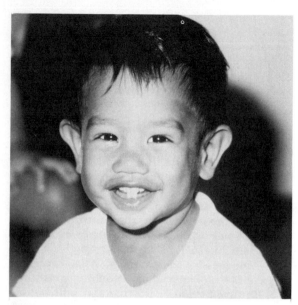

Figure 4. The Filipino child responds to a tension-free environment with friendly caretakers. (Photograph by Brad Powell)

ents. During the interaction, the provider of health care has to contend with cultural attitudes and prescribed roles for children and adolescents, for example, that children are to be seen and not heard, and are expected to give unquestioning obedience to their elders and authority figures. Smooth interpersonal relationships are highly valued, and since Filipino children have many opportunities to observe adult models, they are surrounded by many people who reinforce age-appropriate behavior. In a clinic, when a child is brought for certain treatment, members of the family are usually with the sick child (several members usually). In the hospital, members of the family would stay with the child in the room (this is an accepted practice in Philippine hospitals).

The family and the patient may view the health worker with alarm, confusion, uncertainty, and even fear. Initially, here are important points to consider:

1. *Provide a feeling of acceptance.* Create an atmosphere of friendliness and ease; provide a low-pressure social environment to allow the child and the adults (parents or parent substitute) to feel that they are accepted (Fig. 4). Allow them to re-learn about health care needs of the child. Do not require a greater degree of performance of the child than what he is able to give at

the time. Listen attentively; help the child or his family define the "problem" or need, instead of defining it for them. (Most professionals fail to find time to listen to their clients.) Listen to their beliefs and attitudes regarding illness; avoid expressions such as "you're not supposed to do that," or "that's bad for you." This will require tact and imagination, flexibility, self-control, and patience. Consider individual differences; avoid comparison with other children.

2. *Establish open communication.* Use simple, courteous language. Bluntness or brusqueness is frowned upon. Owing to their upbringing and certain types of behavior expected of them, children will not speak unless spoken to, oftentimes with very brief responses limited to nodding or merely shaking of the head. Sometimes Western observers equate this with shyness. It is important not to "label" this type of behavior pattern. Strive to establish a trusting relationship; ask open-ended questions; help the child and the adults deal with concrete problems; be sincere; and if indicated, teach the child to do things better with the use of visual aids, pictographs, or other forms of creative communication relevant to the situation. Clarify the purpose or the reason for the child's clinic visit or appointment.

3. *Present yourself with self-confidence.* Self-confidence and self-understanding are important therapeutic tools. The nurse must know herself and understand herself; it is the first step in self improvement, and the foundation of meeting her client's needs. She must know the process of trial and error, and the advantages of the objective approach. Explain what nursing intervention can be done for the child's health care needs with expertise (resulting from knowledge and experience).

4. *Strive to gain the patient's confidence.* Once this is established, it is easier to move on into other things, such as exploration of the child's feelings and history of his present illness. Understand that the Filipino child is likely to become very sensitive. Allow him to express negative emotions, the clinic or ward environment is a potential anxiety-producer; quiet acceptance of the child's dislike permits the expression of negative emotions (which is often a healthy sign). Try to keep anxiety factors to a minimum. Avoid feeling-touching maneuvers until a solid relationship has been established.

5. *Strive to become the child's advocate.*

6. *Provide emotional support and reassur-*

ance acceptable to the child and his family. Dependency behavior among Filipino children is accepted in Philippine society; it is encouraged, maintained, enjoyed, and slowly modified through childhood, adolescence, and adulthood. Accordingly, the child has many opportunities to observe adult behavior. He is never alone and is always surrounded by many people who reinforce his feelings of security and sense of belonging. The child therefore will show signs of insecurity when he is left alone in a ward, hospital crib, or treatment room. It is also difficult for a Filipino child to sleep alone, much more so if he is admitted to isolation rooms or an isolation ward. Do not dwell heavily on emotions, but do not ignore them either.

7. *Establish mutually acceptable systems of relationships with the child's family, and teachers, if indicated, regarding his care.* For example, a diabetic child will require observation and special consideration at school: teachers must give snacks at certain times, observe unusual symptoms or possible insulin reaction, and so on.

8. *Understand the child's desire to please.* The Filipino child's development and character formation are designed to please significant others, many others, and they learn to make every effort to respond to the expectations of authority, including those of the health worker.

9. *Understand the impact of sociocultural determinants.* The provider of care must be aware of life-cycle events, folk beliefs, and attitudes of the family regarding health and illness, food preferences, educational background of the child's family, and place of origin.

10. *Bear in mind that the term Filipino represents a diverse cultural background.* These people come from 7100 islands with different languages, sub-dialects, and sub-cultures as a result of historical circumstances, and have experienced colonization and immigration-emigration. It is important, therefore, not to place all the Filipinos into one category; avoid labeling. Despite some differences, the Filipino has needs that are universal to all human beings; do not overemphasize the patient's being a Filipino. Deal with him without being judgmental; certain negative tendencies will create a barrier in the effectiveness of care. Treat him not just as a Filipino, but as a child, a patient, and a human being.

It is not easy to maintain a symmetrical or proportionate relationship with the Filipino; generally the relationships are complementary (e.g., teacher-learner, leader-follower, boss-subordinate). It will be alien to the Filipino mind for a doctor or a nurse to discuss a "mutual approach" with a patient; in the patient's mind, the health worker is an authority with knowledge and expertise, and the patient should do as he is expected to do to cure his illness. If he finds it difficult to conform, he uses a go-between to speak for him.

REFERENCES

1. Cooley, C.H.: *Social Organization.* Scribner, New York, 1922, pp. 273-282.
2. Jocano, L.F.: *Folk Medicine in a Philippine Municipality.* The National Museum of Manila, Philippines, 1973, p.14.
3. Bulatao, J., et al.: "The Manileno's mainsprings." In Lynch, F. (ed.): *Four Readings in Philippine Values.* IPC Papers, No. 2, Ateneo de Manila University Press, Quezon City, 1973, pp. 94-102.
4. Guzman, J.V.: *Psychology of Filipinos.* University of the Philippines Press, Manila, 1967, pp. 3-10.
5. Ibid., pp. 16-20.
6. Kluckoln, C.: "The family and peer groups." In Bell, N., and Vogel, E. (eds.): *A Modern Introduction to the Family.* The Free Press, New York, 1968, pp. 310-320.
7. Vernon, P.C.: *A test for personal values.* Journal of Abnormal and Social Psychology 26:233-248, 1930.
8. Bulatao, R.A.: *The Value of Children.* East-West Population Institute, East-West Center, Honolulu, 1975, pp.20-26.
9. Guthrie, G.M.: *The Filipino Child and Philippine Society.* Philippine Normal College Press, Manila, 1961, pp. 3-28.
10. Pajarillo, R.: A survey of literacy and unemployment rate. Manila Times, 1972.
11. Melendez, H.: *Asians in America.* Twayne Publishers, Boston, 1977, pp. 97-98.
12. Rabaya, V.: "Filipino immigration." In Tachiki, A., Wong, E., Odo, F., et al. (eds.): *Roots: An Asian American Reader.* Continental Graphics, Los Angeles, 1971, pp. 188-189.
13. Jocano, p. 14.

BIBLIOGRAPHY

Agoncillo, T.A.: *A Short History of the Filipino People.* University of the Philippines Press, Manila, 1961.

Bell, N.W., and Vogel, E.F. (eds.): *A Modern Introduction to the Family*. Free Press, New York, 1968.

Bohannan, P.: *Social Anthropology*. Holt, Rinehart and Winston, New York, 1963.

Cabotaje, E.M.: *Food and Philippine Culture*. Centro Escolar University, Research and Development Center, Manila, 1976.

Elmer, M.C.: *Family Adjustments and Social Change*. R. Long and R.R. Smith, New York, 1932.

Gorospe, V.R.: *Responsible Parenthood in the Philippines*. Ateneo Publications Office, Manila, 1970.

Isidro, A.: *Muslim Philippines*. Mindanao State University, University Research Center, Marawi City, 1968.

Keane, P.S.: *Sexual Morality*. S.S. Paulist Press, New York, 1977.

Kephart, W.: *Family, Society, and the Individual*. Houghton Mifflin Co., Boston, 1961.

Lefrancois, G.R.: *Psychology for Teaching*. ed. 2. Wadsworth Publishing Company, Belmont, California, 1975.

Lynch, F.: *Four Readings on Philippine Values*. Institute of Philippine Culture, University Press, Quezon City, 1973.

Pyle, W.H.: *Training Children*. The Century Co., New York, 1929.

Tachiki, A., Wong, E., Odo, F., et al. (eds.): *Roots: An Asian American Reader*. Continental Graphics, Los Angeles, 1971.

Tiglao, T.V.: *Health Practices in a Rural Community*. Community Development Research Council, University of the Philippines, Manila, 1964.

Zabilka, G.: *Customs and Culture of the Philippines*. Charles E. Tuttle Co., Rutland, Vermont, 1963.

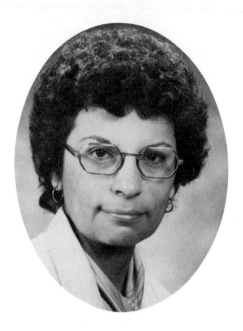

Chapter 8

My parents emigrated from the state of Sonora, Mexico, into southern Arizona as children. My father worked in the copper mines of Arizona all his life until his retirement. The mining community in which we lived was comprised of the laborers (mostly Mexican American) who lived in one part of town, and management (all Anglo) who lived on the "hill." I entered the first grade and was placed in 1B, a section for children that did not speak English or had other "problems." Since my parents were bilingual, I learned English faster than some of my classmates whose parents could not speak English. I firmly believe that the school rule saying that we could not speak Spanish on the playgrounds did nothing to help us to learn English. It only served to make us angry, ashamed, and resentful. My parents were proud of the fact that I was transferred to the 1A section at the second semester and would probably not have to repeat the first grade.

One of the most humiliating incidents that I can remember as a child is that only the Mexican children had their heads examined for head lice every morning. It is easy for me to realize now how I could have felt like a second-class citizen. However, our parents gave us great encouragement and told us time after time that we were just as good as everyone else. My sisters and I were very fortunate to have parents that

had not been beaten down by the system, and who still had a lot left to give to us. We were taught to be proud of our Mexican heritage and proud of our American citizenship, with its guaranteed rights. Our parents, after all, had become naturalized citizens and were well acquainted with the Constitution and the Bill of Rights. We celebrated the 4th of July, cinco de mayo, and el diez y seis de septiembre. We made frequent trips to Mexico to see relatives and they frequently came to see us.

Although our father had no more than a grade school education, he accepted nothing but the best performance from us in our studies. School was a serious business; his aspirations for us were high. The fact that we were girls did not make any difference.

I started my nursing career as a nurse's aide in pediatrics while working my way through college. That seemed to set a pattern for me, as I have worked with children most of my working life. Before obtaining my B.S. in Nursing from the University of Arizona, I also worked in the role of a licensed practical nurse. It was during this time that I vividly remember a Mexican father taking a very ill child home from the hospital because we were sponging him with alcohol and water to reduce his fever. This was in great conflict with his cultural belief of how to treat a fever. He thought the child would die if

The Mexican American (El Chicano)

Marta Borbón Ehling, R.N., M.S.

treated in this way. No one even tried to understand, of course, and I can still remember the comments about the "stupid Mexicans."

In 1965 I received my Masters in Nursing from the University of California in San Francisco. Thereafter, I held teaching positions at the University of Arizona, Howard University, and Arizona State University.

I developed a great interest and concern in day care centers after working for 3 years in a child development program in Merced, California. At present I am contemplating further study in the area of child development.

Together with my husband, Rex, and our children, Leonor, Dominic, and Andre, I presently make my home in Irvine, California.

For the purposes of this chapter, the terms Chicano and Mexican American will be used interchangeably. At the present time, these terms are the most commonly used to describe persons of Mexican ancestry residing in the United States. Other terms used in various parts of the country are Latins, Hispanics, Spanish, and Spanish-speaking.

The term Chicano did not gain popularity until the sixties, with the increase of political activity by the younger Mexican American. This word means different things to different people and many of the older generation do not like to be called Chicanos. During my childhood, the term was viewed as a slang word by some and a derogatory one by others.

Richard Rodriguez, a professor of English at the University of California, Berkeley, describes his feeling in this way:

> When I was young, I was taught to refer to my ancestry as Mexican-American. Chicano was a word used among friends or relatives. It implied a familiarity based on shared experience. Spoken casually, the term easily became an insult.[1]

Alfredo Mirandé describes these terms in the following way:

> Mexican-American connotes greater integration into American Society and is, not surprisingly, the

preferred term of social scientists. Chicano connotes greater ethnic identification and politicization and is more commonly used by Chicanos themselves.[2]

Although not all Mexican Americans like to be called Chicanos, no one can deny that because of the Chicano movement of the sixties, the Mexican American has become more visible and we have all profited from that political movement. Advancement and recognition will come with the increase of political involvement.

Statements made in this chapter are based on the writer's personal knowledge, as a member of the Chicano culture, and interviews of family types that vary according to recentness of migration to the United States, education, economic level, age, and urban-rural locale. Interviews were conducted in California and Arizona. Health professionals and educators working with Chicanos were also interviewed.

My purpose in writing this chapter is to increase the readers' understanding of the Chicano culture, dispel myths and stereotypes that have been perpetuated, and give some insight into some of the problems faced by many Chicano families in this country. This chapter is in no way a complete study of the Chicano culture.

HISTORY

Ancestors of Mexican Americans have lived in this country for centuries and are native to the Southwest. Many have been here since before the land belonged to Spain. The Southwest became part of Mexico when Mexico won its freedom from Spain and became part of the United States after the United States-Mexico War in 1848. Thus many Mexican Americans are not immigrants, but colonized people. A number of writers describe Mexican Americans as an "internal colony."[3] This concept is different from the classic version of colonization in several ways: (1) the land acquired is contiguous, (2) local leadership is removed from power, and (3) the internal colony is not formally recognized.[4]

In 1910 during the Mexican Revolution, many Mexicans fled to the United States. Porfirio Diaz was president of Mexico from 1876 until 1910. The poor man suffered under Diaz. Many small farmers after a bad year had to sell out to a new patron (owner), who allowed them to stay on as farm hands. He treated his peones (farm hands) very much like slaves were treated in the South. There was unrest during the last years of Diaz's term and he announced he would not run again.

Soon there were many candidates running for president, including Francisco Madero, who was proposing reforms. This angered Diaz and he had Madero imprisoned. Diaz decided to run again, but his treatment of Madero had divided the upper classes, who ran the country. Revolution resulted, with Madero factions on one side and Diaz factions on the other. The poor in Mexico wanted Madero as a leader; they were ready for a hero. These people were called Maderistas. The reader interested in life in Mexico at this time is referred to *Barrio Boy*, by Ernesto Galarza. Madero was assassinated and the country went out of control; there was bloodshed everywhere. This is when thousands of Mexicans of all classes fled to the United States. At that time they were welcomed with open arms, since many American men were fighting in the war with Germany, and there were many jobs to be filled.[5] Many settled in the cities of the Southwest in Spanish-speaking barrios (neighborhoods).

As Mexico continues to experience economic difficulty, the number of Mexicans coming to the United States continues to increase. Many of those coming to find work and a better life for their families are "undocumented workers." They are deeply resented by many factions, and to go into these problems is beyond the scope of this chapter.

Most recent figures estimate that there are some 7.2 million Chicanos living throughout the United States, with the greatest concentration living in the Southwest (Fig. 1).

Mexican immigrants are different from other immigrants in that they have close proximity to their native land. This factor along with "inner colonization" seems to have contributed to the retention of the Spanish language and cultural heritage.

THE FAMILY

Much has been written about the Chicano family. It has been characterized as a deterrent to the advancement and acculturation of the Mexican American by many anthropologists and behavioral scientists. Most recently Chicano writers in their efforts to alter this stereotype have gone to the opposite extreme and described the Chicano family in idealistic terms. Chicano families are just as different from each other as are Anglo families. There is no one "Chicano family" that fits the mold. There are, however, certain characteristics that are more likely to occur in Chicano families than in Anglo families.

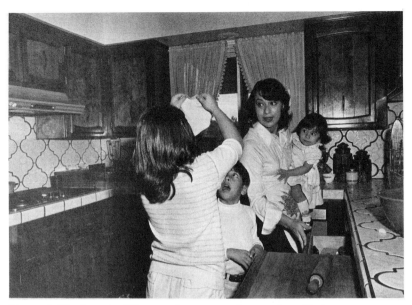
Figure 1. Mexican tradition continues even in a modern kitchen.

The Chicano family has a strong emphasis on familism. There is a dedication to the family, which includes not only the nuclear family but relatives as well. There is a very close bond between aunts, uncles, grandparents, and cousins. First cousins frequently relate to each other as brothers and sisters. The words used to define first cousin in Spanish are "primo hermano" (literally translated it means cousin brother). Relatives usually live close by and there is much visiting back and forth. The family gathers at celebrations and at times of crisis. Much support is gained from family members but this relationship also entails a lot of responsibility. The aged are highly respected and loved. Many times when a parent loses his partner, he will go to live with a son or daughter. Children view their grandparents with much affection and do not see them in a disciplinarian role (Fig. 2).[6]

The family extends to the institution known as compadrazgo. Compadres (godparents) are sponsors in a religious ceremony that establishes a ritual kinship. The most important compadres are the sponsors chosen for a child's baptism.[7] A relative or close friend is asked or asks to be a compadre. This forms a very close relationship between the parents and godparents. The godparents also have a responsibility to care for the child should something happen to the parents. In addition, the godparents, in the Catholic tradi-

tion, are also responsible for seeing that the child has a proper religious upbringing. In many Chicano families, the compadrazgo system appears to have less significance than previously. Historically, the compadrazgo institution dates back to the Colonial Period between 1550 and 1650. It was originally a Spanish custom that was adopted by the Indians of Mexico.[8]

Children are an important part of every Mexican and Chicano family. In most cases, children are desired soon after a couple is married. However, many middle-class Chicano couples, like their Anglo counterparts, are not starting their families right away. Poor families who have family planning available are also beginning to space their children. Since the majority of Mexican Americans are Roman Catholic, the question involving birth control and the Church was asked in the interviews. The answer most frequently given was that the Church did not forbid family planning anymore. Many young women coming from Mexico to California request the "monthly shot" as a means of family planning, according to a public health nurse interviewed. She stated that they are frequently very disappointed when they are unable to obtain it here. The oral contraceptive seems to be the next most acceptable one. As noted by Kay, coitus-dependent methods of contraception are very difficult for the Mexican-American woman to use, since she has

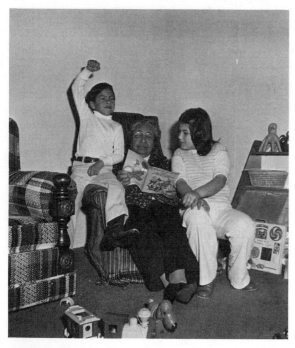

Figure 2. Grandmothers are an important part of the Chicano family.

been taught as a child that masturbation is wrong.[9] Questions asked during interviews in relation to modesty and masturbation were given very definite answers. Many mothers taught their children to be modest at a very early age, and children were punished for masturbating.

Boys are still desired as the first born to carry on the family name. This, of course, is no different from many other cultures. Both Mexican and Chicano families are still large. However, as mentioned previously, more families are beginning to use family planning. The population of Mexico is still growing very rapidly because of the continued high birth rate and the decrease in infant mortality. Recent immigrants to the United States many times find it very difficult to be seen at a family planning clinic. One woman in a large urban area in California, when interviewed, told of her dilemma. She, her husband, and two children had recently come from Mexico just previous to the birth of their third child. She stated that she had been asked about her choice of family planning during her prenatal period. She inquired about this prior to leaving the hospital and was referred to a clinic. She contacted the clinic and was told that there was a 3-month waiting list. She was very frustrated and, not

knowing where else to turn, resigned herself to the fact that she would probably just get pregnant again. She stated that she felt very alone here and really missed her family. There was no one to share in caring for the children and to give her guidance; but, as she said, at least her husband was working and they had something to eat and a roof over their heads.

It has been noted by Komoto and Umbdenstock that, unlike the other fertility patterns of the population in the southeast region of Los Angeles county, women with Spanish surnames continue to reproduce in the later years of the fertility cycle.[10]

It will be interesting to see if this trend continues with the next generation, considering the emphasis on and availability of family planning, the Catholic Church's silence (or perceived silence) on this matter, the effect of the women's movement, increase in awareness of the high risk involved, changes in the cultural attitude toward large families, and increased urbanization.

In the traditional Mexican and Chicano family the mother is the caretaker of the children and the homemaker. However, in the very poor families, both parents and as many children as possible contribute to the family income. One very obvious example is the migrant family that works together in the fields.

Many male Chicanos, however, who have risen above the poverty level, consider it a matter of pride to be able to afford to have the wife stay at home and care for him and the children. Many men find it difficult to understand the women's movement, and the desire to go to work outside the home. As one man said, "She wants to bring in some more money, what I make doesn't satisfy her. Her wanting to work makes me feel like when you give somebody a present and it's not good enough."

The new generation of Chicanos, many of whom have finished high school and college, seems to view a wife's working from a different perspective. They recognize the woman's need to be productive, utilize her talents and to have a feeling of self-worth. Also, they, like couples from many different cultures, find it difficult to make a living without having two incomes. They want to have more for their children, better housing, and so on, and seem to be willing to sacrifice their traditional roles (Fig. 3). Men are seen assisting with formally strictly female chores, such as caring for young children.

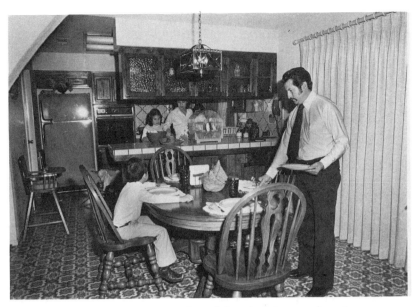

Figure 3. Traditional Chicano male and female roles are changing.

Both parents are usually involved in child-rearing. However, in the early years the mother is the one most involved with the raising of the children. It is only about the time of adolescence that the father gets very involved in the children's upbringing. Members of the extended family usually live close by and share in the child-rearing. When the children are little, they are cuddled and treated with much affection. Children usually go everywhere that their parents go. They go to parties, weddings, funerals, and church. Parents seem proud of their children; when the family has company, the children are always brought out to meet the guest, shake hands, and introduce themselves. Children are taught this regardless of social class. I have worked with children living in the poorest of circumstances, who have been taught these social graces. They are taught at a very early age to respect their elders and to be polite to strangers.

Children are given responsibilities at an early age. Girls are assigned various household chores and also learn how to cook. Everybody has responsibilities, especially in a large family. Boys frequently hold after-school jobs, to assist with the family income. One fifth-grade boy who worked after school was proud of saving his money. When asked about what he planned to do with the money, he said, "Save it for an emergency, for when poverty hits again." This

concept seemed very strange to the middle-class members of his peer group who were all saving up to buy a new toy, or who did not need to save, only to ask. The older children are taught to look after their younger siblings, sometimes when the oldest is only 4 or 5 years of age.

The role of the father is the one most frequently misrepresented in the literature. He is usually portrayed as the ultimate authority in all matters. It is true that the husband does have complete authority in many matters, but he is not the lord and master he is made out to be. He does see himself responsible for the behavior of all family members, and he sees to it that they all stay in line.[11] He also sees himself as the protector of the family, particularly the women in the family. Many women are still not allowed to go out after dark by themselves. A decent man would not allow this. The husband's authority and the wife's submissiveness are both changing, however. If one looks beyond the formal aspects of the Chicano culture, one will see that the male is frequently oblivious to many things going on in the home.[12]

The woman, on the other hand, is expected to be totally devoted to her family. According to a study of Chicano children by Goodman and Beman, the mother seems to be more important to the children than the father.[13] This does not appear unusual, as the mother is around the children most of the time, while the father's long hours at work take him away from the family.[14]

The mother not only meets all the nurturing needs of the children, but she also sets up the ground rules the children have to live by. She teaches, punishes, scolds, and comforts. She is not insignificant as she has been portrayed. True, she does not have the formal status of the male, but the Chicano woman has a warm and affectionate relationship with her children, which the father does not seem to have: "Whereas the father-son relationship is somewhat distant, the mother's relation with her daughter is more intimate."[15]

As the children enter adolescence, the father becomes more of an authoritarian figure. The adolescent girl is protected very carefully. In the strictest traditional families, girls did not date. A beau would ask the father if he could visit the girl. He would come and court her in her home, where the couple was always well chaperoned. If a man wanted to marry a girl, his parents or godparents would go over to the girl's home and ask the father for the girl's hand in marriage. The couple would be fearful that the girl's father might reject him. The girl would have to obey and not marry. Today it is more of a tradition, and couples are likely to elope if the father does not comply with their wishes. Today girls do date but are still accompanied by a chaperone. The parents are very careful with their daughter, lest she lose her reputation and bring shame to the family. The father must give his permission for a girl to go out. Interestingly enough, mothers are known to be helpful in convincing fathers to grant permission.

Obviously the above description is not typical of every family. Not all girls are protected as carefully as described. Much to the distress of many families, social and peer pressure have been too much and girls are dating without chaperones. This has caused much conflict in Chicano homes. Premarital virginity is still considered a virtue, but it is difficult to enforce when there is no chaperone.

With the male adolescent it is different. He is allowed much more freedom and it is understood that this is the time when he becomes a man. (No wonder that girls were guarded so carefully.) He spends a lot of his free time outside the home with his friends.[16] The teen-age boy is very protective of his younger brothers and sisters. He may argue with them at home but he will not tolerate any disrespect for them from outsiders. On the other hand, the oldest brother of the family is respected and looked up to. This entails a great deal of responsibility, as the oldest boy is expected to set an example for his siblings.

The adolescents in the family are expected to show great respect for both parents. If the boys smoke or drink, they will refrain from it in front of their parents out of respect for them. Boys are usually disciplined by their fathers and girls by their mothers. However, if the offense is serious, the girl will be disciplined by the father. The traditional father did not demonstrate much affection when the children became adolescents for fear of losing respect. This too is changing.[17]

In summarizing the Chicano family of today, one must say that it has been subjected to many of the same forces of change as the Anglo family. In addition many families are trying to identify their cultural role. Are they Chicanos or Mexican Americans? Many middle-class families living in urban areas appear to lose many of the traditional features of the family and to become more acculturated. Also, many women, especially in the younger generation, appear to be challenging their traditional role. However, there still remain many Chicanos who are consciously seeking to alter their familial roles while still hanging on to their cultural heritage and refusing to blend into the melting pot.[18]

Maria and Pablo are an example of a Chicano family that has altered its sexual roles and yet has not discarded its cultural heritage. An example of this is that they have not changed their names. They both have been to college and work full time. They have two children of their own, plus a niece that makes her home with them. Grandma lives close by and cares for the children when both parents are at work. Pablo assists with child care and other traditionally female roles, if needed. The children are very important to them and much time is devoted to their care and upbringing. Maria takes the children to a pediatrician when they are ill, but at the same time she consults her mother and mother-in-law for advice. They are very knowledgeable and supportive of her. They have a vast knowledge of herbs that Maria frequently uses. Pablo's mother is known as a curandera. (A curandera is a respected person in the barrio, who is knowledgeable about herbs, and knows how to treat many folk diseases with herbs and prayer. She is not to be confused with a bruja, who deals with witchcraft.) Pablo's mother is very helpful to Maria, who rejects witchcraft because she feels that it is in conflict with her Catholic faith. She still makes tortillas for her family, but not as often as they would like. Beans are a favorite food and the family still has the traditional tamales for Christmas. Both Spanish and English are spoken in the home. Baptisms, compadres, and fiestas are very important parts of their lives. They have recently bought a house in the nice part of town, a dream come true for Maria, who as she describes was born on the wrong side of the tracks and has finally made it.

EARLY INFANCY

The birth of a child is a time of celebration. As previously mentioned, males are the preferred sex, especially the first born. The child is frequently given the name of the saint on whose day he was born. For example, if a child is born on June 24, St. John's day, the child will be given the name of Juan or Juana. The baptism takes place after the compadres are chosen. In the stricter Catholic family, the infant is usually baptized during the end of the first month, since families worry about the infant dying before baptism and being refused admittance to heaven. In less religious families, the baptism may take place anytime during the first year when the time is right for a party. A big celebration is usually held with much food, drink, and music. The child will be taught to address his godparents as ninos. This becomes a very special relationship and the godparents usually remember the child with a gift on special days like Christmas, his birthday, or saint's day.

Presently most babies in the United States are born in hospitals, a real change from the days when midwives did all of the delivering in Mexico. This has caused some modification of cultural practices related to childbearing. According to cultural belief, a woman and infant were not to bathe or go outside during la dieta (a 40-day period after childbirth). A relative usually stayed with her during this time and did all the cooking, cleaning, and caring for children. With hospitalization, women take showers soon after delivery and infants are given a bath. Also the mother and infant are wheeled outside on discharge. Many young women have discarded some "old-fashioned ideas" and kept others. An 18-year-old mother who had recently emigrated told of taking a shower only when her mother-in-law, who was staying with them, was not around. She had an appointment to return to the clinic at 2 weeks postpartum, which caused the grandmother much anxiety. She did not permit her to leave the house until both she and the infant had their head covered to keep out any outside air. This same young woman explained that she had not been able to breastfeed because she ate pork, chili, cabbage, and other foods that were not good for the baby.

Along with the retention of the Spanish language and traditional values, many medical folk beliefs have been retained. It is believed by many that in order to remain healthy one must maintain an even balance between hot and cold. This is based on the Hippocratic doctrine of four bodily humors: blood, phlegm, choler, and melancholia. This doctrine was the basis of Spanish medicine in the sixteenth century. According to this theory, illness resulted from an imbalance of these humors.[19] This appears to be the basis of many Chicano folk beliefs, although most interviewed could not explain it in such terms.

The infant is affected by several folk diseases, the most common being mollera caida (fallen fontanel). This can be caused by pulling out the nipple while the baby is still sucking and by the baby falling. This is one folk disease that most women interviewed had either heard about or believed in. Some mentioned having a curandera treat the disease, but a grandmother who is knowledgeable could easily treat it. Some mothers mentioned taking the child both to the medical doctor and the curandera. Mexican Americans are extremely careful in handling the baby's head and in keeping the head covered, especially when going outside. Olive oil may also be applied on the fontanel to keep the cold out. One 33-year-old mother who had been born in a rural community in California explained how her baby's fontanel had fallen.

I had taken the baby to church and had her sitting in an infant seat. My older child accidently knocked the baby off the bench. My mother-in-law diagnosed her right away as having mollera caida. She could tell because when the baby sucked there was a different sound to it and there was no grip to it. She was then taken to the curandera who cured her by applying pressure on the infant's palate with her thumbs.

Other cures for mollera caida, besides the one mentioned above, are:
1. Holding baby upside down
2. Holding baby upside down over pan of water until the head is barely wet
3. Having adult drink water, then place mouth over fontanel and gently suck

4. Covering fontanel with a mixture of egg and herbs
5. Gently shaking child while holding upside down
6. Gently rubbing forehead and neck with oil (upward motion) and gently applying pressure on palate

Other symptoms of mollera caida besides poor sucking are listlessness, diarrhea, irritableness, crying, sometimes fever, and of course a sunken fontanel. The health professional sees the sunken fontanel as a symptom of dehydration; the Chicano sees it as the illness to be cured.

Another disease that the infant is susceptible to is "mal ojo." This malady is supposed to be caused by a person who really admired the baby and perhaps had envy, but did not touch the baby. It is also caused by people with very strong glances. My mother taught me that while talking to parents and admiring a baby, I should always touch it. To this day, whether in a clinic, pediatric ward, or home, I find myself always touching the infants while admiring them.

Madsen recounts this situation of a public health nurse in Texas:

Mrs. Webster is a kind hearted and devoted public health nurse whose bustling authoritarianism makes her unwelcome when she visits Latin homes. She is greeted politely but her presence is obviously resented. She is unaware of the fact that she has the reputation of possessing the evil eye and spreading sickness among the Mexican American children whom she admires. She is the subject of female gossip throughout the Latin community because she behaves improperly and poses a threat to children. "How can we trust her statements that she understands disease and wants to help us?" Juana asked. "She is either stupid or inconsiderate to admire so many kids when she has strong vision and then not even try to prevent the sickness by touching them."[20]

There does not seem to be much agreement as to the symptoms of a child with mal ojo, except that the child is very unhappy, cries continuously, and cannot sleep. The child may or may not develop a fever. The cure is simply to find the person who is thought to have given the evil eye, and have her touch the baby. The problem however arises when that person cannot be found or the parent is unaware of who it was that caused the illness. According to informants the child is taken to a curandera or someone who knows this art of healing. She rubs an unbroken raw egg over the entire body, then cracks it into a bowl to see if it cured the child. The curandera interprets the findings through the formation on the egg. If it has not worked, she repeats the procedure. The egg is then taken home and placed under the child's bed to complete the treatment. Sandler and Chan from their interviews in a Los Angeles emergency room describe the purpose of the egg under the bed as draining the evil from the body.[21]

The health professional might explain this disease in this way: The mother becomes frightened at a baby's fretfulness, her anxiety is transmitted to the child, and the fretfulness increases. When the child is "cured" the mother relaxes and so does the infant.

Pujos is another affliction that can affect the newborn. The baby is said to be pujon when he makes grunting noises. This is said to be caused by having a pregnant or menstruating woman hold the baby. The treatment is to pin a little piece of clothing (usually a slip from the person responsible for the illness) to the infant's clothing for several days. This malady does not appear to be as well known as mollera caida and mal ojo, and its consequences are not as serious. Many mothers interviewed laughed when pujos was mentioned and attributed it to old-fashioned ideas.

Diarrhea, vomiting, and fever are common in Mexican-American infants, just as they are in others that are part of the culture of poverty. Chicanos, like other cultures, use many different herbs to cure their ailments. There is also much reliance on patent medicine and the pharmacist in a Chicano neighborhood is heavily relied on for medical advice and is highly respected for his vast knowledge of drugs. The pharmacist is placed in this role by many of his customers who come in, describe their symptoms, and expect him to find them a medication for their problem.

A young man in rural Arizona told of his father's total reliance on medicinal herbs. He had never seen a physician but he made frequent trips to Mexico to purchase these herbs. He frequently referred to his Mexican herb books in treating different illnesses.

Olive oil seems to be used quite commonly with infants. For colic or stomach pain, an infant may be given a small amount of olive oil and also have his abdomen rubbed with warmed olive oil. This oil is also used for earaches and is applied to the nose when the infant has a cold.

Yerba buena (mint tea), manzanilla (chamomile), and rosa de castilla (castilian rose) are but a few teas used for stomach ailments. Pepto-Bismol and Kaopectate are commonly used patent medicines. Chicanos usually try all these remedies before ever seeing a medical doctor.

Care of the Infant

As previously mentioned, the infant is thought to be particularly vulnerable to the cold. Outside air is considered bad, but not as bad as night air. The infant is kept tightly bundled, and as one lady said, "We wrap them nice and tight like a tamalito [little tamale]." Children are still being overdressed, much to the distress of public health nurses. Many infants are dressed in an undershirt, shirt, sweater, perhaps another sweater, pants, shoes, socks, and then wrapped in a blanket or two.

When our first child was born in the middle of summer in Arizona, my sister was horrified that we had the baby dressed in nothing but a diaper. She performed her godmotherly duty and proceeded to dress her godchild in socks and an undershirt, and then wrap her in a light receiving blanket. She was particularly concerned as the child weighed only 5 pounds. It was irrelevant that the child's mother was a nurse and her father a pediatrician. After my sister's visit we undressed the child and took her temperature, which was 101 degrees.

Although the fajita (belly band) was traditionally used to prevent umbilical hernia, this practice is disappearing. According to a Chicana public health nurse, new mothers still worry a great deal about the umbilicus, especially with a grandmother in the house who is telling her she should have a band on the baby.

Circumcision of the male infant is on the whole still not acceptable in the Chicano culture, and no need is seen for it. But with the current trend in pediatrics being against circumcision, the Chicano parents are no longer getting pressure from the health professionals.

Unfortunately (in regards to feeding), the bottle has become very popular as a means of infant feeding. A young mother of three children told me of how she was using a bottle for the first time. She had breastfed her previous two children who had been delivered by a partera (midwife) in Mexico. When she came to the United States and the baby was delivered in a hospital, she was asked about her preference. "Almost everyone was going to use a bottle so I thought that was the best thing to do." She stated that she was very sorry she had changed since this baby had been hospitalized twice with diarrhea, was fussy, and did not seem to gain weight. How much better it would have been for both mother and infant if someone had found out how she had fed her previous two children, complimented her, and encouraged her to do the same for this child.

The practice of placing cereal in the bottle is quite common and a fat baby is thought to be a healthy baby. Several health professionals have noticed that Chicano mothers have a tendency to switch infants over to fresh milk as soon as possible, sometimes at 2 to 3 months. Fresh milk is scarce in Mexico and the peasant population does not have refrigeration. People that have a cow or goat and have fresh milk available are fortunate indeed. Perhaps in an effort to do what is the very best for the child, fresh milk is given. Evaporated milk is still used, and sweetened condensed milk is sometimes used to fatten children. The most popular formula, however, seems to be the one sent home with the child from the hospital. Although it is expensive, it is bought in prepackaged ready-to-use nursers that do not require refrigeration. Health professionals need to take many factors into consideration, such as family income, kitchen facilities, and understanding of the germ theory, in counseling parents in what to give their children.

Infants are usually fed on demand and picked up when they cry. In answering the questions on spoiling children and allowing an infant to cry, many mothers answered that they felt like a baby could be spoiled but that they were picked up as soon as they cried. In other words, they "spoiled" their babies and they did not think it hurt them. A few informants mentioned that their mothers told them that it was best for the child to cry a little in order to get some exercise in their lungs. Children are held a lot, since there are usually many relatives or older siblings around. Mothers do their work with the baby supported on one hip. There is much conversation directed to the infant, especially when he reaches the developmental age when he is able to smile. As far as babysitting is concerned, children are cared for by relatives only, and it is only the unfortunate family, which finds itself isolated, that is forced to rely on strangers for child care.

Table foods introduced when a child is about 6 months old may include bean broth, mashed beans, rice, sopitas (macaroni type soups made with chicken or beef broth), and soft cooked eggs.

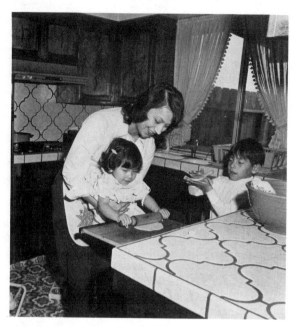

Figure 4. Young children are involved in all aspects of family life.

In giving an infant a bath, one must be careful to wet the top of the head (if one is not going to give a shampoo) in order to equalize the temperature. Alcohol may also be used in the water during winter to close the pores and keep cold from entering. The child is not taken outside after a bath for fear of his getting ill. Also, baths are not given if a child has any nasal congestion, a cough, or appears to be getting ill in one form or another.

THE YOUNG CHILD

Young children are treated with much affection by both parents (Fig. 4). However, in a large family, the baby is soon replaced by another one, which sometimes leads to the toddler becoming chipil. This has been described in the literature as an emotional disturbance caused by the pregnancy of the mother while she is still breastfeeding.[22] However, those people we interviewed used the term chipil to describe the reaction of a child who demands more attention, cries, and regresses when a mother is pregnant or after the new baby comes home from the hospital. It is the acting out of the child's feelings and jealousy that is described in textbooks as sibling rivalry or separation anxiety when a mother and child are separated. The best treatment for this condition was given as extra love and holding, which is consis-

tent with what books on childrearing say to do. However, many mothers do become frustrated with the child's whining and constant demands; consequently the child is taken home by a relative who can give this extra love and attention. It is not a stranger taking the child away, but someone he knows and trusts.

It is not uncommon to see two or three children in the family still drinking from a bottle or using a pacifier. Chicanos do not seem that concerned about early weaning, and it seems to give the children a feeling of security. Unfortunately, the milk-bottle syndrome is quite prevalent, as are dental caries caused by the use of high sugar drinks, instead of the more expensive and nutritious fruit juices. A suggestion by a health professional to substitute water in the bottle, instead of telling parents to take the child off the bottle, might have better results. Explanations as to the cause of caries, milk anemia, and other health problems are helpful to the parent.

Small children learn to eat what the family eats very soon. Needless to say there are no eating problems in poor families. I was always impressed with the way children from the migrant camps used to enjoy the hot oatmeal served for breakfast, while some of the other children in the day care centers would only eat packaged ready-to-eat cereals. Breakfast is pretty similar to the traditional American breakfast. Cooked cereals with evaporated milk are well liked. Chorizo (a spicy Mexican sausage) may be mixed with eggs for breakfast. Children learn to eat this at quite an early age, in spite of the well-meaning advice of many health professionals in telling parents not to feed the children spicy food. This is not to say that a 2 year old is given a hot pepper; discretion and caution are used in introducing all foods to children. Sopas (macaroni type dishes made with chicken or meat broth) are commonly served for lunch, as are sandwiches; soft corn or flour tortillas may be used instead of bread to make a sandwich, burrito, or taco. Dinner usually consists of a dish made from meat, rice or other starch, pinto beans, hot chili sauce, tortillas or bread, and a salad. The most common salad consists of iceberg lettuce and tomato without salad dressing. There are of course a great number of variations in this diet. The common use of beans, cheese, chili peppers, and tomatoes contributes good sources of protein and vitamin C to the diet. As with most groups on the poverty level, organ meats and other inexpensive parts of the animal not commonly used by the more affluent are utilized. Another positive practice in the traditional Mexican diet is the limited use of desserts. Pies, cookies, and cakes are not commonly used. However, carbonated drinks are commonly drunk by all members of the family, including children. Corn, squash, green beans, cabbage, onions, carrots, and spinach, along with tomatoes, cucumbers, and lettuce seem to be commonly used vegetables. Fresh cilantro (coriander) is used in cooking and is eaten fresh as part of a salad. Many a Chicano family has a little patch of cilantro growing in the back yard.

Because families are usually large, it is not uncommon to have the food sitting on the stove, and to have everyone help themselves as they get hungry. This sometimes makes it difficult to know what everyone is eating. If there is room at the table, an attempt is usually made to sit down and eat as soon as the father gets home from work. Some families excuse young children from the table as soon as they finish eating. Others have children remain at the table until everyone is finished. By the time a girl is in kindergarten she is already helping to clear the table and most likely to wash the dishes. Boys usually do not participate in the kitchen.

Discipline for the young child differs from that of the older child. I have often heard that Chicanos do not discipline their children. Chicanos often say that many Anglo children are mal educados (not properly educated in social manners). Discipline is seen in different ways by different cultures and even has different meanings for members of the same culture. Young Chicano children probably have less formal rules set for them than many of their Anglo counterparts. When they are young they are indulged and catered to. Sometimes children are frightened by parents as a means of discipline. There are stories in Spanish with the equivalent of a "boogie man" in them. Also, many a time on a home visit a mother has been heard to say, "If you don't mind me, the nurse will give you a shot!" This, however, does not apply exclusively to Chicano parents. The 3-year-old child jumping about in a home may seem unruly to a non-Chicano, while it may appear as normal behavior to a Chicano mother. As previously mentioned, the Chicano preschooler is taught to introduce himself to strangers, and to be polite and respectful. A Chicano mother once commented on the rudeness of American children, and how they did not ever greet her properly on entering a room.

Toilet training does not seem to be a big issue in Chicano childrearing. Those interviewed seemed to have introduced the child to toilet training around the age of two. When asked about their way of handling an accident after a child is trained, most mothers responded that they would "comfort him." One mother commented, "He felt shame, so I comforted him and told him it happens, nothing to get worked up for."

Children are taught to be modest at an early age. Most informants felt strongly about not letting children walk around the house totally undressed. They felt equally as strong about masturbation. Some responses reflected uneasiness in handling this situation, while others said they would definitely scold a child for masturbating.

The young child's world is comprised of cousins, aunts, uncles, grandparents, and other relatives. He is a participant in many fiestas. The piñata (a colorful papier-mâché animal or figure filled with candy) is part of a Chicano child's memories. The piñata is strung up on a wire or rope, then blindfolded children take turns trying to break it with a decorated club. When it breaks, the candy falls out and the children scamper around trying to pick up the scattered pieces. The grown-ups observing this seem to have as much fun as the children. A piñata is the center of attention at birthday parties and other celebrations.

Health Care

Immunizations seem to be accepted as necessary and parents do not object to them. With an increase in the immunization program in Mexico, many children are arriving in the United States having had immunizations for diptheria, tetanus, pertussis, and measles.

Children in the preschool age are likely to suffer from a folk disease called empacho, although it can occur at any age. It is most commonly described as a ball of undigested food that adheres to the stomach or intestinal lining. It is sometimes thought to be gum that a child has swallowed. This indigestion may also occur if a person eats when he is upset or when he is forced to eat. The symptoms are anorexia, abdominal pain sometimes accompanied by vomiting, and diarrhea. The treatment varies somewhat but most often consists of a laxative and massaging of the back along the lower part of the spinal cord. The skin along the lower part of the spine is pinched and pulled in an effort to dislodge the ball of food. The abdomen may also be rubbed with lard or oil. This treatment is continued until a certain noise is heard in the abdomen and the ball is dislodged.

Laxatives and enemas appear to be commonly used. They are given to a child if he does not want to eat. Enemas are also used for fever control with the herb malba used in the enema water. Sauco, another herb, is brewed as a tea and also used for fever control. It is said to be of particular value in chickenpox and measles, where it hastens the breaking out of the rash. One informant told of sweating out the fever. Her method was to mix aspirin and Vicks, apply to joints, then apply hot cloths over joints. Vicks rubbed on chest and back, which are then covered with a warm cloth, is also a good remedy for a chest cold. Cold air is thought to cause pneumonia; one informant reported that she had just given her 2-year-old daughter a bath, when somebody opened the door and let the night air in. The child became ill that night and was later diagnosed as having pneumonia.

Susto is a kind of fright sickness that can affect children as well as adults. It may occur as a result of a frightening experience or simply being scared. Susto is used interchangeably with the word espanto by many Mexican Americans, although many members of the older generation differentiate between the two words. Susto is attributed to a natural type of traumatic experience while espanto is caused by a supernatural force. Whatever the cause, symptoms are thought to be nightmares, loss of appetite, restlessness, and exhaustion. On noticing these symptoms, the family usually tries to determine if a frightening experience took place. Treatment can be done by a grandmother or someone knowing the remedy. However, if the condition is considered serious, a curandera is summoned. There are many variations of treatment, but the one most commonly mentioned was the sweeping of the body with a holy palm or escobilla while reciting prayers. This is supposed to drive the undefined evil out of the body.[23] Most Chicanos would not share their belief in susto with a health professional for fear of being ridiculed. Up to 20 years ago, many people felt that tuberculosis was the result of susto that had not been treated; however, this was not mentioned by any of the informants.

THE SCHOOL-AGE CHILD
Children in this age group are still pretty much involved with the family. Playmates are usually cousins or friends of the families living close by. The children are not allowed to venture out too far, particularly the girls. In poorer families the children have plenty of chores to do and have little playtime. As mentioned before, boys frequently have jobs after school.

Going to school can be quite traumatic to the Chicano child, depending on how much he has ventured away from the family, his knowledge of the English language, and the awareness and desire of the school to meet his needs.

Luis Valdez, the playwright, on being interviewed on television, described his feelings when going to school in the following way:

> When I left home for school, the taco my mother prepared was warm and it represented warmth, home, and mother. At lunch time, all the Gringo kids were eating their scientifically white square sandwiches. All of a sudden you are ashamed of your taco. It is cold now and it represents all that you are ashamed of.

Children coming to school from a background of poverty are found to have a greater number of problems than children coming from homes that are above the poverty level. Many of them come to school poorly fed and clothed. They have more health problems and develop a poor self-image when they are unable to compete with children from middle-class homes. Chicano children come to school with a different cultural and often linguistic background than the majority of those in the classroom.[24] It is only recently that courses on Chicano culture have been offered in schools of education, and California has required teachers to have a cross-cultural experience during their practice-teaching experience.[25] There is much controversy over bilingual programs offered in some schools and the money being spent on them. In addition there is much controversy over Title VI of the Civil Rights Act of 1964, which barred discrimination under any program receiving federal funds.[26] But this is beyond the scope of this chapter and will not be discussed. Statistics clearly show that failure and drop-out rates are very high for Chicanos and that the educational establishment has failed them.[27] Consider the case of a kindergarten child who enters school already with knowledge and skills learned in the home. However, when he arrives at school this knowledge has no value and even the language that he learned is either ignored or considered sub-standard. Think of what this does to a child's self-esteem and his desire to learn. In many cases the teachers have very little knowledge of the culture and are unable to help these little children. Most things learned in the classroom are related to the Anglo culture and the Chicano child quickly falls behind.[28] This situation is changing in some areas of the Southwest, but it is hopelessly slow in others. One can walk into most school libraries these days and find some books in Spanish for the child who reads this language.

Other cultural differences that may be viewed in a negative way by the classroom teacher are that children are taught to respect their elders and be polite to strangers. Many children have difficulty participating in class discussion and volunteering answers, perhaps because of this or because they are afraid to be ridiculed by their peers especially if they have a Spanish accent. I have observed that much overt discrimination still exists. Recently I overheard some Anglo children from a sixth grade calling the Chicano children "Beaners." Children of this age group are known to be quite clickish and sometimes not very nice to each other, especially if they are a little different from them.

Acuna, in his book *Problems of the Mexican American*, states that children are taught not to look into the eyes of a person punishing you, as it is a sign of disrespect. In the Anglo culture, it might have a totally opposite meaning. He also mentions that a boy is taught to defend his honor. A teacher disciplining a boy in front of his friends is making him lose his honor, which may result in the boy fighting with the teacher in order to uphold his honor.[29]

It was noted by a Chicano teacher that none of the Mexican-American children in his class were going to participate in an outdoor recreation class that entailed sixth graders being away from home for a week. Most of these children were first generation or immigrants. He felt that many of the parents thought the children were too young to be away from home for that length of time, and many of the children had never been away from their parents.

The subject of modesty has been mentioned previously and has some implications in regard to communal showers found in some junior high schools, high schools, and universities. Children are many times pressured to shower unclothed in front of their peers. If they are uncomfortable, they usually find ways to avoid this, such as missing physical education, refusing to undress, or dropping out of school altogether.

Health supervision in this age group usually consists of immunizations that are required for school. Since he is in school, the child would be screened for hearing and vision problems. The school-age child is susceptible to colds, communicable disease, dental caries, and accidents. The economically poor Chicano child has more health problems than the child from a higher economic level. He frequently has to have dental extractions because he has had no dental care; he may have hearing loss because of repeated untreated ear infections. He may also have very poor vision in one eye because of previously undetected amblyopia, and he may be more susceptible to strep infections and rheumatic fever because of crowding, poor nutrition, and lack of treatment. These are but a few of the health problems that may face the Chicano child.

It was noted in the interviews that many Chicanos were still treating their own sore throats with antiseptic mouth washes and Vicks. One remedy given for tonsillitis was to take hot tomatoes and apply them to the soles of the feet. The heat was to go through the body and relieve the sore throat.

As far as discipline is concerned, the school-age child is being prepared for the hard task of adulthood. As mentioned previously, the Chicano child has many responsibilities. They frequently start when they are very young and they have to start caring for their younger siblings. These responsibilities are equated with establishing positive traits of discipline, while at the same time increasing a child's self-worth.

ADOLESCENCE

Adolescence is a difficult age for most children and parents. The Chicano parent and adolescent are no different. In the traditional family puberty is treated quite differently for boys and girls.

The male is allowed much more freedom and usually has a strong peer group that he identifies with. The male adolescent spends a lot of time outside the home with the boys or what is frequently referred to as the *palomilla*. The word means moths that gather around a light at night.[30] Palomillas are not to be confused with gangs found in some urban areas. Gangs are more frequently associated with violence, and fights over property or "turf." There is much being written about gangs and some organizations are working towards turning them into something positive for themselves and the community. Many feel that gangs are a result of weakening of the Chicano family caused by

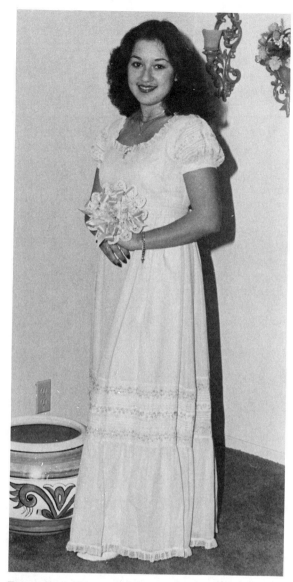

Figure 5. A Chicana celebrates her Quinceañera.

thority figure. At the present time there is much revolt by young males against their fathers. It is difficult for the father to maintain his traditional role when his children are being exposed to different values in the society.

The Chicana adolescent faces a similar struggle with her mother in regard to dating practices. When a Chicana girl has her fifteenth birthday she is given a very special birthday party. If her parents can afford it, they give a large party with food, drink, and music. This occasion is called a Quinceañera and is equivalent to a coming out party or debut (Fig. 5). With the Chicano movement and the rededication to the culture, Quinceañeras have increased in popularity. The girl usually dresses in a white dress (like a bride), carries flowers, and is accompanied by 14 couples to a church service. Middle-class acculturated parents who are trying to hang on to parts of their cultural heritage are also having Quinceañeras for their daughters. In Mexico this meant that a girl was ready to be courted in her home. Although some Chicano families still hold on to this tradition, most have been forced to relax their standards by the young girls who are rebelling against this authority. The old and new generations are clashing and parents are no longer able to keep young Chicanas within the confines of the home. In some urban areas, they are even going out into the streets and forming their own social clubs, much like the palomillas of the teen-age male.[31] They are challenging the traditional male-female relationship, which has given them very little flexibility in their roles. At the same time many Chicanas are advancing changes that advocate positive cultural values.[32] This is not true of all families and many still maintain extremely strict rules of conduct for the daughter. Mothers and daughters continue to be close in most cases, with the daughters doing many of the household chores and caring for the younger children.

Menstruation is viewed as a necessary evil. Many girls are still not prepared for it, although with sex education in the schools this is much less likely to happen. The theory of hot and cold applies to menstruation; many cold foods are avoided during this time. Sour foods, such as lemons and pickles, are avoided as are chilled drinks. These are thought to cause menstrual pain and to coagulate the blood. Many herbs are used for the relief of menstrual cramps, with the most common being mint tea, chamomile, and

urban pressures and weakening of family roles. This is a phenomenon that will not be dealt with in this chapter.

The palomilla, then, is a harmless peer group that serves a need for the Chicano male. This is where he receives his sex education, and not surprisingly most of the discussions center around girls. There is not much discussion in the home in regard to sex education. Any discipline the boy might get will be given by his father. It is at this time that the father becomes a very strong au-

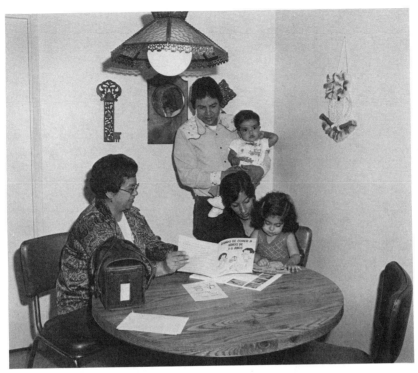

Figure 6. A Mexican-American public health nurse discusses diet.

cumin. A girl is taught to take it easy on those days and to avoid bathing or shampooing her hair. This restriction, along with the one after delivery, seems to be disappearing. Chicano girls see Anglo girls taking a shower and nothing happens, so they try it.

Most parents want their children to do better than they did in a career goal. A study of Hoppe and Leon on coping and non-coping parents showed that parental aspirations for children in coping families were high. They attached a high value to education and saw it as a means for the children to do better in life than they had done. They at least desired that their children finish high school, as most of the parents had to drop out of school for reasons of family finance or illness. The non-coping families in the study had lower aspirations for their children, including in education. According to this study neither group of parents voiced higher hopes for sons than for daughters, as had been expected.[33]

Fifty percent of our informants felt that they wanted their children to go to college, while the other fifty percent said they wanted their chil-

dren to finish high school. Most parents indicated that it would be the child's choice and that they would accept average grades if that is all that the child could do.

IMPLICATIONS FOR THE HEALTH PROFESSIONAL

A major part of this chapter has been devoted to a discussion of Mexican-American traditional customs, values, and beliefs. This was done in order to further understanding of the Chicano of today.

The Chicano culture is in a state of fluctuation. With the recent trend towards involvement and politicalization, Chicanos are hanging on to their culture and rediscovering it, while others are being assimilated into the melting pot.

In working with the Mexican American, the health professional might find it helpful to assess each individual client as to birthplace, recentness of migration if appropriate, urban or rural locale, level of education, and belief or disbelief in folk diseases and herbs. The health professional might keep in mind that many folk diseases are only different names for the same illnesses and may be treated simultaneously by physician and curandera without hurting the child. Many herbs used by the Chicano culture have been found to have a pharmaceutical effect and have been used since before modern medicine.

There are many strong points in the traditional Chicano diet such as beans and cheese for protein and chili and tomatoes for vitamin C (Fig. 6).

Mexican-American people are more likely to return to a medical clinic if they are treated with respect. A handshake and an introduction go a long way in showing that respect.

Chicanos value the family, which includes aunts, uncles, cousins, and compadres. Health professionals need to acknowledge the importance of the family instead of treating them as a burden. Remember that the family has afforded protection, security, and comfort in the face of oppression.

Do not stereotype the Chicano male and female. Political familism has brought about a considerable change in Chicano families.

Chicano families take their children everywhere. In planning health education meetings, include the children.

The Chicano likes to have big fiestas. Remember that this serves a purpose for him: it allows him to maintain his ties with his culture.

Many Chicanos have been here since before parts of the Southwest were part of the United States. They are not immigrants.

Chicano families may need some anticipatory guidance on how a toddler is feeling when a new baby comes into the home.

Health education is needed in the area of the infant's immature temperature control mechanism, in regard to overdressing.

More Chicano health professionals are needed, particularly nurses at the baccalaureate and masters levels, since this is the only way they will be placed in decision-making positions, when it comes to serving Chicanos. Colleges of nursing need to make a greater effort to recruit and *retain* Chicano students.

ACKNOWLEDGMENTS

The author wishes to thank Maria Rubalcava and Norma Arvizu for assisting with the interviews, and Linda Umbdenstock and Phyllis Jones from the Southeast Health Services Perinatal Project in Los Angeles County; Ramona Torres, public health nurse; Steve Miranda, educator; and Rex Ehling for contributing to the writing of this chapter.

REFERENCES

1. Rodriguez, R.: *On becoming a Chicano.* Saturday Review. February 8, 1975, p. 47.
2. Mirandé, A.: *The Chicano family: a reanalysis of conflicting views.* Journal of Marriage and the Family 39(4):747, 1977.
3. Acuña, R.: *The Story of the Mexican Americans, the Men and the Land.* American Book Company, New York, 1969, p. 134.
4. Goodman, M.E., and Beman, A.: "Child's-eye view of life in an urban barrio." In Wagner N.N., and Haug, M.J. (eds.): *Chicanos: Social and Psychological Perspectives.* C.V. Mosby, St. Louis, 1971, pp. 111-112.
5. Nava, J.: *Mexican Americans—Past, Present, and Future.* American Book Company, 1969, pp. 66-67.
6. Mirandé, p. 753.
7. Madsen, W.: *The Mexican Americans of South Texas.* Holt, Rinehart and Winston, New York, 1964, pp. 46-47.
8. Ibid.
9. Kay, M.: "The Mexican American." In Clark, A. (ed.): *Culture, Childbearing, Health Professionals.* F.A. Davis Company, Philadelphia, 1978, p. 106.
10. Komoto, S., and Umbdenstock, L.: *Perinatal and Selected Health Indicators with Projection Source Book.* Southeast Health Services Region, Los Angeles County, California, Charles R. Drew Postgraduate School, April 1978.
11. Madsen, p. 51.
12. Mirandé, p. 752.
13. Goodman and Beeman, p. 112.
14. Ibid.
15. Mirandé, p. 753.
16. Madsen, p. 54.
17. Mirandé, 754.
18. Ibid.
19. Madsen, p. 71.
20. Ibid.
21. Sandler, A.P., and Chan, L.S.: *Mexican American folk belief in a pediatric emergency room.* Medical Care 16:9, 1978, p. 782.
22. Madsen, p. 74.
23. Ibid.
24. United States Commission on Civil Rights: *Toward Quality Education for Mexican*

Americans. Report VI: Mexican American Education Study, February 1974, p. 41.

25. Ibid., p. 38.
26. Ibid., p. 49.
27. Ibid.
28. Ibid., p. 68.
29. Acuña, p. 167.
30. Madsen, p. 54.
31. Mirandé, p. 754.
32. Murillo, N: "The Mexican American Family." In Wagner, N.N., and Haug, M.J. (eds.): *Chicanos Social and Psychological Perspectives.* C.V. Mosby, St. Louis, 1971.
33. Hoppe, S.K., and Leon, R.L.: *Coping in the barrio: case studies of Mexican-American families.* Child Psychiatry and Human Development 7 (4):270, 1977.

BIBLIOGRAPHY

Anderson, J.G., and Evans, F.B.: *Family socialization and educational achievement in two cultures: Mexican-American and Anglo-American.* Sociometry 39(3):209-222, 1976.

Calvert, P.: *The Mexicans, How They Live and Work.* David Challer, Newton Abbot, London, 1975.

Farge, E.J.: *Medical orientation among a Mexican-American population: an old and a new model reviewed.* Social Science and Medicine 12:277-82, July 1978.

Galarza, E.: *Barrio Boy.* University of Notre Dame Press, Notre Dame, Indiana, 1975, pp. 140-141.

Hayes-Bautista, D.E.: *Chicano patients and medical practitioners: a sociology of knowledge paradigm of lay-professional interaction.* Social Science and Medicine 12(2A):83-90, 1978.

Heller, C.S.: *Mexican American Youth: Forgotten Youth at the Crossroads.* Random House, New York, 1966.

Howard, J.: *Mexico, the Land and Its People.* Macdonald Educational Ltd., Holywell House, London, 1976.

Kagan, S., and Ender, P.B.: *Maternal response to success and failure of Anglo-American, Mexican-American, and Mexican children.* Child Development 46(2):452-458, 1976.

Kearns, B.J.: *Childrearing practices among selected culturally deprived minorities.* Journal of Genetic Psychology 116(2):149-155, 1970.

Peón, M.: *Cómo Viven Los Mexicanos en Los Estados Unidos.* Impreso en Mexico, Talleres de B., Costa-Amer., Editor/Mesoner, 14, Mexico (1) D.F., 1966.

Sears, R., Macoby, E., and Levin, H.: *Patterns of Child Rearing.* Harper & Row, Evanston, Illinois, 1957.

Zinn, M.B.: *Political familism: toward sex role equality in Chicano families.* Aztlan-International Journal of Chicano Studies Research 6(1):13-25, 1975.

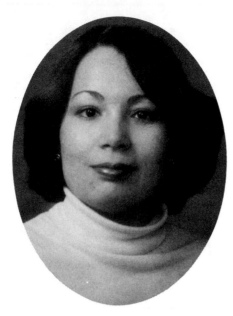

Chapter 9

I was born Gloria Ivelisse Lopez in Ponce, Puerto Rico, at the height of the 1950s (1952) mass Puerto Rican migration to the United States. Ponce, the largest city on the southern coast, is Puerto Rico's principal shipping port. It connects with San Juan via a recently built major highway.

My father, having spent most of his youth in rural Adjuntas, moved to the Playa de Ponce (Ponce Beach) where he met and married my mother. They resided in "La Playa" until financial conditions prodded them toward a decision to migrate in search of better economic opportunity.

In April 1953, when I was 5 months old, the Lopez family joined the "exodus" that had overtaken the Island by that time. Arriving in New York City, we were met by concerned relatives who saw to our needs until my father obtained employment and we were settled in our own home. We soon moved to an apartment in Brooklyn. Accounts from my parents of those first days in New York characterize the hardships, frustrations, and cultural shock evident in the lives of the Puerto Rican migrant family. I have always admired the stamina with which my parents have confronted and prevented these obstacles from weakening our family unit.

I come from the family-oriented environment typical of Puerto Rican culture. My parents have always been protective and nurturing toward their children. Memories of my early childhood bring back the security and contentment of being surrounded by aunts, uncles, and cousins. I remember my late grandfather, Papa Felipe, the love and patience he taught us, and the great void he left in our family circle when he passed away. I see my childhood as a deeply gratifying experience.

I decided to become a nurse at the age of five. I remember the encouragement I always received as a child toward educational and professional achievement. I attended the New York Public School System for 12 years and in 1970 entered the Hunter College-Bellevue School of Nursing, from which I graduated in 1974 with a Bachelor of Science in Nursing. I have since been employed on the Medical-Surgical staff of the Bronx-Lebanon Hospital Center, on the Pediatric staff of the Institute for Rehabilitation Medicine in New York City, and for the past 3 years have been a Public Health Nurse with the Maternity, Infant Care-Family Planning Project of New York. I am assigned to the Brownsville Center in Brooklyn where I do prenatal and family planning conferencing and teaching.

My husband, Gerard, and I are now expecting our first child, so that, initially, the prospect of writing on Puerto Rican childrearing

The Puerto Rican in Mainland America

Gloria Lacay, R.N., B.S.N.

without parental experience took me slightly aback. However, upon undertaking the project, I was amazed at the wealth of information that was available to me from just having been a product of Puerto Rican childrearing. Interviewing Puerto Rican mothers and observing their behavior with their children has been an enlightening and fulfilling experience. My experience as a nurse working frequently with Puerto Rican patients has brought me awareness of myself as a Puerto Rican health professional. I have become more keenly attuned to the distinctive needs of the Puerto Rican individual involved in the American health care system. It is my hope that the observations and suggestions that follow will help bridge some of the gaps that exist between the health care professional and the Puerto Rican parent.

THE GREAT MIGRATION

The Puerto Rican people began arriving in the States in small numbers in the 1800s in search of economic betterment. By 1910 there were Puerto Ricans residing in 39 of the States, and by the middle of the twentieth century 4000 people were migrating from the Island yearly. The end of World War II saw a boom in Puerto Rican migration, taking the yearly number to 50,000. Statistical evidence shows that migration waves vary with the economy, thus the increase ran reciprocally with the post-war job market improvement.[1]

In the 1950s the air route between San Juan and New York became known as the "air bridge" in light of the massive migratory activity that had gripped the Island at the time. One major reason for the exodus was the arrival of inexpensive air fare. This, coupled with the intense waves of job propaganda reaching the Island from the States prompted the decision for the large majority. In 1968 there were 1 million Puerto Ricans living in the United States. It has been predicted that by the year 2000 5 million Puerto Ricans will have migrated to the United States.[2]

Many of the Puerto Rican migrants were agricultural workers who, finding themselves unemployed following the sugar cane season, migrated to the U.S. once a year during the fall harvesting season.[3] Others remained in the U.S. either out of

211

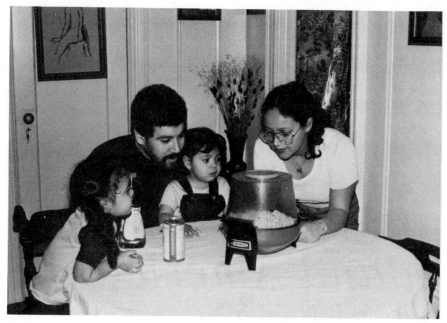

Figure 1. The family occupies a central place in Puerto Rican culture. (Photograph by Gerard Lacay)

determination to reach their economic goals or out of financial inability to return. There are many who after attaining some economic success have returned to the Island to purchase their own homes and in some cases set up their own businesses.

A great number of the migrants settled in cities such as Philadelphia, Cleveland, and Chicago, but the majority were drawn to New York City. Most settled on the Lower East Side and the Upper West Side, where Spanish Harlem was born. The Puerto Rican migrant arriving in New York describes his experience as being one of physical and emotional shock. He has left an island of green vegetation, tropical warmth, and close family and friendship ties to meet head on with an island of aged gray buildings, northeastern temperatures, and the impersonality and anonymity of a large city. It is no wonder that some have been unable to cope with such disorientation and have abandoned the ideals of the Island to succumb to idleness, crime, and drug addiction, factors that were almost nonexistent until the advent of mass migration. The latter group, however, constitutes the Puerto Rican minority. The Puerto Rican culture has been described as having "a certain resilience, a certain capacity for survival and resistance,"[4] and it is

this attribute that has allowed and will continue to allow the family along with its ideals to survive the threats of depersonalization and loss of cultural identity.

THE TRADITIONAL FAMILY

The family has always occupied a central theme in the Puerto Rican culture, as it has in most other Hispanic cultures (Fig. 1). Traditionally, it consists of the nuclear family (mother, father, and children) and the extended family (grandparents, grandchildren, brothers, sisters, aunts, uncles, and cousins). In years past it was common for nuclear and extended family members to reside within the same household. The extended family provides the availability of help in time of need and the provision of a social milieu.

The traditional nuclear family comprises a husband who has complete authority over his wife and children. He is the sole family provider and decision-maker. The wife is "reduced almost to the status of a child"[5] and not expected to rise above her role of meeting her husband's demands and caring for the children. Such a distinctive line separating the roles of the spouses leaves little room for communication between them.[6]

The sexual double standard is very much a part of the culture. The woman is expected to be a

212

virgin at the time marriage takes place, and absolute fidelity to the extent of not being seen talking to other men is expected. The husband, however, is expected to maintain his macho image. Premarital and extramarital sexual activity is accepted as part of a man's nature. While a man may leave his wife and children without suffering too much social disapproval, a woman who does likewise may never be able to regain social approval.

Conception is viewed as the consummation of a marital union and is expected to occur soon after marriage takes place. The childless marriage is looked upon with either disapproval or pity and not expected to last long. Producing a child gives the mother the satisfaction of fulfilling her physiological and social role as a fertile woman and the father of fulfilling his role as a virile man. In a culture in which emphasis is placed on social approval, childbearing often occurs as the result of social pressure. The first born should preferably be a male and has much to do with the patriarchal family structure. Traditionally, the number of children desired is irrelevant. Children are seen as a gift of God and are to be accepted into the family at any cost. The family economy has no influence on the number of children produced.

The Puerto Rican child is traditionally brought up to obey and respect (respeto) his parents. Love is considered to be secondary.[7] The child is fondled and enjoyed during his first 2 years of life but is afterwards subjected to the "demands for obedience and respeto."[8] Corporal punishment is the traditional means of ensuring obedience and respeto; it is mainly considered part of the father's role and when carried out by the mother is done in the father's name. Rewarding good behavior is frowned on for fear that the child will lose respeto for his parents.

Both males and females are brought up to be dependent on their parents throughout life. They are taught to turn to their parents in times of need even as adults, and the demands for obedience and respect continue. Children are expected to remain with the parents until they are married. The latter expectations, however, vary in degree according to sex.

The little girl is kept constantly clothed. She is closely guarded and taught to be submissive. She is allowed to play with girls only and discouraged from playing typical male games. As she grows she is taught to help mother with household tasks such as house cleaning, dish washing, and cooking. As she enters puberty and adolescence she is guarded more closely. Mixed male-female activities are carefully chaperoned by a responsible adult. Boys interested in her must come to the girl's home and gain her parents' approval. Courtship (noviazgo) occurs under strict chaperonage. Marriage usually occurs without prior dating experience. Rosario states that "noviazgo is a period in which the woman learns to submit her will to that of the man. It is not a time for the couple to get to know each other and set up roots for future compatibility."[9] Sex education is considered to be part of the husband's role after marriage, the parents being completely relieved of the responsibility.

The little boy is less closely guarded. He is allowed to go about without clothes. He is encouraged to be more aggressive and is allowed to play outdoors without supervision. He is, however, expected to play with children of his own sex and is discouraged from playing typical female games. Household duties may involve doing errands or helping the father, but the demand for carrying these out is much more lenient for the male. Puberty and adolescence place less of a strain on the male than they do on the female, for the male is considered to be more capable of defending himself. Less pressure toward marriage is placed on the male.

These are the roots of the Puerto Rican family tradition. It will be interesting to note the changes that have occurred on the Island and Mainland as a result of American influence.

THE FAMILY TODAY

Throughout its history the Puerto Rican family has had to deal with constant invasion from numerous other cultures. Assimilation has, in many instances, been its only means of survival. Today, most of the traditional values instilled by the influence of past Spanish rule are being challenged by the influx of American culture into the lives of those living on the Island and Mainland.

Cultural values and the degree of assimilation into the American culture vary greatly from class to class and from Island to Mainland. The lower classes have a tendency to hold on more closely to traditional values, whereas the middle and upper classes, because of higher educational levels, are better able to absorb other cultural values and incorporate them into their own value system.

The nuclear and extended family concept has experienced conversion into what Safilios-Rothchild terms "the modified extended family." The latter "involves residential separation of the nuclear family" while maintaining "a close relationship . . . between the couple and their parents."[10] Although this has occurred on the Island to some extent, the greatest change has been observed on the Mainland, where the American value of autonomy has a greater influence. Where family residences are separated by a great distance, close contact is generally maintained through periodic visits, correspondence, and telephone calls. Puerto Ricans on the Mainland generally enjoy visiting their homeland as frequently as financial conditions allow.

The nuclear family has undergone much change throughout the years. There appears to exist more communication between husband and wife and the establishment of a more democratic marriage and household. The husband still has a tendency to remain the higher authority, but he now more frequently looks to his wife for support and approval. Women are frequently employed outside the home, acquiring more independence and self-assertion. Although the care of the children is still mainly the wife's responsibility, the husband now takes more of an active part in their upbringing. Older children are now often contributing to the family budget and becoming part of the decision-making process.

The ideals of courtship and marriage have undergone a drastic change from the traditional. On both the Island and Mainland dating is now allowed unchaperoned. Although the opinions of the family continue to influence the girl's choice of marriage partner to some extent, the girl is now generally allowed to make her own decision regarding marriage. Non-commital dating is no longer frowned upon. Following marriage the couple is still expected to soon produce a child, but their decision to put off childbearing for 1 or 2 years is often respected. There appears to be less of an emphasis on the first born being a male. Children are still seen as a gift of God, but economic conditions now play a major role in family limitation. Many young couples today are satisfied with one or two children.

The changes that have occurred within the Puerto Rican family have not taken place without some deleterious effects. Migration has played a significant role in the deterioration of many family ideals. The family arriving in the States has had to face the confusion of being surrounded by people who do not understand their language. Exploitation by merchants and employers because of this has reduced many a Puerto Rican's sense of dignity and self-worth. Children have been placed in lower grades simply because they do not understand the language being spoken. They have been exposed to the strange new world of racial prejudice—a factor that was almost non-existent on the Island. Nuclear and extended families have been separated for years and family ties have been drastically weakened. Parents have had to contend with defiance when they have tried to impose traditional Puerto Rican values on children who are growing up in an American world.

Yet, in spite of all these obstacles the Puerto Rican family continues to thrive on the Mainland. The family continues to be the core of Puerto Rican existence. The Puerto Rican has managed to learn the English language, become educated, succeed in American society, and assimilate certain values without losing his Puerto Rican identity.

CHILDREARING

The Puerto Rican culture has shown its greatest resilience in its patterns of childrearing. Childrearing has, perhaps, presented one of the biggest challenges for the Puerto Rican parent residing on the Mainland. The parent has had to incorporate American values into his own value system in order to meet the demands of living in an American society. Although American childrearing practices have filtered into the Puerto Rican household to some extent, Puerto Rican ideals continue to occupy a central place in the process of childrearing. The reader must bear in mind, however, that variance in educational levels, economic conditions, and geographical and environmental factors has resulted in diverse versions of the basic traditional practices of childrearing. The following are observations of some childrearing patterns found in the Mainland Puerto Rican family as the child progresses from infancy through adolescence. The parent's perception of health and disease and the implications of such concepts and behavior patterns will be considered in relation to the health care professional.

The Young Infant (Birth to 6 Months)
The birth of a child is a celebrated occasion in the Puerto Rican culture. Entering the status of parent is seen as prestigious and considered an indication of maturity. The occasion involves the parents as well as grandparents and other members of the extended family. The family cus-

214

tomarily displays their approval at the couple having fulfilled their childbearing role through paying them increased attention, being extremely helpful, and presenting the infant with gifts.

The birth of a child is a religious occasion in most families and is usually preceded by a ceremony. The Protestant parent presents his child to the congregation, where an elder prays over the infant, asking God that he might live a peaceful life in God's will. The Catholic has his child baptized in order that he may be protected from evil and guaranteed entry into heaven. A godmother (comadre) and godfather (compadre) are chosen for the child. The "compadres" are expected to help out in time of need and to care for the child should anything happen to the parents.

The baptism ceremony is usually followed by a reception at the home of the infant and is attended by family and friends. Food, drink, music, and dance permeate the atmosphere. Baptism often occurs regardless of the parent's involvement in the church. I have observed that although a parent is not an active church member, much concern is displayed over the child's religious instruction. This is evident in the many Puerto Rican parents who enroll their children in Catholic school although they themselves have no religious affiliation. It is generally believed that religion plays a significant role in the child's moral and emotional development.

The father is often supportive of his wife and may be helpful with household duties and other children in the event of an infant's birth. The maternal grandmother, however, appears to be the young mother's major source of support. The husband usually accepts the role of his mother-in-law during this time because he is able to continue to work with the assurance that his wife has the help she requires during those first days. The Puerto Rican mother displays a great deal of concern toward her daughter and grandchildren. She is usually available at the birth of a grandchild to help out with household duties and the care of other children. The mother will often travel to the Mainland or the daughter to the Island for the birth of a child so that the child's grandmother can perform what she sees as her role. The mother's supportive role continues throughout the daughter's childbearing years. It is to her that the young wife and mother turns for guidance and advice, and it is she who is the preferred babysitter.

Years ago in Puerto Rico breastfeeding was the customary method of feeding the infant.

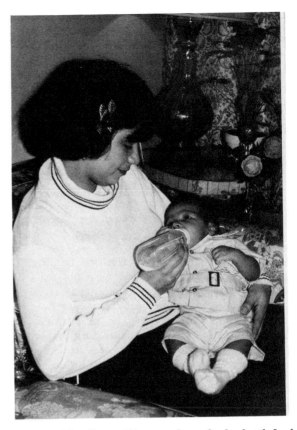

Figure 2. Most Puerto Rican mothers of today bottlefeed their infants. (Photograph by Gerard Lacay)

American influence on the Island and migration to the Mainland have served to almost obliterate this custom in the Puerto Rican culture. The Puerto Rican mother today generally bottlefeeds (Fig. 2). I have encountered very few Puerto Rican mothers who breastfeed, and the few that do, receiving little or no encouragement from their families, often abandon the practice in their early post-partum period. Possible reasons for this reaction may include:

1. Improved economic conditions making it possible to purchase prepared formula.
2. The mother's desire to follow modern American trends.
3. The Puerto Rican woman's sense of modesty and reluctance to expose herself in public.
4. The increase in the number of working mothers, for whom breastfeeding is inconvenient.

Most new mothers will keep their infants on the infant formula they were started on in the hospital. Some, for economic reasons, will change to evaporated milk soon after they are home from the hospital. Many will have their infant on whole milk by the end of the sixth month. The infant is generally fed on a 3- to 4-hour schedule.

Solid foods are usually introduced by the second or third month in the form of cereals and commercial baby foods. Years ago mothers in Puerto Rico would feed their children home-prepared foods, among them mashed yautia (a tropical vegetable), potatoes mixed with milk, or barbecued or grated plantains made into a puree. Mothers today heed more closely the doctor's and nutritionist's advice regarding infant feeding. Foods are generally introduced to the child with a spoon, or on occasion placed in the bottle with the infant formula.

The cup is generally introduced at 5 to 6 months. Mothers appear to be patient in this area, the cup being encouraged but not forced on the child. Meals continue to be supplemented by the bottle. There appears to exist the same type of attitude with the handling of feeding problems. Foods are introduced gradually and not forced on the child. Foods not accepted by the child are often mixed with those that are.

The Puerto Rican mother is generally very protective of her children, an attitude which appears to remain a part of her throughout life. A cry will bring the mother to the child's side to check for signs of danger or discomfort. The latter reaction, however, is counteracted by the fear of spoiling the child. There is often much ambivalence in this area for the desire to hold and cuddle the child is suppressed by the fear of spoiling. Interacting with the child through talking, singing, and play usually will occur while primary care is being given and for short intervals throughout the day as the child grows older. The infant is kept in the parents' room for the first few weeks of life and then moved to his own room or into a room with a sibling.

The pacifier appears to be the accepted aid in comforting the child among most Puerto Rican mothers. Some, however, do feel that it is damaging to the mouth and gums.

Daily bathing of the infant is very important to mothers. A sponge bath is usually given until the umbilical stump falls. Thereafter a daily tub bath is customary. Infants are usually dressed slightly warmer than the adult, but are not overclothed. The amount of clothing varies with the weather and the mother's own perception.

Propping a child up to sitting position prior to the third month is frowned upon by many Puerto Rican mothers, for they believe that this will result in deformity of the child's back. For this reason young infants are often held in an erect or semirecumbent position. Younger mothers who have been raised on the Mainland and been exposed to American infant literature tend to abandon this belief.

The concept of health and disease plays a major role in Hispanic culture. Health is often accepted as a sign of God's approval, illness as either the result of God's disapproval or the operation of evil forces in one's life.

Belief in "mal de ojo" or the evil eye prevails throughout most of the Puerto Rican culture. It is believed that a person who admires a child inadvertently exposes him to the evil eye. A child who has been afflicted with the evil eye is believed to become irritable and restless, to experience loss of appetite, vomit, and have fever and diarrhea.[11] The death of an infant is often attributed to "mal de ojo." To prevent the effects of the evil eye, the admirer customarily adds "God bless you" to his remark of admiration.

The "azabache" is often pinned to the child's clothing or worn on a chain around the neck or wrist to ward off the evil eye. It is an amulet made of coral or jet shaped into a small fist with the thumb protruding between the middle and index fingers.[12] Many mothers, although stating that they do not believe in the evil eye, continue to put the azabache on their infants.

Reactions to the ailments of early infancy vary with the length of time the mother has lived in the U.S. The longer the time on the Mainland, the stronger the tendency to turn to the physician for advice and treatment. Mothers who have been raised on the Island and those recently arriving on the Mainland have a tendency to employ home remedies prior to consulting a physician. If the home remedy is not effective the physician will then be consulted. Following are some of the more common infant ailments and the corresponding treatments often used for their alleviation:

Colic—the abdomen may be massaged with a warm oil and salt mixture; "te de anis" (anis tea) or "te de oja de naranjo" (orange leaf tea) may be placed in the bottle.

Hiccups—a piece of string is removed from the infant's clothing, rolled up, and placed on the child's forehead.

Constipation—believed to be caused by the ingestion of foods with "hot" qualities so that

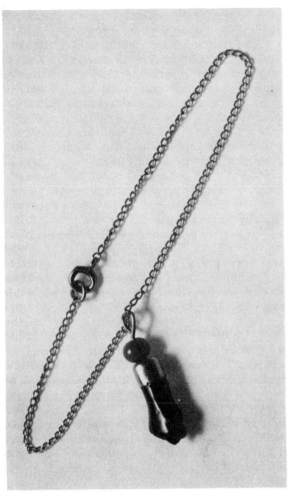

Figure 3. The azabache wards off the evil eye. (Photograph by William Soler)

fruits, believed to have a cooling effect, are given to neutralize the effects of the hot food.

Heat rash (calor)—believed to be caused by the ingestion of hot foods is neutralized by giving teas made from native plants believed to have cooling qualities (alumbre, tautua, flores de sauco).

Fever—believed to be caused by the ingestion of hot foods; given cooling teas as in heat rash.

Diarrhea—"te de oja de tartago" (tartago leaf tea, a tropical plant) or "agua de cal" (lime water) may be given.

Insomnia—"te de lechuga" (lettuce root tea) may be given.

The concept of "hot and cold" foods prevails throughout the Hispanic world and is evidenced in much of Puerto Rican folklore. It reflects the Hippocratic humeral theory that health is dependent on the balance between hot and cold in the body. In Hispanic culture foods are considered to be either hot or cold, the terminology being "independent of such observable characteristics as form, color, texture, and physical temperature, and it is descriptive only of the effects which a substance is thought to have upon the human body."[13] Foods considered to be cold include most fresh vegetables, fruits, dairy products, bottled milk, corn, sugar cane, avocado, white beans, pork, chicken, and mavi (an iced beverage). Hot foods include canned milk, vitamins, penicillin, aspirin, chocolate, coffee, green peas, pepper, garlic, onions, cinnamon, ginger, kidney beans, cod liver oil, rum, wine, anisette, beef, fish, cloves, pigeon peas, and foods containing iron.[14] Lubic, in her article on the Puerto Rican family, includes an interesting observation made by Dr. Alan Harwood in his study of the Puerto Rican mother. He felt that the early switch from formula to bottled milk undertaken by many Puerto Rican mothers could be attributed to their belief that the early infant skin rash is caused by canned milk (a hot food), necessitating the ingestion of bottled milk, which has cooling effects.[15] Dr. Harwood also felt that the high incidence of diarrhea in Puerto Rican children has much to do with the hot-cold concept.

The purpose of the hot-cold concept is not to omit certain foods from the diet, but rather, to maintain a balance between the ingestion of hot and cold foods. It is believed that both heat and cold must be taken into the body in order to ensure homeostasis. For this reason, cooling remedies are given to restore the balance rather than to remove the hot qualities. For example, heat rash, an imbalance believed to be caused by the ingestion of heat, is alleviated by balancing it out with the coolness of alumbre tea.

Empacho is an ailment believed in by many Puerto Ricans and other Hispanic cultures. It is believed that food that is not properly digested by the child remains attached to the wall of the stomach, forming a ball. The symptoms of empacho may include abdominal distention, pain, vomiting, and diarrhea. Empacho may result from eating against one's will, eating hot bread, overeating, or having an unpleasant emotional experience. It is a disease that can occur at any age but is believed to be more common in children.[16] Treatment for empacho may include the ingestion of teas, such as ginger tea (te de jengibre). Curanderas (healers) are sometimes employed. Their method of treatment consists of special massage of the abdomen with oil, followed by the pinching of the skin along the spine. The treatments are aimed at softening and dislodging the hardened undigested food and permiting proper digestion.[17]

The process of assimilation has done much to vary the degree to which these cultural values and behaviors are adhered to. Younger mothers, who have spent their youth in the U.S., continue to turn to their mothers for support and advice, but have more of a tendency to consult the physician immediately at the sign of illness. Older mothers and those recently arriving from the Island tend to turn to home remedies and the advice of family prior to consulting the physician. Both groups appear to respect the physician's position and show an interest in trying to follow medical advice as closely as their cultural convictions will allow. Puerto Rican mothers generally display a sincere interest in the health and development of their children. Taking their children for their immunizations is considered an important part of mothering. What may appear as lack of interest in some mothers in this area may be more the result of a language barrier and a lack of understanding of the American health care system owing to recent arrival from the Island. I have generally found mothers responsive in my clinical experience when I have taken the time to translate and explain procedures in Spanish. When a Spanish-speaking staff member is not available, understanding the above factors may help to alleviate some of the health professional's frustration, allowing him to function in a more effective capacity in the care of the patient.

The Infant (6 Months to 1 Year)

Mother continues to be the major care provider and her protective attitude continues throughout the remainder of the first year and subsequent years of life. More time appears to be spent during this time period protecting the child as his motor activity and mobility increase. Mothers find the walker and playpen very helpful. The walker is employed as soon as the child is able to sit up by himself. The child is allowed to crawl on the floor with supervision, usually being restricted to one room in the house. More time is spent by the mother in play activity with the child. Father also often takes an active role in entertaining the child when he is home. Toys and television are found to be very helpful when mother is busy.

Mothers become even more conscious of the possibility of spoiling the child now and may tend to let the child cry for longer periods.

Most mothers have begun to give the child small amounts of table foods, such as rice, small pieces of meat, mashed potatoes, eggs, and vegetables. Baby foods and the bottle of milk continue to be the major sources of nutrition. Mothers prefer to have their children spoon-feed rather than finger-feed. A more structured feeding schedule takes form about this time. Meals are divided into three daily feedings and children are usually fed just prior to the rest of the family. Snacks and a bottle of milk may be given in the mid morning or afternoon. The bottle of milk will usually accompany a child to bed.

For teething discomfort some mothers will place honey on the infant's gums. The teething ring is commonly used.

Discipline during this age period usually consists of scolding. Most mothers appear to feel that spanking at this time is cruel.

The Toddler (1 to 3 Years)

Feeding during this period becomes characteristically more difficult.[18] The child's increased motor activity necessitates much patience and ingenuity on the part of the mother or other care provider. Puerto Rican mothers, being overly concerned with the child's proper food intake, are willing to try several approaches. Some will force the child to sit still during the meal, the high chair being very helpful. Many mothers appear to incorporate mealtime into play activity. Television is often used to distract the child and feeding undertaken during a favorite television program.

Feeding problems are handled as in the other stages, replacing or mixing disliked foods with those that are liked. Throughout life the Puerto Rican mother has a tendency to cater to her children's food preferences. Many will later complain that the child is a picky eater. During these years children are encouraged to feed themselves and to use the cup with supervision.

Sleeping habits tend to vary with the child's place among his siblings. Parents show a tendency to impose stricter curfew on their first born and to become more lenient as subsequent children are born. Naps during the day continue through 3 years of age.

Toilet training is usually started around the eighteenth month. The training chair or potty is often used. Mothers will observe the child for signs of a desire to eliminate and place them on the potty. Many will do this at various intervals throughout the day. Success is customarily praised. Failure during the early stages is handled by reasoning with the child and giving him encouragement. Mothers admit feeling more anxious around this time, and as the child grows older will tend to scold them when accidents occur. Puerto Rican mothers are very concerned with the child's developmental progress, and delays or what may appear to be regression can often cause excessive anxiety in many mothers.

Diapers are worn to bed at night but usually omitted during the day. Bed wetting at this time is either handled by comforting the child or scolding him. Reactions in this area appear to vary with the mother's educational level.

After the first year mothers generally feel that spanking is necessary for good discipline. Scolding usually precedes spanking. During this stage mothers state that they experience an increase in anxiety in relation to the child's increased motor activity and what the mother perceives as being misbehavior. The Puerto Rican mother's preoccupation with instilling obedience and respect in the child may cause her to see this change in behavior as the beginnings of the defiance the child will display toward her when he is older. They are threatened with the fear that the child is already losing respect for them.

Sexual modesty appears to remain a part of the Puerto Rican method of childrearing on the Island as well as on the Mainland. Little girls still have more of a tendency to remain dressed at all times while this is not stressed for the boy. Boys are expected to play with boys and imitate Daddy and girls are expected to play with girls and imitate Mommy.

The Preschooler (2 to 5 Years)

The child at this age is generally eating with the rest of the family at the table. The eating schedule consists of three meals a day with snacks in the mid morning and afternoon. The bottle is generally discouraged at 3 years of age and the child encouraged to drink from a cup. This, however, is not strictly adhered to. If the child refuses, the bottle continues to be a supplementary source of nutrition and reassurance. Table manners are encouraged but not strictly enforced and children are usually allowed to leave the table once they are through with their meal.

Children at this stage are generally eating the foods eaten by their parents. Although many American dishes and cooking techniques have been introduced into the Puerto Rican household,

traditional Puerto Rican foods (comidas criollas) typical of the culture continue to predominate in the Puerto Rican diet. Following is a list of foods most commonly prepared on the Mainland:

Rice (arroz) in its various forms
blanco (white rice)
con habichuelas (with beans)
con pollo (with chicken)
con salchichas (with sausages)
con bacalao (with cod fish)
con gandules (with pigeon peas)
con garbanzos (with chick peas)
con leche (with milk)
Meat in its various forms
chuletas de cerdo fritas o asadas (fried or roasted pork chops)
pernil asado (roast pork)
biftec frito con cebollas (fried beefsteak with onions)
costillas de cerdo asadas (roast pork spareribs)
pollo frito, guizado o asado (fried, stewed, or roasted chicken)
Other dishes
pasteles (rectangular patties made of grated plantains, green bananas and other tropical vegetables, stuffed with meat and wrapped in green banana leaves or special paper—papel de pasteles—and then boiled)
alcapurrias (grated yucca, green banana or other tropical vegetable formed into a ball, stuffed with meat, and deep fried)
empanadillas (flour patties stuffed with meat and deep fried)
rellenos de papa (mashed potatoes mixed with flour, stuffed with meat, formed into a ball, and deep fried)
bacalaitos fritos (codfish patties)
tostones de platano (fried plantain)
gazpacho (salad consisting of codfish, onions, peppers, tomatoes, avocado, spices, oil and vinegar—other ingredients may be added)
asopao (rice soup prepared with chicken, ham, beef, pork, beans, or chick peas)
sancocho (soup consisting of meat and balls of grated plantain and other tropical vegetables)
arroz con dulce (rice pudding)
Drinks
malta (non-alcoholic black beer)
cafe (coffee)

219

mavi (iced tropical beverage)

refresco de tamarindo (iced tropical beverage)

te de jengibre (ginger tea)

This list is limited, for the Puerto Rican kitchen is so replete with typical dishes that a book dedicated to the subject could not cover all its recipes and their variations. Puerto Ricans on the Mainland have tended to mix American recipes with those of the Island, producing some very unique results. Puerto Rican children will accept many of the Puerto Rican foods, but their diet most often consists of a combination of both American and Puerto Rican foods.

At this stage, bouts of crying during the night because of nightmares or fear of the dark are handled by comforting the child and leaving a light on in the child's room. A child will occasionally be allowed to sleep with his parents when ill or in distress, but this is generally not encouraged.

Toileting accidents will more often evoke anger in the mother at this time, who sees it as an act of disobedience in a child whom she has accepted as being toilet trained. Mothers interviewed stated that accidents during these years were infrequent, so that they were not considered a problem. Bed wetting is included in this category. In cases in which bed wetting was viewed as a problem (persisting through 5 to 6 years of age), mothers appear to express much anxiety over the child's emotional development.

Children are now expected to understand what is expected of them, so that misbehavior is less tolerated. Spanking is common at this stage. Punishments, such as being confined to bed or the withdrawal of privileges, are used often by mothers on the Mainland. A threat that Father will take care of the matter when he returns home is often effective and may circumvent the need for spanking.

Mainland and Island mothers feel that the child should receive recognition for his success and obedience. This is usually done verbally or through the granting of special privileges.

The mother continues to be very protective throughout this stage. Children are generally not allowed to play outdoors or visit friends without parental supervision. They are expected to be friendly and courteous toward adults and other children, but socialization outside the home does not appear to be of great concern to parents. Playmates are most often siblings and cousins.

Attitudes toward nursery school and kindergarten vary. Non-working mothers and those who have been raised on the Island will often keep their children home with them until they are school age. The thought of leaving their children with strangers produces anxiety. These mothers are likewise reluctant to leave their children with babysitters other than close relatives. Working mothers and those who have been raised on the Mainland have a more relaxed attitude toward preschool programs. Many of these mothers are especially concerned with the child's social and intellectual development. The mother's interest in educating the child at home varies with her educational level. Many mothers enjoy providing their children with books and other educational materials and toys and encouraging them to watch educational programs.

The Puerto Rican child growing up on the Mainland learns to speak both English and Spanish at an early age. The degree of fluency in either language during the preschool years depends on the fluency of the parents. Children whose parents have been raised on the Island and who are not fluent in the English language will have Spanish predominate in their vocabulary. A few English words and phrases will enter his vocabulary through television and persons visiting the home. The child whose parents have been raised on the Mainland tends to have English predominate in his vocabulary, with a few Spanish words and phrases entering his vocabulary through grandparents and other relatives. Many young Puerto Rican parents, owing to increased awareness of their Puerto Rican identity, are now taking the time to teach their children both languages. Educational television programs are now being presented bilingually so that children in all situations learn both languages simultaneously. Puerto Rican parents, although preferring to hear their children speak Spanish at home, take great pride in the child who is able to speak fluent English. This is especially true in those parents who are not fluent in the language.

The issue of language becomes a problem when the child moves permanently or temporarily to the Island and is unable to communicate with relatives, teachers, and peers. Bilingual education on the Island and Mainland has served to alleviate this problem to some extent, but the child's inefficiency in communicating in either language often results in ridicule from his peers.

Influence from the English language has resulted in the evolution of Puerto Rican Spanish into what is known on the Island as "Spanglish" and in New York as "Nuyorican." Miguel Algarin describes this language quite vividly in the following passages.

> The experience of the Puerto Rican on the streets of New York has caused a new language to grow: Nuyorican. . . . pressures of getting a job stimulates the need to master a minimal English usage. But really it is the English around you that seeps into your vocabulary. Everything is in English in the U.S.A., yet there is also alot of Spanish, and Spanish is now gaining. The mixture of both languages grows. The interchange between both yields new verbal possibilities, new images to deal with the stresses of living on tar and cement.[19]

He adds:

> Nuyorican is full of muscular expression. It is a language full of short pulsating rhythms that manifest the unrelenting strain that the Nuyorican experiences.[20]

Nuyorican or Spanglish is a mixture of Spanish and English, so that what often appears to be Puerto Rican terminology is in actuality Hispanicized versions of English terms. Some examples of these are tineyers (teen-agers), biftec (beefsteak), bar, record, standard, ticket (these four terms being pronounced in Spanish but retaining their English spelling), coctel (cocktail), and okey (okay). Sentences often contain a mixture of both languages, such as "dame half pound de chuleta" (give me a half pound of pork chops) or "un momento Mister, no speak to me de esa manera" (one minute Mister, don't speak to me that way).[21] Mixtures of both languages usually occur between Mainland children and their parents. The parents will speak to the child in Spanish and often receive a response in English. This appears to occur even though both parties are fluent in both languages. Communication taking place in this manner appears to establish a certain degree of familiarity between the two individuals who are interacting, a factor that appears to be important to most Puerto Ricans. I find myself establishing more of a rapport with my patients when I express myself in this manner.

The School-Age Child (5 to 12 Years)

The child at this stage is expected to have acquired more stable eating habits and is expected

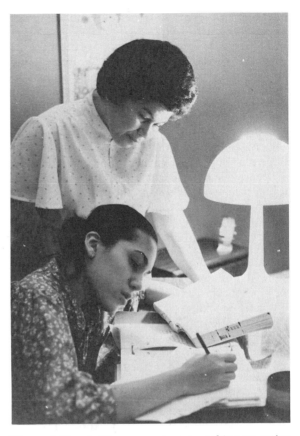

Figure 4. Puerto Rican parents enjoy taking an active part in their children's education. (Photograph by Gerard Lacay)

to eat his meals with the rest of the family. The problem here occurs when the child begins to refuse traditional Puerto Rican foods, turning instead to hamburgers and french fries. The mother's attempts at trying to satisfy the child's tastes often bring complaints from the father, who prefers his traditional rice and beans. Mothers often end up preparing two separate meals for husband and children.

A definite line is seen at this stage separating the sexes. The female is distinctly treated as being the more vulnerable sex and is overprotected. She is expected to be like mother in character and to participate in household tasks typically female. She is also expected to remain in the home and to have her friends visit her there. The male, however, is allowed to play outdoors and visit friends unescorted. There is less of a demand on the male in carrying out household duties. The male child is expected to have the macho character of his father and should be aggressive and assertive.

Children are expected to clean up after themselves and to keep their rooms moderately clean, but specific household chores are not usually assigned. The mother is generally preoccupied with the latter and will pick up where the child leaves off.

Good behavior is expected from the child in school. Misbehavior usually causes the Puerto Rican parent shame and anger and the child may be severely scolded or spanked. Mothers appear to feel that it is very important for the child to maintain a favorable image before his teachers and peers. The child is encouraged to have a good grade average, but excelling is not usually overstressed. The typical Puerto Rican parent feels that his child should take advantage of the educational opportunities offered him so that he will not have to work as hard as his parents. A better future for his children is of prime importance to the Puerto Rican parent. For this reason parents enjoy taking an active part in the child's education by making sure they do their assignments and helping them when they can (Fig. 4). This attitude exists in the parent regardless of the number of years on the Mainland, for these ideals are a part of the Puerto Rican parent wherever he may be residing. Parents arriving from the Island with their children may find it very difficult to deal with this area. Language barriers may place the children in lower grades. Inability to communicate with teachers may cause many parents to stay away from the schools, and they will often be mislabeled as unconcerned.

Discipline takes on added meaning for this age group. An obedient school-age child is of extreme importance to the Puerto Rican parent. The threat of losing the child's "respeto" becomes more of a reality at this stage and becomes stronger as the child approaches puberty and adolescence. Arguments may begin to occur between parent and child and punishment may take the form of removal of privileges.

Sex education at this stage varies. Most mothers state that they are guided by questions initiated by the child, but will not initiate discussion of the subject themselves. Discussion most often occurs between mother and daughter. Males will rarely bring up the topic with their mothers and the father takes on a very passive attitude in this area. Many parents prefer that sex education take place in the schools.

The child's social character becomes more of a concern to the parent at this time. Boys are encouraged to go out and play with friends; girls are encouraged to bring friends home. Playmates may be of any race and color so long as they appear to be obedient and respectful children.

Children during these years may undergo further religious instruction. The Catholic child will go through his First Communion and Confirmation. The Protestant is expected to attend Sunday School and to begin thinking about spiritual matters.

The Adolescent (13 to 17 Years)

Puerto Rican adolescents on the Mainland grow up with many of the same ideals as their Anglo-Saxon counterparts. They are expected to be responsible, care for themselves, pursue their studies, and go on to college or pursue a trade. The latter expectations, however, are intermingled with many of the traditional Puerto Rican ideals, resulting in added conflicts between parent and child. Here parents become increasingly conscious of the dilemma involved in raising a Puerto Rican child in an American society. The child who is already going through the identity crisis typical of early adolescence must deal as well with his Puerto Rican versus his American identity. The child's experiences outside the home teach him that he is an American, while his experiences at home teach him that he is a Puerto Rican. In school he is discouraged from speaking Spanish; at home he is expected to use his native language. The conflict widens as the independence and self-assertion that is taught in school is viewed by his parents as defiance and revolt against parental authority.

The Puerto Rican male approaches adolescence with aspirations of becoming an independent man. Parents, however, continue to demand respect and adherence to parental authority far into adulthood. The parent likes to see his son grow into a responsible adult, yet feels that the child should not override parental authority. Dependency is especially encouraged by the mother, who continues to cater to the young man's tastes in food and continues to clean up after him. He is expected to do well in school and to either enter some sort of career or obtain a good paying job. The Puerto Rican child is taught from an early age that he must work hard to realize his goals.

Males generally begin dating at an earlier age. Parents prefer to know the dating partner, but will not object if this is not the case. He is expected to date several girls before he makes a decision to marry. The marriage choice should preferably be someone of the same culture, but other cultures are very well accepted into the Puerto Rican family. The son is expected to bring the girl home to meet his parents. Several visits by the girl prior to marriage are expected so that the parents can get to know her. Conversations may revolve around the girl's family background. An instant bond is often formed if the girl or her family are from the parents' home town. This is often followed by having the girl's parents meet the boy's parents, bringing the relationship to a more serious plane.

Independence to a degree is more accepted in the male than it is in the female. The son is allowed to be absent from the home for longer periods without causing much alarm on the part of the parents. The female who does the same can disrupt an entire household.

As has been previously mentioned, the female is as a rule overprotected. Although expected to be successful in school and career, she is expected to remain close to home while realizing these goals. The father is especially protective of his daughter, often imposing excessive restrictions on her. The female is expected to be more dependent on the parents. It is almost mandatory that dating partners be introduced to the parents. The marriage partner here should, again, preferably be of Hispanic background to facilitate communication between him and the girl's parents. Boys dating the daughter are customarily scrutinized by the parents, whether or not they are steady partners, in order to determine the daughter's degree of safety with the individual. Although chaperonage has become rare, the traditional belief in male aggression and female weakness prevails in many Puerto Rican homes. Women are still often seen as "incapable of defending themselves against male sexual aggression, while men are incapable of internally imposed self discipline."[22] When a female begins to see a certain partner on a steady basis, he is expected to visit her home frequently and to be conversant with the girl's family.

Interpretations of the marriage relationship vary in the Puerto Rican culture. Ideally, a period of engagement should be followed by a formal wedding ceremony and reception. It is important to the parent that the daughter wear a white gown with crown and veil so that society may see that she is chaste and respectable. In many families, however, the common law marriage is ac-

cepted. This is particularly the case in those families where financial conditions do not allow for a formal wedding. Although the young adult is granted the freedom to choose the marriage partner, family opinion tends to have a great influence on the relationship. Pressure from either of the two families is often enough to create discord in the marriage.

Attitudes toward sex and the adolescent also vary. As a rule, sexual activity should not occur outside marriage. The female is expected to be a virgin at the time of marriage, but this is not stressed for the male. The adolescent will most often obtain his sex education in school and from his peers. The mother and daughter continue to be the ones who discuss sexual matters in the home. The father continues to be passive and the son excluded almost completely from home discussion in this area.

The parent's involvement in the child's health care is mostly geared toward nutrition, physical illness, and emotional problems if some appear to exist. Although many parents continue their all-out effort to continue the child's preventive health care, the child's resistance results in less stress in this area at this time. Parents are often more involved in dealing with the conflicts that arise during this stage of development. Parents who were accustomed to an obedient and respectful child may now be faced with what they see as a rebellious and disrespectful teen-ager. Many parents may experience feelings of failure during this period. Father, in particular, may experience a threat to his authority and self-esteem when his son's interests and opinions differ from his own. These differences may be great between a father who has seen his youth in Puerto Rico and a son who is seeing his on the Mainland.

Parents prefer that their children remain in the home until they marry. A son's or daughter's decision to obtain a separate apartment may be offensive to the parents, who feel that they are no longer appreciated or respected. When marriage does occur the family appears to go through a period of adjustment, during which frequent visiting takes place between the couple and their parents. Families still often reside in close proximity to each other.

The ultimate dream of the Puerto Rican parent is to see his children attain educational and professional success, establish a stable marital relationship, and bring forth grandchildren. Grandchildren are seen as a reward for the years of striving to raise their children properly. The

Mainland Puerto Rican strives for self-fulfillment in an attempt to regain that serene and complacent character typical of the Island Puerto Rican. It is very possible that this desire plays a significant role in the persistence of the parent in trying to get his children to comprehend the value of Puerto Rican ideals.

IMPLICATIONS FOR THE HEALTH CARE PROFESSIONAL

Knowledge of the culture in question has much bearing on the quality of communication existing between the member of the culture and the health care professional. The health care provider's behavior, attitude, manner of speaking, and terminology does much to enhance or deter the promotion of health care planning. Brownlee presents many factors and suggestions that should be considered when involved in a cross-cultural situation. She states that "outside health workers who have a poor understanding of their own culture, that of the society where they are working, and the differences between them are likely to give 'assistance' that may actually do more harm than good."[23] She points out that every society has its visible parts (housing, food, dress) and its invisible parts (values, attitudes, traditions), the latter being often unconsciously misconstrued by the health worker as being identical to his own.[24] Understanding of family organization, power structure, and economy contributes significantly to the establishment of a valid communication pattern between patient and health care provider.[25] Brownlee suggests that "health workers or students should also focus on their own cultural background, their biases and preconceptions, and the health program itself."[26]

Communication poses many problems for the health care provider whether or not he is dealing with someone of another culture. The professional's frequent attitude of superiority very much influences the patient's response. The terminology used by the health care provider may often be too technical for the average layman to grasp. Disinterest or detachment displayed in reference to the patient's immediate situation may accentuate the barrier. The care provider's disapproval of the patient's appearance or language may become evident in his manner, and time with the patient shortened.

When two different cultures interact, the barriers encountered may be twofold. In addition to the above possibilities the problem may be complicated by foreign language, values, and cultural attitudes. Following are some of the barriers that may exist between the health care provider and the Puerto Rican patient. Suggestions have been made that may aid in alleviating some of the barriers that exist and in preventing further barriers from developing.

Language differences may be one of the more obvious problems encountered between the health care professional and the Puerto Rican patient who is not fluent in the English language. Rapport becomes extremely difficult when the non-Spanish speaking health care worker attempts to communicate instructions in limited Spanish. Misunderstandings in regard to treatments very frequently occur. The patient's anxiety level, raised by the inability to communicate effectively, may be so high that even simple instructions will not be fully grasped. The patient's health history and that of her children may often be incomplete because of this problem. I encounter this often in Hispanic patients in my clinical experience. Often the presence of an interpreter in the examining room does little to resolve this problem, for the patient will wait until she is conversing with someone in Spanish to communicate the relevant information. For this reason interdisciplinary communication is vital when working in a cross-cultural setting. Where an interpreter is not available, time should be taken with the patient, whenever possible, to clarify misunderstandings. Literature printed in Spanish can be very helpful if the patient is literate.

The use of an interpreter may not completely obliterate the possibility of communication problems. Problems unique to this situation may include lack of fluency in either language on the part of the interpreter. The interpreter's own biases may transform the information communicated into something entirely different. Brownlee refers to this particular type of interpreter as "the gatekeeper." The interpreter in this case censors or transforms the information into what he feels the health care worker would like to hear or into responses that are more socially acceptable.[27]

The language problem is not unique to non-Spanish-speaking personnel, but may exist as well between Spanish-speaking staff and patients. The professional's desire to express his superiority may lead to the use of formal Spanish terminology that the patient is unfamiliar with. Differences in dialect may also result in the misunderstanding of certain terms and phrases.

Possible means of approaching these problems could involve observing staff-patient communication within the clinic setting. Discussing difficulties with staff and exploring possible solutions may prove to be helpful.

The person's perception of the world around him becomes quite evident in his language. Brownlee demonstrates this by quoting Lyle Saunders regarding the Hispanic individual's perception of time. For the Anglo-Saxon individual, time runs, whereas, for the Hispanic individual, time walks (el reloj anda). The Hispanic individual, then, has a tendency to live his life at a more leisurely pace, a characteristic that is often misinterpreted by the American society as laziness and irresponsibility.[28]

The family organization has much influence on the Puerto Rican individual's ability to absorb information. The health care worker must be observant as to where the power within the family lies and who the decision-maker within the family is. Brownlee points out that "health personnel who do not have sufficient knowledge of the typical authority and decision-making structure within the family . . . may direct instructions, health education advice, and other efforts of persuasion toward the wrong family member."[29] In the Puerto Rican family power may lie in different areas with different families. In the family where the husband is present, he will most likely be the decision-maker and the wife may be reluctant to carry out medical instructions without consulting him. In homes where the husband is absent, the woman may be the decision-maker or the authority may be delegated to an older family member such as her mother. Teen-age girls will most often look to their mothers for guidance in regard to their own health care and that of their children. Mothers recently arriving from the Island and who are unfamiliar with the English language and the American health care system may look to relatives or friends who are more acquainted with these areas. Younger mothers who have been raised on the Mainland appear to be more independent in the decision-making process and will often make decisions prior to consulting with other family members.

Taking the mentioned possibilities into consideration, the health care professional should observe and become receptive to the patient's degree of understanding and willingness to comply with medical regimens in order to be able to determine the capacity in which the patient's decision is being made. The question must be asked as to whether the patient is agreeing with the intent of carrying out the instructions or whether she is agreeing with the intent of consulting with another person prior to carrying out the advice. This can be done by questioning the patient and observing her responses.

Another factor that may influence communication between Puerto Rican patients and the health care professional may be the Hispanic's traditional use of diplomacy and tactfulness in communicating with others. Murillo states that "concern and respect for another's feelings dictate that a screen always be provided behind which a man may preserve his dignity."[30] For this reason, the Hispanic individual may often appear to understand or agree with information or advice, when in reality such is not the case. This is done in order that the informant not be offended. The practice of having the patient repeat instructions may help to alleviate misunderstandings in many cases.

In addition to observing family structure, the health care provider must consider the Puerto Rican's sense of family privacy. Although health care is frequently sought outside the home, the health care professional's attempts to investigate the family situation may often be met by resistance. The Puerto Rican generally prefers to keep existing problems within the family circle and may often view questions regarding the family situation as impudent. Patients will often deny problems in the home in order to avoid involvement by the health care professional. The Puerto Rican generally feels that the family is responsible to itself and that outside parties should not enter the family circle unless there is no other alternative. I have on occasion observed seemingly cheerful Puerto Rican patients suddenly burst into tears, stating that they can no longer handle the home situation. Such displays are often followed by apparent shame and embarrassment at having disclosed personal family information to outside individuals.

A tendency to seek treatment in the form of folk remedies may cause delays in seeking medical treatment in many instances. The health care provider may interpret this behavior as irresponsibility or aloofness. It is important that the health care worker lay aside his biases and seek information from the patient regarding his reasons for the delay, his approaches to the problem at home prior to seeking medical consultation, and his attitudes toward the provider's recommendations. It is well to note some of the more commonly used folk remedies and to be constantly aware of the culture's tendency toward reliance on home treatment. The health care professional needs to become aware of the fact that the Puerto Rican culture is health oriented. This orientation may not always involve the health care system, but nevertheless it is there in the form of folklore, folk remedies, and religion. The health care provider's demonstration of respect for these cultural characteristics may help to make the patient more susceptible to professional advice, for the patient will have less of a tendency to feel that his culture is being threatened.

The influence of religion on the Puerto Rican's view of health and disease cannot be ignored. The fact that health and disease are seen as products of good and evil has a great bearing on the individual's motivation to seek medical attention. Many may delay seeing a physician because they feel that they must see through their punishment or chastisement for some act of disobedience. Religion plays a major role in the complacent attitude that many Puerto Ricans display toward illness. The religious attitude appears to exist in most Puerto Ricans in different degrees. Even individuals who rely strongly on institutional medicine tend to look at health and disease as part of God's will.

CONCLUSION

The study of the childrearing patterns of a culture is applicable to all health care professionals and not only to those individuals employed in a pediatric capacity. It is through the patterns of childrearing that the seeds of a culture are planted, allowing it to continue to exist and thrive. The study of a given culture must begin with the health care professional's awareness that there is a significant difference between his own cultural values and that of the patient. With this as the cornerstone, communication levels can be built and barriers torn down.

The Puerto Rican culture, because of its past and ongoing involvement with other cultures, possesses myriad versions of the childrearing practices presented in this chapter. Class, educational, and environmental differences within the culture result in many variations of the traditional childrearing practices. The health care professional dealing with the Puerto Rican people must maintain an unbiased mind at all times and not judge or evaluate every individual by the same standards. The limited presentation of childrearing practices outlined in this chapter is meant to serve more as a guideline to more extensive study on the subject. It is the duty of the individual health care professional to explore within his own clinical setting cultural practices unique to the specific population he is working with and to share these observations with other providers, so that the quality of health care for this cultural group can be improved.

In conclusion, then, let us keep in mind that the use of interpreters in the care of the Puerto Rican is not the ultimate solution to the problem of cross-cultural communication, but merely a tool. It is the orientation of the health care professional toward the culture that is the key to the solution. Puerto Rican mothers will continue to produce children with varying levels of Puerto Rican and American orientation and it is through ongoing study and exploration that the health care worker will come one step closer to grasping the essence of the Puerto Rican parent and child and be able to apply it to his own growth as a health care provider and human being.

ACKNOWLEDGMENTS
I would like to extend my sincere thanks to Betty Carrington, Administrator of the Nurse-Midwifery Service at Brookdale Hospital, for her guidance and encouragement; and to the mothers who so graciously participated in the interviews.

REFERENCES
1. Wagenheim, K., and Jimenez de Wagenheim, O.: *The Puerto Ricans*. Praeger Publishers, 1973, pp. 293-94.
2. Ibid., p. 393.
3. Ibid., p. 295.
4. Maldonado-Denis, M.: "Puerto Ricans: protest or submission." In Cordasco, F., and Bucchioni, E.: *The Puerto Rican Experience*. Littlefield, Adams, and Co., Totowa, N.J., 1973, p. 225.
5. Mintz, M.W.: "Puerto Rico: an essay in the definition of national culture." In Cordasco, p. 62.
6. Ibid., p. 63.
7. Ibid., p. 65.
8. Ibid.
9. Ibid., p. 61.
10. Safilios-Rothschild, C.: *Trends in the family: cross-cultural perspectives*. Children Today 7:38-44, March/April 1978.
11. Foster, G.M.: "Relationships between

Spanish and Spanish-American folk medicine." In Arguijo Martinez, R.: *Hispanic Culture and Health Care*. C.V. Mosby Company, St. Louis, 1978, p. 191.

12. Ibid.
13. Currier, R.L.: "The hot-cold syndrome and symbolic balance in Mexican and Spanish-American folk medicine." In Arguijo Martinez, p. 138.
14. Watson Lubic, R.: *The Puerto Rican family.* American College of Nurse Midwives 14:104, November, 1969.
15. Ibid.
16. Baca, J.E.: "Some health beliefs of the Spanish speaking." In Arguijo Martinez, p. 96.
17. Holland, W.R.: "Mexican-American medical beliefs: science or magic." In Arguijo Martinez, pp. 103-104.
18. Ilg, F.L., and Ames, L.B.: *The Gesell Institute's Child Behaviour.* Harper & Row, New York, 1955, p. 72.
19. Algarin, M., and Pinero, M.: *Nuyorican Poetry: An Anthology of Puerto Rican Words and Feelings.* William Morrow and Company, New York, 1975, p. 15.

20. Ibid., p. 16.
21. Ibid.
22. Mintz, p. 74.
23. Brownlee, A.T.: *Community, Culture, and Care: A Cross-Cultural Guide for Health Workers.* C.V. Mosby Company, St. Louis, 1978, p. v.
24. Ibid.
25. Ibid., p. 81.
26. Ibid., pp. vi-vii.
27. Ibid., p. 54.
28. Ibid., pp. 73-74.
29. Ibid., p. 85.
30. Murillo, N.: "The Mexican American family." In Arguijo Martinez, p. 8.

BIBLIOGRAPHY

Leach, P.: *Your Baby and Child: From Birth to Age Five.* Alfred A. Knopf, New York, 1978.

Senior, C.: *The Puerto Ricans: Strangers—Then Neighbors.* Quadrangle Books, Chicago, 1965.

Steiner, S.: *The Islands: The Worlds of the Puerto Ricans.* Harper & Row, New York, 1974.

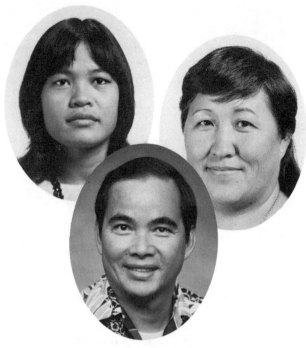

Chapter 10

I, Lorraine Chiyeko Suzuki Stringfellow, was born on Maui, one of the major islands of Hawaii. I am the eldest of seven children born to a second-generation Japanese couple. My father was employed by a pineapple company. Although the language spoken at home was English, much of the conversation I heard at family and community social events was in Japanese. A few of the traditions and cultural practices that survived the acculturation process in my early childhood and adolescent years, which were simultaneous with the difficult times of World War II, are still remembered, valued, and practiced when appropriate. My recollections relating to childrearing as I experienced it are generally very positive and happy ones. As the eldest, I had many responsibilities for housework and care of my younger siblings. I was expected to be a good example for them in the areas of academic performance, a good play supervisor, a model chore doer, and to be able to assist in cooking and laundering. My father was the disciplinarian. He gave approval and meted out punishment, but he was also the rewarder. My mother was often the advocate for us to help get approval for certain activities. She also frequently rewarded good behavior with her warmth, clothes, special foods and other treats. Life with my husband, who is a Middle-American Nebraskan of English, Dutch, and German background, has required surprisingly little cross-cultural adaptation. We have two sons and a daughter who are examples of the blending of races that results in the bright and beautiful faces of the children of Hawaii. Our favorite recreations as a family include swimming, diving, fishing, and surfing in the warm Pacific waters that bathe the shores of the islands.

My professional career began at The Queen's Hospital School of Nursing in Honolulu. I continued my studies at the University of Washington School of Nursing in Seattle, from which I graduated with honors, and I did graduate work at the University of Hawaii and earned a master's degree in public health. I have been teaching in the Maternal and Child Health Program of Hawaii's School of Public Health for a number of years. Throughout my career I have been aware of, and sensitive to, the ethnocultural aspects of patient care and health care delivery. This interest has been an especially important factor in the health care of the many new immigrant groups that are constantly moving to Hawaii. All the problems of adapting to a new community are magnified when English is a second language. Knowledge of the background of such groups is always of great value to the health care provider.

The time and effort that I have invested in

The Vietnamese in America

Lorraine Stringfellow, R.N., M.P.H.,

Nguyen Dang Liem, Ph.D., and

Linda Diep Liem, R.N., M.P.H., B.S.N.

the preparation of this chapter have made for a fascinating and enriching experience. The credit for much that is presented here should be given to the Vietnamese who so willingly shared their knowledge and experience in the hope of helping some of their own people scattered throughout the United States.

My name is Nguyen Dang Liem. I was born in Cho-Lon, South Vietnam, on February 6, 1936. My father was a civil servant, and my mother was a housewife and small businesswoman. I was the eldest in the family, with two sisters.

I went to elementary schools in Saigon, now called Ho Chi Minh City, and in Rach Cat, a small town 10 miles south of Saigon. During World War II and the fighting between Vietnamese nationalists and French troops after it, I could not go to school for 3 years.

In 1950, I entered Petrus Truong Vinh Ky Lycée, a public high school, and was of the last class where French was the language of instruction. Like other public high schools, Petrus Truong Vinh Ky Lycée had entrance examinations that were highly competitive. In the early 1950s, the Lycée was also the headquarters of the Binh Xuyen army. As such, it was the ground for heavy fighting between the Binh Xuyen troups and the Ngo Dinh Diem army in 1955, and it was not unusual for us to have no

classes for months because of the armed conflicts. Also, when we had classes, we were not allowed to stay on school grounds after school hours. As a result, we had no extracurricular activities. Because of the instability in the country, we students felt that we had to burn all our energies to succeed in our examinations.

From 1956 to 1959, I went to the Faculty of Letters of the University of Saigon, where I graduated with a License-ès-Lettres in French Language and Literature. From 1959 to 1961 I attended the University of Michigan, where I graduated with an M.A. in English Language and Literature, and an M.A. in Linguistics. From 1961 to 1963 I taught on the Faculty of Pedagogy of the University of Saigon. From 1964 to 1967 I went to the Australian National University, where I received a Ph.D. in Linguistics. I joined the University of Hawaii in 1967, where I am now Professor of Southeast Asian Languages and Literature at the Department of Indo-Pacific Languages.

The influx of refugees from Indochina in 1975 to the United States prompted me to get involved in community services. I am presently co-investigator of RICE (Refugees of Indochina Culture Education, a mental health training program), and I am advocating bilingual-bicultural education for Indochinese refugee children.

Being a child during war time, I did not profit from normal Vietnamese childrearing practices. My research on Indochinese mental health and education convinced me that the traditional values in the Vietnamese culture, which is composed of an amalgamation of Buddhism, Confucianism, Taoism, and lessons from nature, should be preserved among the Vietnamese in the United States. Yet, these values should not dictate the way of life of these people, as they are at times in conflict with American values. In terms of Vietnamese childrearing in this country, I advocate a degree of authority given to parents, but at the same time flexibility, freedom of choice, and individualism accorded to children. I advocate something in between the strict hierarchy of the traditional Vietnamese family, where the parents have total control, and complete anarchy. I believe in the teaching and educating role of parents.

I, Linda Diep Liem, was born in 1946 in Tay Ninh, Viet Nam, a small town near the Cambodian border. Our family moved to Saigon when I was 3 months old. My father was an architect and my mother a trained midwife. She at one time had a five-bed home where she delivered babies. She had a physician to call on when it was needed. I eventually became the eldest sister to three brothers, three sisters, one half-brother, and one half-sister.

My father had strong authority in our family. He expected all his daughters to marry, but he also wanted them to have professional careers. Although he believed traditionally that sons were more valuable to have than daughters, he gave us all the same educational opportunities.

My education began at 4 years of age when I went to a French school. I received a high school diploma from that same school in 1963 and attended medical school for 5 years. My life came to a turning point after Tet (Vietnamese New Year) of 1968, when the Viet Cong temporarily took over all major cities in South Vietnam. I decided it was more important for me to join my fiancé in Hawaii than to finish medical school. Hawaii, with its blue skies and waters and its lands full of fragrant blossoms, was paradise to me compared with the barbed wires, the moist heat and dust, and above all the human miseries of the city I left behind. I got married in the Honpa Hongwanji Temple in Honolulu. My higher education continued in the School of Public Health where I studied Maternal and Child Health from 1968 to 1970. After receiving a master's degree in Public Health, I devoted the next 5 years to my family, which included by then two growing children, a son and a daughter. I returned to the University of Hawaii in 1976, this time attending the School of Nursing, and earned a B.S.N. in 1978. I have worked at Kapiolani Children's Medical Center as a staff nurse and am presently a public health nurse in the Headstart Program.

Our family roles have evolved over the years. When I was a full-time housewife and mother, all the household chores and childrearing responsibilities were mine. Now that I am working full-time, they are shared equally according to who is available to do what at a certain time. My husband and I do have different ideas about childrearing. Oftentimes we end up with compromises after our discussions. We have not set ideas about what our children should be when they grow up. Of course, we would like them to be happy and successful in whatever field they choose, and we are providing them with the best education available. We encourage them to develop their fullest potential. We may be one of the very rare families of Vietnamese ethnicity to begin sex education for our children in their preschool years. I answer my children's questions about sexuality honestly and give them all the facts in a language they can understand. My 4-year-old daughter knows how babies are made and born. My 8-year-old son has never been scolded for playing with himself in the privacy of his house.

This open attitude towards sexuality has not come overnight. My own sex education was left to friends, books, and high school science classes. My mother kept her midwife textbooks locked in a closet, which did not keep the children from looking at them whenever we could get hold of her keys. In this age of changing attitudes about sex, I do have my personal beliefs, but respect each individual's choice of life-style.

As a family, we do not plan to have any more than two children and I am looking forward to having a satisfying and rewarding career while enjoying my childrearing responsibilities at home.

After the fall of South Vietnam in April 1975, 140,730 refugees found homes in all 50 states, American Samoa, and Puerto Rico.[1] California sponsored 26,850 refugees, the highest number in any one state. About half the adults spoke some English when they arrived, with a fourth of them reporting some university education.[2] The population was relatively young with many women and children separated from husbands and fathers. Many were government workers, officers, and enlisted men. About one third were reported to be Catholics. The impression is that most of the refugees were urban and semi-urban residents who were already acquainted with some of the American style of living.

Scattered reports throughout the media identified no major health problems among the refugees, although more tuberculosis cases were reported. The most common medical problem noted was the need for dental care. The priority of need was to learn to speak English and obtain employment. There is limited literature available in English on the people in Vietnam in contrast to the many volumes on the war and against the war.

Since 1975, about 141,000 refugees have settled in the United States. There have since been additional refugees arriving in smaller numbers. The refugee population have been relatively young with many nuclear families separated from each other. Many have relocated near extended family members.

In the process of adaptation to life in the United States, the problems with communication and the lack of understanding of traditional beliefs and practices in childrearing of the Vietnamese presented barriers to nurses and other health professionals who try to help them. Well and sick child care needs family involvement and support (Fig. 1).

Nurses and other health workers with knowledge and sensitivity of specific cultures can develop patterns of intervention that fit the client or patient.[3] Since each individual varies from the next, familiarity with cultural backgrounds and assessment of the acculturation process of the individual is important to health workers in the development of their plans for intervention.

Leyn recently related her ability to give more effective health care to Southeast Asian refugee families when she had learned more about their cultural beliefs and practices and developed ways to overcome the language barrier.[4] Dr. Nguyen Dang Liem has described the need for

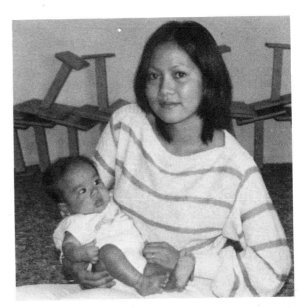

Figure 1. Child care needs family involvement and support.

mental health services among the refugees.[5] His background in the culture facilitates health workers in their approach to help Vietnamese to cope and adapt to their new life in Hawaii. Le-Thi-Que in her interviews describes many cultural behaviors that are helpful to health professionals.[6] However, none of the work done so far gives adequate detail relating to Vietnamese childrearing. The comments related to Vietnamese childrearing made by Stringfellow are based on a small sample.[7] Therefore, the survey of a larger sample was undertaken and findings will be presented later in this chapter.

In order to better understand their special needs in adjusting to life in the United States, a brief description of the history and traditional life of the Vietnamese is presented.

HISTORY

Vietnam is one of three countries located on the Indochinese peninsula of Southeast Asia. It occupies the whole 1200 to 1400 miles of coastline from the Chinese border on the north to the Gulf of Siam on the south. It is bordered on the west by Cambodia and Laos and by the Gulf of Tonkin and the South China Sea on the east. The total land area is 127,000 square miles of beautiful mountains, plains, deep valleys, and small deserts. The green is that of jungle, trees, bushes, and cultivated rice fields along the Red River in the north and in the Mekong delta in the south.

The climate is tropical with greater seasonal differences in the north. Northern winter lasts from November to April, when the average temperature is 60°F, and its summer is from May to October, when there is heavy rainfall and typhoons and when the average temperature is 86 to 89°F. The monsoon climate in the south has an average temperature of 77 to 86°F. The wet season is from May to October and the dry from November to April.[8,9]

Population figures in the late 1960s estimated 15 to 16 million lived in the south and 16 to 17 million lived in the north. The distribution and density was wide in range, with five to six per square mile in the mountains to 1000 to 3000 per square mile in the river delta.[10]

Vietnam is in a strategic location for trade and military efforts. It is a crossroad of the Asian world. Vietnam was known by other names—Tongking (north), Annam (central), and Cochinchina (south)—while under French rule until 1946, when it finally appears in the literature as Vietnam.[11]

Crawford presented a simplified history of dates and events by dividing them all into five eras.[12]

2879 B.C. to 111 B.C.—Establishment of a nation
111 B.C. to A.D. 938—Chinese domination
939 to 1883—The great national dynasties
1883 to 1954—French domination
After World War II

The first era is described in legends. It is important that the Vietnamese emigrated from central China. The second era characterized by Chinese domination is significant for the great influence the Chinese had on the culture of the Vietnamese, whose earliest formal records and literature are recorded in Chinese. The teachings of Confucius underlie much of the culture of Vietnam. The end of this era was a time of revolt. One of the early rebellions was led by two sisters, Trung Trac and Trung Nhi, who established a brief period of independence. When defeated by Chinese forces, they dramatically committed suicide by jumping into a river. During the era of the dynasties, especially during the eleventh-century Ly Dynasty, the country was unified, and cultural development and Buddhism were established. Although the country was divided again, it was unified before the French administration. During the French administration,

French was established as the second language and great advances were made in the areas of medicine, architecture, administration, and education. In the later part of this era, as France fell in World War II, the Japanese occupied and exploited the country while still maintaining the French colonial administration. As the Japanese and the French were reducing their involvement, the independence of Vietnam was realized. Ho Chi Minh established the "Democratic Republic" in Hanoi, while a National Government was organized in Hue. However, the Allies gave Indochina back to France. The attempt of France to reinstate her colonial regime forcefully and the Vietminh decision to oust them from Hanoi started the war that began a "duel between world 'communism' and 'democracy.' "[13] The final withdrawal of the French in 1954 also began the refugee movement, when a million people were allowed to go south. In that final era the United States became involved with aid to help settle refugees.

The fall of South Vietnam in April 1975 started a new era, with thousands of Vietnamese who no longer live in their own land.

THE PEOPLE

The Vietnamese are described as the gentle type who are shy, patient, and polite, yet outgoing with foreigners (Fig. 2).[14]

Language

Crawford stated that there is no agreement on the origins of the Vietnamese language.[15] The Chinese characters were used for official transactions, correspondence, and literature. When the missionaries came, they romanized the spoken Vietnamese and saw it established as the official language.

Religion

There is no official religion. Although not a true religion, Confucianism, which presented a way of life with a code of ethics and morals, provided a tremendous influence on the lives of the Vietnamese. It instructed man to maintain an even temper, to be just and fair, to adapt to life around him, gain honor and respect by improving oneself, and to practice ancestral worship.

Buddhism was reported to have 10 million followers, with an additional 40 percent of the remaining population known to be nominal followers. Its major concepts are:

1. Moderation and the middle path is best.

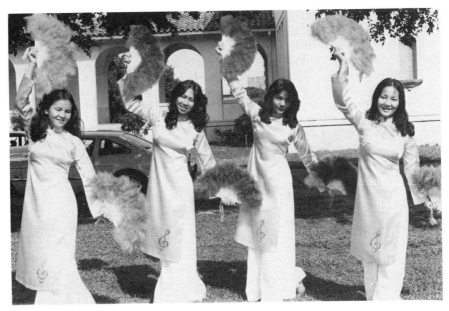
Figure 2. Artistic form is valued by the Vietnamese.

2. Self-denial is as bad as overindulgence.
3. Reincarnation is basic.
4. Life is a succession of suffering caused by desire for happiness, riches, and power.

Taoism, derived from the writings of Lao Tzu, is vital to the Vietnamese philosophy of life. The belief is based on how man participates with universal order. This order is exemplified by the equilibrium of yin (negative) and yang (positive) elements, such as rest and motion, liquid and solid, light and darkness. The material world is based on the duality of nature. Therefore, man tries not to disturb this order and appears to be passive and uncaring. He essentially seeks contentment in nature, quietness, and a peaceful mind. Combination of these three forces provides the Vietnamese with a philosophy of life that influences their behavior. Buddhism promises future happiness after life in Nirvana; Confucianism and Taoism offer happiness in the present life with moderation, balance, and harmony.[16]

The introduction of Catholicism in the seventeenth century produced the second largest population of Catholics in Southeast Asia after the Philippines. It is estimated that ten percent of the population in the south is Catholic.[17]

Education
Formal education consisted of study of Con-fucian texts. Scholarship was directed at a more perfect repetition of the past rather than toward invention and progress.[18] This formal education consisted of an unsystematic collection of stories and precepts, concerning such virtues as patience and humility.[19] Success in education will bring honor to the family.[20]

The Family
The three major Vietnamese institutions are the family, the village, and the state. Since the model for all three is the family, there is only one type of organization.[21] The child grows up to accept the authority of certain people: son to father, wife to husband, and Mandarin to his emperor.[22] However, when there is a lack of trust that expectations of security and loyalty will be fulfilled by the high authority, ambivalence grows in the civil servant as it does in like manner between father and child. Fathers may appear to be stern, cold, and distant, while mothers are seen with warm and easygoing attitudes.[23]

The early development of cohesion in the family and the community organization with the same model provided (1) the economic base of life; and (2) the social organization to administer the state. This cohesiveness helped the Vietnamese people retain their identity during the steady movement south.[24]

Large families were desirable and boys were

especially welcome to carry on the family name and contribute manpower on their farms. At one time families with only girls were thought to have done something wrong and to have been punished.[25] If there was no son, families adopted in informal procedures the second son or other young male of the husband's lineage. Another alternative was the adoption of a son-in-law. Sometimes a poor family received money for the adoption of a son into a family in which his opportunities would have greatly improved. Girls were also adopted, but less frequently.[26]

Family names always appear first in a Vietnamese name, which usually consists of three names. The second name usually refers to sex, that is, *van* for males and *thi* for females. The given name is the final name.[27] However, nicknames are commonly used by family and friends. This practice results from the belief that since the given name is equivalent to one's soul, it is unwise to use the real name, as it might catch the attention of the spirits. So, nicknames are used to confuse them.[28]

Children were also valued for the protection they would provide the parents in their senior years. Therefore, adoption was an important alternative.

Marriage

Marriage is one of the most important events in the life of a Vietnamese villager.[29] The male has the opportunity and obligation to continue the family line and ensure his immortality. The ideal age for marriage is 21 for a male and 17 for a female. Since a proper feast is necessary at the time of marriage and the couple needs to be able to support themselves, children of poor parents may have to wait until they are able to save enough money. The couple is usually expected to reside at least temporarily with the groom's family. The bride is expected to perform servile tasks without complaint. The husband is expected to turn over all cash to his wife. She budgets it to (1) provide food, clothing, and other necessities, (2) save some, and (3) give her husband an allowance for food and drink with his friends while he is away from home.

Although fewer marriages are arranged today, the practice persists in the rural areas of the country. This is less true in the cities, and it may be even less likely among the refugees (immigrants).

Only rarely is divorce acceptable. The reasons allowed are sterility, theft, jealousy, and incurable diseases, such as leprosy.[30]

234

Health

Health is the concern of the family. Ill health is perceived as preventable, as illness is a direct result of disharmony with the universe. There are techniques to prevent ill health. Rituals are aimed at requesting a deity to protect one or at appeasement of evil or errant spirits.[31]

One must not touch only one shoulder of another because that would disturb the genie, so the other shoulder must be touched as well to offset any bad luck. The head is also to be left alone, as it is linked with one's ancestors.[32]

Skin conditions such as pustules and pox are caused by ill winds; therefore, wrapping a scarf over them is adequate before playing with other children. This is typical of families who prefer to try home remedies before consulting a physician for what appears to be a minor condition.

Western medicine is associated with innoculations. Hospitals are to be avoided if at all possible, since one would be in the hands of strangers and, moreover, will not be properly fed. If it becomes necessary to go to the hospital, a member of the family must remain close and cook for him.[33]

Mental illness requires sorcery to exorcise evil spirits. Amulets are used. The victim's upper arm or tongue is cut to obtain blood to write a special formula to frighten the evil spirits away.[34]

Herbalists, or pharmacists, are important in the folk-medicine practices and are associated with minor aches and pains.

A proper diet is important to prevent sickness. The basic diet, which is based on a staple of rice, includes the following preferred foods: fish, pork, soups with noodles, coagulated blood from animals, spices, hot peppers, fish sauce ("nuoc mam"), soy bean sauces, vegetables, fruits, and green tea. The usual adult intake is about 2490 calories per day. Soups are viewed as excellent snacks anytime and anywhere. Sweets are popular with the children, as expected.[35]

Special foods are included for specific reasons. A bitter melon (kho qua) is necessary periodically to refresh the stomach and intestines. Frequent consumption of red chili peppers prevents worms. To "refresh" the heart, one chews areca or betel, and to promote robust health, one drinks from among many alcohol preparations, which might include items like porcupine belly or snake. Glutinous rice is used for any gastrointestinal ailment.[36]

The Survey

An interview schedule was developed, translated into Vietnamese, and pretested by the coauthors. The selected sample of 42 respondents included three males. A total of three interviewers obtained all the data.

The sample had an age distribution of 19 respondents in their twenties, 10 in their thirties, 7 in their forties, and 6 in the 50 to 70 age group. Of the 19 who gave their marital status, 15 were married and 5 were single, separated, or divorced. Their average number of children was two. Seventeen of twenty-four who reported their point of origin said they came from South Vietnam.

The findings will be presented in the following discussion of children in various age groups.

CHILDREARING
Infancy and Toddler Years
The newborn is, of course, the responsibility of the mother. She is assisted and advised by the grandmother and older aunts. Most mothers expect to nurse their infants unless they need to return to their jobs. Of the 42 respondents to the question about how often babies should be nursed, 36 (86%) recommended nursing every 3 to 4 hours rather than on demand. Regarding a night feeding, 16 (38%) thought that they should stop at 3 to 6 months of age and 22 (52%) thought they should stop at 6 to 12 months of age. Infants should be weaned to a cup by about 1 year of age according to 31 of 40 (78%) responses to that item.

The addition of solid foods to the infant's diet occurs at about 5 months, according to 9 respondents (23%); or 6 months according to 30 respondents (51%). Foods they would add first (ranked in order of highest frequency of total responses) were fruits and vegetables, meats, and cereals.

These Vietnamese parents did not appear to approve of thumbsucking or the use of pacifiers. Thirty-one (79.5%) of 39 said they thought thumbsucking should not be allowed, and 28 (63.3%) of 41 respondents said pacifiers were not allowed.

It is interesting to note that 100 percent of 41 respondents thought that babies should be fat.

Generally speaking, a majority, 74 percent (28 of 38), of the selected sample of adults feel that nudity for infants and toddlers should be discouraged or not allowed, and 79 percent (30 of 37) want children fully clothed after age 2 years.

There were 41 respondents to a question asking when toilet training should start. Eleven (26.9%) thought they should start before the end of the first year. Ten (24.4%) thought 1 to 2 years

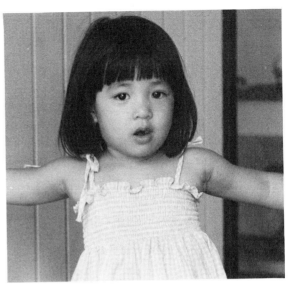

Figure 3. Discipline is not addressed until the child is about 3 years of age.

was a good time to start, and twenty (48.8%) felt ages 2 to 3 years of age was early enough to start.

When a baby cries, 22 of 48 respondents (45.8%) said to pick it up; 19 (39.6%) said feed it; and 7 (14.6%) said baby should be left alone.

In regard to health care, the doctor is reportedly the first to see the child, according to 38 (86.4%) of the 44 total responses.

Mother has the responsibility for early socialization and educational skills. Thirty-three (39.3%) of 84 responses agreed that this was the mother's responsibility. Twenty-one or 25 percent said the father had the same responsibility.

Discipline is not addressed until the child is about 3 years of age (Fig. 3). Up until that time, they believe that there is no harm in "spoiling" children.

Preschool Years
Family food practices among the Vietnamese do not seem to be "foreign." According to 26 (62%) of the 42 respondents, children should be fed separately. They are expected to have acquired good table manners around age 5 or older, according to 25 (60%) responses. An additional 14 (33%) expected good manners between 3 and 5 years of age. When children refuse to eat certain foods, 19 parents said the child should be forced to eat it; 15 thought they should be spanked; and 15 thought they should be sent to their rooms. Important foods for children were listed in response to an open-ended question. They are listed from high-

235

TABLE 1. Important foods children should eat

Foods	No. of Responses
Meat	31
Vegetables	26
Fruit	24
Fish	23
Rice	9
Cereal	4
Eggs	3
Total	120

est number of responses to the least in Table 1.

In the area of toilet training, 14 (34%) of 41 respondents said that children should be at least 30 months or older. On the other hand, 5 (12.1%) thought they should be spanked; and 15 thought between birth and 1 year of age. Most parents essentially watched for signals and toileted the children and encouraged them with running water and other imitative sounds and posturing. When asked about the parent's response to success or failure, 23 (57.5%) of 40 praised success and scolded failure, whereas 11 (27.5%) said they praised success and ignored failure. Of the 41 respondents, 15 (36.6%) said they would comfort, 11 (27.5%) scold, and 9 (22.5%) shame the child when an accident occurred.

In regard to the behavior of bed wetting, the mean age for remaining dry all night was 3 to 3½ years. Of the 37 who responded to a question of what they did about a wet bed, 17 (45.9%) scolded the child, 10 (27%) comforted the child, and 4 (10.8%) ignored the incident. The rest spanked, shamed, and/or teased the child.

It was interesting to note that parents were permissive about letting children of both sexes toilet, dress, and bathe together at about 2 to 3 years of age. They permit children of the same sex to bathe and dress together up to age 10, but all of these activities with both sexes are terminated by 5 years of age.

Parental behavior in response to masturbation by children unanimously requires parents to scold, forbid, threaten with "bad" consequences, or spank. Even if the behavior is unnoticed by others, 33 of 35 respondents said they would not allow it. Only 7 (22%) of 32 parents indicated that mother should stimulate erections during infancy, only to insure capacity as an adult male. Twenty-five (78%) said that this is not a desirable behavior of parents.

In the area of discipline, 21 (52.5%) of 40 respondents said that their children did not usually have to be asked to do something more than once. Immediate obedience was important to 23 (63.8%) of 36 responses, while 34 (87.2%) of 39 responses said that their spouse thought it was. Only 2 (5.7%) of 35 responses indicated that it was all right to let it go when a child is disobedient, and 15 (42.9%) said it was all right to let it go sometimes. When these parents were asked, "Do you think a child has a right to be angry with you?" 13 (31.7%) of 41 respondents said yes and 28 (68.3%) said no. When a child is disobedient, 24 (38.1%) of 63 responses said the child should be deprived of something he likes, 22 (34.9%) said he should be spanked, 11 (17.5%) said he should be scolded and told he is a "bad boy (girl)," and 6 (9.5%) said he should be sent to his room. There were 59 responses to the item asking about punishment. It is interesting to note that 23 (39.0%) said that mother should spank, 12 (20.3%) said father should spank, 8 (13.6%) said older siblings may spank, and 5 (8.5%) said teacher may spank. The body part to be spanked is the buttocks. When a child does well, 30 (58.8%) of 51 total responses said he gets a great deal of praise, 13 (25.5%) said he is rewarded with sweets, and 3 (5.9%) said he is paid money. One response was no reward and four indicated he may be given something else.

Socialization and school readiness skills are important and encouraged by the parents. It seems that the major responsibility usually rests with the mother of the child, though other members of the family contribute. Out of 84 total responses to this item, 33 (39.3%) thought the mother should help the child begin to learn to read and write. Father, older siblings, and grandparents in that order were most frequently thought to share in this responsibility.

Health and illness are still related to spirits and fate. When a child becomes ill, sometimes offerings are made to special spirits. Most parents seek out the traditional remedies and the traditional medicine man first. When this is not successful, they go to the Western doctor. Their expectations are that he will give pills (55.5%), injections (33.3%), or other treatments (11.1%). When asked what they did to prevent illness, out of a total of 112 responses, they checked the following most frequently: 36 (32.1%) give the proper foods; 29 (26.0%) give immunizations; 28 (25.0%) keep the child clean; and 19 (17.0%) take him to the doctor for regular check ups.

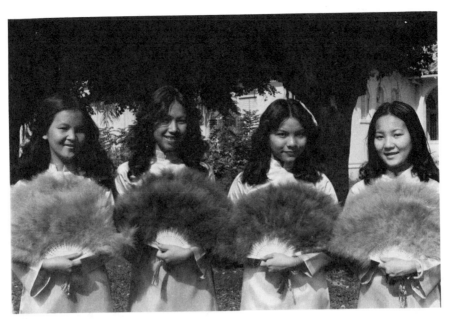

Figure 4. The traditional practice of choosing a mate for a daughter is giving way to allowing young people to choose their mates.

Childhood and Adolescent Years

During this highly accelerated period of physical and personal growth, children are learning to be independent and developing an identity. Children spend more time with their peers and more time away from home and from parental supervision. Sex information, sexuality behaviors, and career goals become important areas of focus.

The parents who were surveyed reported thoughts and feelings not unlike those of many American parents. Many young women start wearing lipstick and sexy clothes in their early teens. Of 36 respondents to this item, 27 (75%) thought their young women should not wear lipstick and sexy clothes until they are 18 or 19 years of age. Only 3 (8.3%) thought they could be as young as 14 or 15 years old when they start. One hundred percent of the 21 responding to an item about when children should be taught that sexual intercourse might result in pregnancy said that they should be at least 16 years old. Sixteen (40%) of 40 respondents thought that information should be given by doctors or nurses, 10 (20%) by the mother, 6 (15%) by the teacher, and a few listed other children, fathers, and older siblings. Regarding sexual intercourse and marriage, 32 (91.4%) of 35 respondents felt that intercourse should occur only after marriage. A movement away from traditional Vietnamese

practice is demonstrated by 22 (61.1%) of 36 respondents, who thought that young people may be allowed to choose their marriage partners (Fig. 4). Twelve (33%) maintained that this is permitted only if approved by elders in the family. In the event that a teen-age woman becomes pregnant, 13 (35.1%) of 37 respondents thought she should marry, 10 (27%) thought she should have an abortion. An interesting tendency noted on this item was that the younger respondents thought abortion was the best way to deal with the teen pregnancy. While none made any response to the items requiring the baby be adopted, 8 (21.6%) thought she would be allowed to keep the baby, and would receive help from the family to raise it. As for the putative father, 27 (84.4%) of 32 respondents thought he should marry her. Other responses indicated he should help in making decisions and supporting her.

Career goals for both girls and boys are considered important to the parents surveyed. Fifty-seven responses were made for girls and forty-seven were made for boys. The general pattern was the same, but the interesting differences in percentages are presented in Table 2.

LIMITATIONS OF THE STUDY

The interview schedule was an abbreviated, modified Sears form, translated and pretested

TABLE 2. Career goals for young Vietnamese girls and boys

Career Choice	Girls		Boys	
	No.	%	No.	%
Doctor	11	19.3	14	28.6
Government Worker	9	15.8	11	22.4
Teacher	7	12.3	5	10.2
University Professor	4	7.0	4	8.2
Nurse	4	7.0	2	4.3
Secretary	4	7.0	3	6.1
Lawyer	1	3.5	3	6.1
Sales Person	3	5.3	4	8.2
Other	13	22.8	3	6.1
Total	56	100	49	100

among Vietnamese. Three interviewers completed all the interviews. Reliability among interviewers was controlled by the interviewer trainer. The sample was selected by availability and willingness of the Vietnamese to participate, with the clear intention of the coauthors to get an age distribution of respondents having current childrearing experiences as well as those who are older and had traditional and earlier experiences in childrearing. The respondents may have answered questions so that they would be "right," rather than answered what they actually believe or actually do. The findings of the study are not representative of all Vietnamese. However, the coauthors hoped that this effort will help health professionals to be aware of and more sensitive to childrearing issues among Vietnamese.

IMPLICATIONS FOR HEALTH CARE PROFESSIONALS

The major barrier to providing comprehensive services to Vietnamese is communication (Figs. 5 and 6). Some patients speak very little English and may need an interpreter during medical and nursing interviews. To facilitate communication when the interpreter is not available, a set of flashcards with Vietnamese words and their English translations can be used. Words that focus on activities of daily living (sleep, eat, body motions) and symptoms of illness (pain, headache) are most helpful. Sign language with pointing, mimicking, and other forms of body language are invaluable aids to communication. Leyn described her unique approaches.[37]

The Vietnamese philosophy of life presented earlier in the chapter described the basis of their stoicism. The degree of stoicism varies with the individual. Some Vietnamese patients may scream with pain or sob with anguish as other patients from different ethnic and cultural backgrounds do. Others may tend to endure pain and discomfort in silence. Here is an example of such a situation in a labor and delivery suite. A young Vietnamese woman did not utter a word or a groan during the whole time she was in labor. The nurse who took care of her, however, noticed that she was tossing around in her bed and that her face was distorted with pain. When asked if she was in pain, she nodded and accepted her pain medication with obvious relief.

In those instances where intense emotions are suspected, such as fear or grief, the nurse and other health professionals should anticipate them and guide their patients towards the expression of those feelings. Too much questioning and probing may cause the patient to "clam up," but a concerned and caring attitude will be greatly appreciated.

Many Vietnamese are shy, especially women and children. Out of respect for the person they are dealing with, they may always nod their heads and say "yes" even though they may completely disagree or may not understand a word of what is being said. An example of this is described here. On a post-partum floor a young first-time Vietnamese mother wanted to nurse her baby. When the nurse asked her if she knew how to breastfeed, she said, "Yes." Without further exploration, the nurse left her with the baby. When she returned, the young mother was

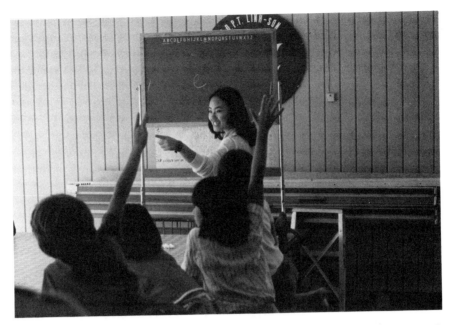

Figure 5. Learning the English language is of prime importance to the new arrivals.

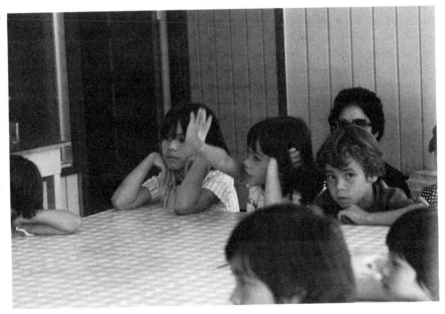

Figure 6. Re-learning the Vietnamese language is also valued by the parents.

standing and leaning over the bed to give her breast to the baby who was lying on the bed. She wondered if that position was the one used by Vietnamese women breastfeeding their infants. She learned that Vietnamese women nursed either sitting up with the baby in their arms or lying down with the baby on their side, as women from other cultures do. This young mother simply did not know how to nurse and was too shy to ask for help.

This episode emphasizes the need to be alert to look for non-verbal cues of hidden messages given by facial and body expressions. A bland or puzzled look along with the head nod would indicate the need for further checking about what the patient has understood of the message given. The best way to validate good communication is to have the patients repeat instructions, demonstrate the procedure that is being taught, or summarize the situation as they see it. Do not take a "yes" for a "yes!"

Although many families are embarrassed about their current living arrangements and might be reluctant to receive health professionals into their homes, home visits can be a part of their health delivery system. They will respond to a friendly and interested attitude and manner. Use of good English spoken slowly and establishment of a feedback pattern to insure good communication will facilitate the relationship with the family.

The Vietnamese receive and give strength to each other in their extended families. Their valuing of children, education, good health, and responsibility for each other will influence their positive response to any efforts by health professionals to help them. Establishing and maintaining a close, supportive relationship with primary caretakers of children will make it possible to monitor any questionable practices used, such as home remedies prescribed by their traditional healers.

Although not specifically addressed in the survey, dental health is an important service for the Vietnamese children. The change in their diets as Americans, the increased availability of sweets, and the practice of rewarding good behavior with sweets by some parents all contribute toward the development of increasing dental caries, loss of teeth, and problems of malocclusion and peridontal disease.

The need for preventive and early identification for mental health services cannot be over-emphasized. The stresses of moving whole fami-

lies, unresolved grieving for those left behind or lost, adapting to a new country, new way of life, new language, new jobs, new schools, new friends, new institutions, new health professionals, and loneliness can be overwhelming. Identification with Vietnamese associations and their network of resources can be invaluable to isolated individuals or families.

Sexuality and family planning information and services need to be implemented much earlier than survey respondents indicated. Maternal and child health professionals should be sensitive to this and involve parents to educate them about the need for youth to have this important information much earlier and integrate it into "normal" well-child care services.

The interdisciplinary health team approach should be the model of choice for health care delivery, where maximum utilization of resources can be mobilized for comprehensive preventive, acute, and rehabilitative services for the childrearing Vietnamese families.

REFERENCES

1. *Refugees no longer wards of U.S.* The Sunday Star-Bulletin and Advertiser, Honolulu, December 21, 1975, B-2.
2. Fitzgerald, F.: *The refugees: hope and trial.* Honolulu Star-Bulletin, January 1, 1976, E-13.
3. Clark, A.L.: *Culture Childbearing Health Professionals.* F.A. Davis, Philadelphia, 1978, p. 16.
4. Leyn, R.B. *The challenge of caring for child refugees from Southeast Asia.* American Journal of Maternal Child Nursing May-June 1978, pp. 178-182.
5. Nguyen, D.L., and Kehmeier, D.: "The Vietnamese in Hawaii." In McDermott, J.F., Wen-Shing, T., and Maretzki, T. (eds.): *Peoples and Cultures in Hawaii.* University of Hawaii Press, Honolulu (in press).
6. Le-Thi-Que: *Changing Structure of the Vietnamese Family from 1925–1975.* East-West Population Institute, University of Hawaii, 1975 (mimeo report).
7. Clark, p. 180.
8. Buttinger, J.: *The Smaller Dragon.* Praeger, New York, 1958, p. 18.
9. Crawford, A.: *Customs and Culture of Vietnam.* C.E. Tuttle Co., Rutland, Vermont, 1968, pp. 23-27.
10. Ibid.
11. Buttinger, pp. 22-52.

12. Crawford, pp. 34-40.
13. Buttinger, p. 454.
14. Crawford, p. 49.
15. Ibid., pp. 61-63.
16. Nguyen and Kehmeier.
17. Ibid., pp. 65-66, 88-89.
18. Fitzgerald, p. 12.
19. Ibid., p. 18.
20. Crawford, p. 91.
21. Fitzgerald, p. 15.
22. Ibid., p. 22.
23. Ibid., p. 112.
24. Buttinger, pp. 41-43.
25. Crawford, p. 121.
26. Hickey, G.C.: *Village in Vietnam*. Yale University Press, New Haven, 1964, p. 109.
27. Ibid.
28. Ibid., p. 80.
29. Ibid., p. 99.
30. Vassal, G.M.: *On and Off Duty in Annam*. W. Heinemann, London, 1910, p. 132.
31. Hickey, pp. 117-118.
32. Crawford, p. 110.
33. Ibid., p. 120.
34. Hickey, p. 80.
35. Crawford, p. 52.
36. Hickey, pp. 117-118.
37. Leyn, pp. 178-182.

Index

Self-orientation, middle childhood and, 24-25
Sensitive period, 17, 20
Sexual practice, middle childhood, 22-23
Shichigosan Festival, 124-125
Spanglish, 221
Susto (fright sickness), 204

TABOOS
  postpartum, 10
  pregnancy and, 13-14
Thematic Apperception Test, Filipinos and, 173
Thonga, male initiation rites of, 25-26
Toilet training, 22
Touching, adult-child, 21
Traditionalists, matrix America and, 48-50

VENTING systems, 12
Vietnamese
  adolescent, 237
  childhood of, 237
  education of, traditional, 233
  family of, 233-234
  health and, 234
  health care and
    dental, 240
    family and, 240
    family planning and, 240
    language and, 238
    mental, 240
    shyness and, 238-240

stoicism and, 238
history of, 231-232
immigration of, 231
infancy of, 235
language of, 232
marriage and, 234
preschool
  discipline and, 236
  food and, 235
  health and, 236
  masturbation and, 236
  socialization and, 236
  toilet training and, 236
religion of, 232-233

WEANING
  sense of separation and, 21-22
  time of, 4
Woman
  American, loneliness and, 12-13
  role of, 7-13
  self-concept of, 11
  support groups for, 12-13

YONSEI, 100

ZAMBIANS, adult-child contact and, 40-41
    sleeping habits and, 218
Zar Cult, 12